MANY SLEEPLESS NIGHTS

OTHER BOOKS BY LEE GUTKIND

Bike Fever
The Best Seat in Baseball, but You Have to Stand
God's Helicopter (a novel)
The People of Penn's Woods West
Our Roots Grow Deeper than We Know

LEE GUTKIND

MANY SLEEPLESS NIGHTS

THE WORLD OF ORGAN TRANSPLANTATION

University of Pittsburgh Press

Published by the University of Pittsburgh Press, Pittsburgh, Pa. 15260
Copyright © 1988, 1990 by Lee Gutkind
All rights reserved
Reprinted by arrangement with W. W. Norton & Company, Inc.
Baker & Taylor International, London
Manufactured in the United States of America

Library of Congress Cataloging-in-Publication Data

Gutkind, Lee.
    Many sleepless nights : the world of organ transplantation / Lee Gutkind.
        p.   cm.
    Reprint. Originally published: 1st ed. New York : Norton, c1988.
    ISBN 0-8229-5905-4 (pbk.)
    1. Transplantation of organs, tissues, etc.—United States—History—20th cen-
tury   2. Transplantation of organs, tissues, etc.—England—History—20th century.   I. Title.
    RD120.7.G88   1990
    617.9'5'009—dc20   89-40585
                                                                             CIP

*To those patients who lived, and to those who died
fighting; to their families, who suffered with them and
the families of their donors, who suffered differently,
but equally.*

*And to those members of organ transplant teams around
the world—surgeons, nurses, coordinators, social workers,
procurement specialists—without whom so many sick and
dying people would have been forever denied their fighting
chance.*

Contents

Acknowledgments

I wish to express my deep and sincere appreciation to the Maurice Falk Medical Fund for its generous support, to Patricia Park, RN BSN, for her invaluable technical and editorial assistance, and to the medical centers and transplant teams around the world, whose cooperation and enthusiasm made this very difficult project possible:

In Great Britain, Cambridge University; Addenbrooke's Hospital, Cambridge; Papworth Hospital, Papworth Village, County of Cambridgeshire; Freeman Hospital and the Royal Victoria Infirmary in Newcastle Upon Tyne. In the United States, Stanford University (California); Columbia-Presbyterian Hospital (New York); Charlotte Memorial Hospital (North Carolina); The Texas Heart Institute (Houston); Johns Hopkins University (Baltimore); the Pittsburgh Transplant Foundation; University of Pittsburgh (Pitt) School of Medicine, and its clinical affiliates, Children's Hospital, and Presbyterian-University Hospital.

It is to "Presby" that I owe the most significant debt, for that institution was always open and available to me in every possible way, above and beyond anything I, as a journalist, had expected. From the first day I began my work there, and for the four years I have continued to return, no person was inaccessible, no question was too difficult to answer, no answer too complicated to explain. No doors, night or day, were ever closed to me, anywhere. I was welcome to observe, to probe, and to report from the operating rooms, the patients' rooms, or the board rooms. I wandered and listened, at my own convenience. As time passed, I was accorded similar privileges at Pitt and at Children's. But without Presby's initial trust and cooperation, the thoroughness of this book, the extent to which I have probed, would not have been possible.

No pseudonyms have been used in this book, no composite characters. Everyone who appears in this book is real. They have contributed their stories generously.

A scientific discovery is never the work of a single person. Each of those who collaborated in it has contributed many sleepless nights.

—Louis Pasteur,
French chemist and bacteriologist

Introduction

Despite its generally conscientious coverage, the media has presented society with a rather skewed portrait of the world of organ transplantation.

Watching TV news and scanning headlines, viewers and readers often glimpse transplant surgeons at press briefings announcing successful and innovative procedures. But years of laboratory experimentation, hundreds of practice operations on animal subjects and many failures have preceded that moment in the limelight. In fact, surgery is the easier part of the battle, while the danger to the patient after surgery—the immune system's natural tendency to "reject" the implanted organ—has been a much more difficult and challenging area to conquer. Over the past thirty-five years, two generations of surgeons and scientists have attempted to unravel the secret of "immunosuppression," with as yet limited success.

Transplant surgeons have periodically tested and expanded society's moral and ethical boundaries—and paid heavily in the process. In 1984, when doctors transplanted the heart of a baboon into a dying infant, Baby Fae, the surgeon, Dr. Leonard Bailey, was soundly criticized by many, including colleagues. One surgeon observed that the child's chances of survival would have been equally served if Bailey had dispensed with the baboon—and sewn in an alarm clock.

Such cynicism must be put into perspective. Baby Fae lived

twenty days, and surgeons learned a great deal about the feasibility of *xenografting* (transplantation from one species to another)—a notion that may well become more palatable if the organ donor shortage is not somehow eased: more than 40 percent of infants and young children on transplant lists will die in 1988 while awaiting a suitable organ match. Bailey's work might be compared with the experimentation of another young surgeon two decades earlier, Dr. Thomas Starzl, who was criticized with equal harshness for repeatedly transplanting human livers from brain-dead donors into adults and children who died within days, weeks, or months.

Today, liver (and heart and kidney) transplantation are well-accepted therapy, covered by private insurance companies, Blue Cross and Blue Shield organizations, Medicaid, and (in some instances) Medicare programs. Coverage is just one indication of how far transplantation has traveled. State and federal laws have been passed prohibiting the sale of donor organs. A transplant bureaucracy has been created and funded by the federal government, requiring hospitals to offer the option of donation to families and potential donors. The U.S. Department of Health and Human Services will deny Medicare or Medicaid reimbursement to institutions that do not comply.

In addition to the surgeons and researchers, nurses, social workers, and procurement coordinators have contributed generously to early pioneering efforts. But it is the patients—recipients of heart, kidney, and liver transplants—who should be singled out for their courage. It might not be completely accurate to call patients "heroes," but the earliest ones in particular were willing to endure tremendous pain and suffering essentially for the sake of those in similar circumstances who might someday follow in their footsteps. This willingness to contribute continues today, not only for the heart-lung and pancreas recipients—transplants that are still considered experimental—but also for the even more complex attempts at lifesaving, such as xenografting and multiple organ (pancreas, liver, spleen, and intestines) procedures.

Perhaps the most frequent misconception concerning the transplant experience as it is today is the assumption that once the procedure is successfully completed, the patient can return to a normal life. This is often not true. Rejection of the transplanted organs is a never-ending threat, only partially controlled by great quantities of medications, which recipients must take for the remainder of their lives. Even if rejection remains in check, the side effects from the medications are often so severe that a return to normalcy is virtually impossible. The three major immunosuppressants currently used—cyclosporine, azathioprine (Imuran), and steroids—have caused, among many other problems, kidney failure, lymphoma, osteoporosis, cataracts, gout, hypertension, and severe mood swings. Because a recipient's immune system is severely weakened by the immunosuppressive drugs, such minor infections as the common cold can become threatening. Medications will cost the transplant recipient anywhere from $7,000 to $10,000 annually. The onus of having been transplanted, combined with the physical limitations caused by the drugs, often makes it difficult for recipients to find employment. These emotional and financial hardships have destroyed many families. Ironically, the disease that originally triggered the transplant can also return—or the implanted organ can one day fail—necessitating retransplantation.

Yet the value and importance of transplantation is certain. In the four years in which I have been intimately involved in the transplant world, primarily in Pittsburgh, but also at many of the other major transplant institutions in the United States and England, I became convinced that this view predominates. Thousands of patients, dying from incurable liver, heart, and lung disease, have been returned to productive lives because of organ transplantation. Children have been given the opportunity to experience adolescence and beyond. Families have been torn apart by the hardship of transplantation, but many also have been further united by the experience.

Today, forty-three-year-old Brian Reames of Greenville, Pennsylvania, a former army career officer, who was essentially confined to his bedroom for the three years prior to his 1982 heart transplant, has helped raise his three children, while establishing TRIO, Transplant Recipients International Organization, and attending graduate school to retrain himself. Winifred (Winkle) Fulk of Kansas City, Missouri, also forty-three, with four children, is now working on a second master's degree while teaching part time at a community college. In 1985, Winkle required an oxygen bottle to breathe and a wheelchair to move about the house. Doctors gave her weeks, a couple of months at most, to live—unless she received a heart-lung transplant—her one and only remaining option for survival.

Brian, Winkle, and the many other recipients whose stories are told in this book, realize as do the surgeons, such as Thomas Starzl of the University of Pittsburgh and Denton Cooley of the Texas Heart Institute, that organ transplantation is not an ultimate answer. But despite the difficulties, most recipients are wholeheartedly appreciative. Transplantation has provided them with the opportunity to contribute to society, to watch their children grow, and to experience the many simple joys and gifts that life provides.

"I opened my eyes one morning, and it was raining," said Terry Avery, an aeronautical engineer from Seattle, Washington, whose life before and for months after transplantation had been frequently endangered. "And I remember thinking that that was kind of amazing. I mean, I knew that without transplantation, there was a good chance that I would have never seen the rain again."

P A R T   I

THE SURGEONS

Chapter 1

THE BIRTH OF A DREAM

It began as a myth, which originally inspired artists—not surgeons.

In the sixth century in Rome, a desperate man, his leg riddled with cancer, is said to have slept for a night in the Church of St. Cosmos and St. Damian, two brothers, both Syrian physicians, who had been made patron saints of medicine. During that night, the dying man saw the brothers emerge from the shadows. One brother surgically removed the diseased leg, while the other went to a nearby cemetery and amputated the leg of a black man—an Ethiopian—who had recently been buried. He brought the leg back to the church, grafted it to the white man's stump. The following morning, the white man opened his eyes, stood up, and walked away on a healthy black leg, while his cancerous leg was found lying beside the black man in his grave. Today, more than 1,500 paintings, drawings and other representations of this story have been counted in churches, galleries, and private collections throughout the world.

Approximately fifteen centuries later, at the turn of the twentieth century, Dr. Alexis Carrel of France solved what had heretofore been considered an impossible surgical mystery by creating a method of joining two blood vessels together. Carrel's technique for the "anastomosis" (from the Greek words *ana* or "to," and *stoma*, which means "mouth"; together "joining mouth-to-mouth") was simple and logical:

he developed a clamp for the artery to keep blood from leaking out, and a technique whereby three guide sutures or "loops" would hold the arteries in place to be sewn with a specially designed needle and thread. In the future, the transplant surgeon could sever the vessels connecting diseased organs to the body, and then subsequently *anastomose* them to the bare ends of vessels coming from the donor organ.

But although his anastomosis techniques had basically made transplant surgery a viable possibility, Carrel and other scientists soon recognized that they would nearly always be defeated by the inevitable aftermath of the transplant procedure—the phenomenon known as "rejection." Whether in animal or in man, the body's immune system would not accept—it would automatically *reject*—the organs implanted into it.

To understand the rejection process, one must first understand how the body defends itself against invasion of foreign substances. Scientists believe that B lymphocytes, which are found in white blood cells, are the first line of defense; they produce proteins called antibodies, which destroy harmful antigens (viruses or bacteria) leaked by foreign invaders. B lymphocytes are usually effective, but if and when they do not work, the body triggers its second line of defense—T lymphocytes, known as "killer" cells, which penetrate the antigens and directly attack the foreign invader.

Under a microscope, you can see the immune system in action soon after the transplant. Immediately, the B lymphocytes approach the antigens of the transplanted organ. Contact occurs—and the immune system must make a decision: Is this an invader, or does this belong? Self or nonself? Us or them? When it is determined that the transplanted organ is a foreign object, the B lymphocytes will joust with and attempt to repel the antigens. T lymphocytes begin to multiply and go into action only after the B cells have failed to do the job . . . if and when the transplanted organ has been strong enough to fend off the B cells and establish itself in the body. This is not too dissimilar to a panoramic Pacman game: a beautiful new heart, pink and beefy, but defenseless, appears on a TV screen. Suddenly an army of killer T cells, clad in black, storm onto the screen and swarm all over the heart, causing the heart to swell uncontrollably from infection—and die.

The chief problem is that the immune system lacks the ability to make value judgments, to distinguish between good and evil. Thus, if it perceives foreign tissue, whether it is a friendly foreigner like a transplanted heart, or unfriendly, the B lymphocytes will go after the antigens, and failing that, the killer T cells will attack. Rejection could occur in nine days or nine months, but Carrel and others realized that sooner or later it would always occur. Rejection was part of the transplant process. For transplantation to work, rejection had to be controlled.

During World War II, Dr. Peter Medawar, who in peacetime was a lecturer in zoology at Oxford University, became a member of a surgical group commissioned by the British government to examine and develop methods of skin grafting for soldiers and civilians burned in bombing raids. Medawar, who eventually won the Nobel Prize for thirty years of work in immunology and was knighted by Queen Elizabeth II, discovered that "homografts," transplantation from one species to another member of that same species [of skin in this case] was not a generally successful method of covering burns— except when the grafts were made between identical twins. With these facts established, Medawar and others reasoned that perhaps a kidney could be transplanted into a sick twin from a healthy identical sibling. People have two equally capable kidneys, while the body requires the use of only one kidney for normal functions; the second serves only in an emergency or back-up capacity.

There were other scientists and surgeons who had blazed the transplant trail before and immediately after his vital discovery. In 1936, Dr. U. Voronoy, a Russian surgeon, performed the first kidney transplant on a human; his patient, however, died in two days. In the early 1950s, there were no fewer than eight failed attempts at renal (kidney) transplantation in France. In his book, *Transplant*, Dr. Francis D. Moore, a respected transplant pioneer from Peter Bent Brigham Hospital in Boston and Harvard University, reports that Dr. Richard Hufnagel, a surgical fellow at "the Brigham" in 1947, was asked to transplant the kidney of a dying patient into a young woman who, while pregnant, had developed an infection in the uterus.

Hufnagel recalls that the patient's condition appeared extremely critical and because of this "there was some administrative objection to bringing the patient to the operating room. In the dark of the night—about midnight—when the kidney had been obtained immediately after the death of the donor, our little group proceeded to one of the end rooms on the second floor, and by the light of two small gooseneck student lamps prepared to do the transplant. . . ." It proceeded perfectly.

The transplanted kidney was only temporary, removed in two or three days, but it had successfully kept the woman alive while she recovered from her infection and until she regained efficient use of her own kidneys. Seven years later, in 1954, Dr. Joseph E. Murray, a young surgeon from "the Brigham," along with a colleague, John P. Merrill, proved that, under the right circumstances, transplantation could work, perhaps indefinitely.

It began with a physician, David Miller, serving at the U.S. Public Health Service in Boston, who was treating a twenty-four-year-old Coast Guardsman, Richard Herrick, for severe end stage renal disease. During the course of treatment, Miller had met Herrick's brother, an identical twin. He knew of Medawar's work during the war, demonstrating the feasibility of skin grafting in identical twins, and he knew that only a few months at most separated the young sailor from death. It could be assumed that with identical twins there would be no biological factor, and thus no rejection. Miller referred Herrick to Murray's surgical group and recommended that he be considered for transplant. David Miller may not have known it then, but he had sparked a climactic event—his idea to help a dying patient was the last link in a series of ideas beginning at the turn of the century with the work of Alexis Carrel.

Before agreeing to attempt the transplant, Murray, trained as a plastic surgeon, employed Medawar's research, when he grafted skin from one brother to another to guarantee that they were indeed identical—not fraternal. It took a number of weeks for the skin graft to take, during which time Herrick was kept alive on Merrill's adaptation of an artificial kidney (dialysis), the prototype of which was developed by an ingenious Dr. Willem J. Kolff under extraordinarily difficult circumstances during World War II in Nazi-occupied Holland. Kolff continued his work after the war at the Cleveland Clinic, where he utilized a tub from a Westinghouse ringer washing machine for the chamber of an improved method of dialysis. Today, Kolff teaches at the University of Utah, where he inspired the work of Robert Jarvik, creator of the world's heretofore most successful version of the artificial heart.

It is impossible to exaggerate the importance of Kolff's artificial kidney in launching the transplant era, for it provided surgeons with a wide range of flexibility in experimentation. Not only did Kolff's creation extend the lives of thousands of people, but it offered the secure knowledge that patients could usually be returned to dialysis if the transplant didn't take. No such "back-up" device existed for the early pioneers working in the extrarenal (other than kidney) transplant field. Once committed, heart and liver transplant surgeons shouldered the full burden of the lives of their patients. There was no second chance, no turning back.

Although twenty-five years ago, scientists were accorded considerably more freedom than today for experimentation, unhindered by government regulation and control, history illustrates that each major step in the evolution of transplantation has stimulated a corresponding legal and/or ethical development or decision that has helped put science into public and social perspective. The legal and ethical evolution began less than two years after the Herrick procedure, when Murray and his team at "the Brigham" were asked to consider a similar procedure for Leon Masden, who was dying from a chronic kidney ailment, and his healthy brother, Leonard. In significant contrast to the twenty-seven-year-old Herrick twins, however, Leon and Leonard were nineteen, which, in the state of Massachusetts, meant that they were minors.

It was a practice in hospitals then, and it is now, that consent be obtained from adult patients prior to surgery. For minors, consent is required from a parent and/or guardian, but in this instance, the hospital questioned the family's ability to be fair and objective. Potentially, the transplant could save Leon's life. At the same time, Leonard would lose one of his two kidneys. What if his remaining kidney was someday jeopardized by accident or illness? With virtually no legal precedent established, hospital attorneys sought a declaratory judgment from the Supreme Court of the Commonwealth of Massachusetts.

At the hearing, Supreme Court Justice Edward A. Counihan, Jr., heard testimony not only from the consenting parent and from Leon, but also from a psychiatrist who had examined the twins and determined that, "if the operation was not performed and the sick twin were to die, it would result in a 'grave emotional impact' on the healthy twin." Thus, the court ruled that the hospital could proceed with surgery. The following year, a similar scenario was followed in two other cases involving twins, one set of which was fourteen, and the other, sixteen. These rulings, the first in particular, which transplant surgeon Thomas Starzl has called "the legal (and probably the moral) basis for living donations," established an important and long-standing precedent for living-related organ donation.

At that time, the only real hope for long-term survival with kidney disease was transplantation involving identical twins, but throughout the next decade, as surgeons became more practiced and sophisticated in transplant techniques, other family members, as well as friends and distant relatives, were included as voluntary kidney donors. Experiments involving the *cadaveric*, or unrelated "brain-dead" donor, were also becoming increasingly successful—an area of particularly special interest to Starzl, who experienced a change of mind concerning the ethical acceptability of living-related donation midway through his career.

"The most compelling argument against living-donation is that it is not completely safe for the donor," Starzl has explained. The percentage is very small, but he can recall nearly two dozen living-related donor fatalities. "The deaths have been caused by anesthetic complications, postoperative pulmonary emboli [an air bubble or blood clot obstruction in the artery], postoperative hepatic [liver] dysfunction, and technical surgical complications. When deaths have occurred, they have had a devastating effect on everyone even remotely associated with the case. The heartbroken surgeons to whom I have talked, including one whose patient died twenty-three years ago, have told me that the donor deaths represented the most terrible moment in their lifetime, and I suppose it might be fair to say that this kind of suffering pales beside that of family members themselves."

Starzl's objections extend to psychological and moral grounds. "I have seen examples of donor abuse within families. If a prospective donor is deficient in some way, usually intellectually, the family power structure may focus on him or her on the basis of their presumed expendability. I have seen refusal of donation lead to ostracism within a family, or alternatively, donation could be a reluctant sacrifice offerred to someone for whom there was little or no affection." Starzl is also concerned about the "donors who may not possess their full civil rights"—children, "who must answer to their parents and are thus captive." He added: "Although I was one of the first to use living donation, and have never had a donor die, the concept remains troubling to me, and I have not operated on a living donor since 1972.

"In my opinion, however, the modern era of renal transplantation could never have developed without living-related donor transplantation. The results with nonrelated donors, for the most part cadaveric, were so poor from 1962 to 1972 that the great effort often was hardly worthwhile. The only real option [for surgeons and scientists] at that time, was the living-related donor."

It was certainly the only conceivable lifesaving option in Boston two days before Christmas, 1954, when Dr. Joseph E. Murray and his surgical team transplanted the kidney of his identical twin, Ronald Herrick, into U.S. Coast Guard Seaman Richard Herrick. After a long and difficult recuperative period, Herrick lived a healthy life for eight years. He died in 1962 of a heart attack, probably never realizing that the courage he and his brother both displayed during a time when transplantation was considered by many to be antireligious

and totally impossible has since paved the way for the improvement and preservation of hundreds of thousands of lives.

Murray commented recently: "The longest survivor is Edith
Helm, whom we transplanted in 1956. Edith is a mother,
the first transplant recipient to complete a pregnancy, and
last year Edith became a grandmother. She has normal renal
function and leads an active life as wife of a rancher in Oklahoma."

From an historical perspective, Murray's surgery on Richard
Herrick was extremely significant in the evolution of organ
transplantation. But its impact, especially upon the public's
perception and interest in transplantation, is miniscule compared to a sudden and completely unexpected event that occurred nearly fourteen years later and halfway around the
globe.

Chapter 2

THE HEART OF THE MATTER

As an undergraduate, Dr. Norman E. Shumway, now Chairman of the Department of Cardiovascular Surgery at Stanford University School of Medicine, attended the University of Michigan with the intention of studying law, but when World War II erupted, he was quickly drafted and assigned to the infantry, completing basic training. "Since at the time nobody knew how long the war might last, the army decided that they needed more trained personnel. So they took everybody with a certain IQ—and it was not very high, believe me— and sent them to engineering schools throughout the country, thinking they might need more engineers."

The army also recognized a need for trained physicians, and all the engineering students were also asked to take a special medical aptitude test. Later, Shumway and a dozen other budding "engineers" were transferred into pre-med. He received his M.D. from Vanderbilt University (Tennessee) in 1949. After his hitch in the army and a fellowship at Minnesota, he joined Stanford's Department of Cardiovascular Surgery in 1958 and immediately began experiments with animals; his intention being to explore open-heart surgical techniques. As an offshoot, Shumway decided to see what would happen if an animal's heart was removed from the body and then sewn back in again. "It worked," said Shumway, "the heart functioned."

Subsequently, Shumway and a cardiovascular resident, Dr.

Richard Lower, together developed the surgical techniques and the immunosuppressive protocols (suppressing the immune system was essential to combatting rejection) for cardiac transplantation. Some of the dogs experimentally transplanted by Shumway and Lower could, within weeks, run and play with almost as much vigor as before, although their lives could not be sustained indefinitely, primarily because of rejection. Back then, Shumway knew that someday he would attempt a heart transplant in man, but it wasn't a priority; in the field of cardiac transplantation, there were many more problems and puzzles than answers and solutions. But after all, there was no real hurry—or so Shumway thought.

Lower soon completed his residency and accepted a position at the Medical College of Virginia at Richmond, joining another prominent transplant pioneer, Dr. David Hume, who previously had "scrubbed" with Merrill at Harvard. Early in 1967, Lower and Hume were visited by a South African surgeon, Dr. Christiaan Barnard, a classmate of Shumway's at Minnesota. Barnard told Lower and Hume that he was interested in Richmond's kidney transplant program, but according to Shumway, Barnard apparently observed Lower performing heart transplants in the animal laboratory, and "simply decided that it was going to be a lot more interesting to do a heart transplant."

Barnard returned to Groote Schuur Hospital in Cape Town, South Africa, assembled a transplant team of surgeons, nurses, and other specialists and, late in 1967, shocked the world by taking a heart from the chest of a twenty-five-year-old woman killed in an automobile accident and implanting it into a fifty-five-year-old grocer, Louis Washkansky, who, upon awakening just hours after the surgery, proclaimed, "I am the new Frankenstein."

Within three weeks, Washkansky died of complications from surgery, but it was Barnard's second patient, a young dentist named Philip Blaiberg, transplanted a few months later, whose extended survival of seventeen months stimulated the unprecedented rash of transplant activity that followed. Dozens of surgeons from throughout the world quickly copied Barnard, prompting cardiologist Irvine Page, that year's recipient of the American Medical Association's "Outstanding Physician Award," to comment: "There ensued what appeared to be an international race to be a member of the me-too brigade." Dr. Denton Cooley, of the Texas Heart Institute in Houston, the esteemed pioneer of open heart surgery, became the undisputed leader of the pack.

Ironically, Cooley had initially claimed to be staunchly opposed to the idea of heart transplantation, maintaining in a symposium in Louisiana on May 2, 1968, that the medical community had been wrongly rushed into heart transplantation, that more study and research were necessary and that the aura and the hoopla (Barnard was constantly on television, hobnobbing with movie stars and heads of state) surrounding the procedure was in poor taste.

Back in Houston, twenty-four hours later, Cooley performed his first heart transplant on a forty-five-year-old accountant, Everett Thomas. Forty-eight hours after that, he performed his second heart transplant, and forty-eight hours later, he performed his third heart transplant. And by August 15, the man who had so recently criticized colleagues for irresponsibly following Christiaan Barnard's lead, had performed ten heart transplants—more than anyone else in the world. There was a photograph published in a Houston newspaper at about that time, of the tall, handsome, slightly silver-haired Denton Cooley surrounded by six happy survivors of his transplant procedures. The photographer had captured a magic and fleeting moment in the history of transplantation, however, for soon after, these six smiling men and women, who, by Cooley's own admission, regarded him as "some kind of a deity," began to return, one-by-one, to the scene of the surgery where they had been given a second chance at life.

It began on November 3 with Everett Thomas, who suddenly could not button his trousers because his abdomen had gotten too large, and who was depressed. "I feel punk," he said. Two days later, Thomas was joined in the hospital by Louis Fierro, a used car salesman who had been Cooley's fourth transplant recipient. (Cooley had once told Thomas: "You are the only used car salesman who ever had a change of heart.") Their symptoms were almost identical: an overabundance of fluid in the chest above the heart, a loss of EKG voltage, difficulty in breathing, swelling in the liver, a general feeling of depression. Thomas and Fierro deteriorated rapidly. First they were confined to bed. Then they were put on oxygen. Thomas was re-transplanted on November 20, but it was much too late. By Christmas, both men were dead.

By Christmas of the following year, 1969, all of the eighteen patients Cooley had transplanted, beginning in the spring of 1968, had expired. Even Barnard's survival success, Philip Blaiberg, had died by then. (Barnard himself was first to realize that Blaiberg was an aberration, and he quickly curtailed his transplant attempts.) By Christmas of 1970, a little more than three years after Barnard's "Miracle at Cape Town," 166 heart transplants had been attempted, worldwide, but according to the American Heart Association, only 23 of those patients were still alive—an embarrassing overall mortality rate of 85 percent.

The failure of the most active transplanter during that period, Denton Cooley, was no surprise to Norman Shumway at Stanford, who had also followed Barnard into the transplant arena. But at that point, because of his research and experience in the laboratory, Shumway had succeeded in helping nine of his attempted twenty-six heart transplants to survive—the only program in the United States with any survivors. Shumway, who usually avoided the eyes of the media, could not help being critical of Denton Cooley. "It's [transplantation] not a surgical business, primarily," he said. "If it were merely a surgical exercise, they'd all have survived." Then Shumway quoted and criticized a recent statement by Cooley, who had said: "The prescription for success in heart transplants is 'cut well, tie well, get well.' "

"That's naïveté," said Shumway. "The problems come after surgery. They're not surgical problems."

Shumway's declaration is supported by history and emphasized by transplant specialists throughout the world. Without a doubt, the real challenge of transplantation centered upon the dilemma of rejection—the same problem that had stymied Alexis Carrel back at the turn of the century, and the same problem that had caught up with Philip Blaiberg after seventeen months of relatively good health. The transplant world had not yet learned how to manage the body's complicated and disconcerting immune system, although a few dedicated scientists were beginning to make progress in unraveling the riddle.

The first step, at least as scientists had perceived it in the late 1950s, was to devise a way to stall or hold off the immune system until enough time had elapsed for the transplanted organ to establish itself in the body and come to be accepted. There was a second equally challenging part of the problem. If scientists immobilized the body's immune system for any length of time, then the body would be vulnerable to the hundreds of other invaders it naturally and normally repels. The condition of people suffering from AIDS (Acquired Immune Deficiency Syndrome) is a prime and tragic example of what happens to a body deprived of its immune system. The AIDS virus destroys the T lymphocytes, leaving the person helpless, susceptible to all manner of infection and disease.

To deal with the problem of rejection, some patients initially underwent whole body irradiation, but the few successes that were registered with this procedure hardly justified the obvious danger of radiation poisoning. David Hume, who left "the Brigham" and preceded Richard Lower at the Medical College of Virginia, was one of the few transplant specialists who maintained a belief in irradiation. As late as 1969, he told a group of physicians at a seminar in atomic medical research that transplant patients would soon be wearing a type of plastic bracelet that would provide irradiation to destroy selectively the white killer T cells—a prediction that has not yet come true.

Recent preliminary studies have indicated that small and repeated doses of radiation do in fact reverse the immune system back toward a fetal or nonresponsive state. At this point, so theorists speculate, the body can be "re-educated" to permanently accept the new tissues, quite an important point, because, back in Hume's day, scientists were beginning to realize that their original assumption that the body would eventually and *permanently* accept a transplanted organ was in error. T cells, they discovered, were relentless. Thus, the transplanted patient would have to be regularly subjected to radiation for the remainder of his life.

The search for pharmacological agents—"immunosuppressive" drugs—to control tissue rejection in transplant patients can be compared to an ongoing and frustrating detective saga that spans three decades (and still continues)—a story with many characters, plots, and subplots, each of which seems to bring the scientist-sleuth closer to an understanding of his problem, immunosuppression, but never quite close enough to develop a permanent solution.

Researchers first turned to the realm of oncology, attempting to combat rejection of transplanted organs with chemotherapeutic agents, particularly azathioprine (trade name Imuran), a product that kills replicating or "multiplying" cancerous cells, which are similar to those cells or lymphocytes that cause rejection. The initial research with azathioprine was done in the early 1960s in conjunction with John Merrill at Harvard by a young British research associate, Dr. Roy Calne, whose name was to become extremely prominent in the hepatic (liver) transplant field. ("Sir" Roy Calne was knighted by Queen Elizabeth in 1981.)

Concurrent with Calne's research, another young surgeon, Dr. Thomas Starzl, at the University of Colorado, was experiencing some success in the use of steroids—chemical relatives of hormones made by the human adrenal gland—such as cortisone, or a laboratory-developed derivative, prednisone. Steroids differ from azathioprine, which destroys all of the cells it contacts, by being more selective, killing only cells that primarily affect the immune system. Based upon his own research and Calne's, Starzl created the concept of what became known as "cocktail" therapy or, in this case, "double-drug" therapy, combining steroids with azathioprine. This was a complementary package in that azathioprine functioned as a maintenance immunosuppressive—the patient used it daily to safeguard himself from rejection. But if he did develop rejection, heavy dosages of steroids were prescribed to reverse it.

Starzl launched a long series of kidney transplants between 1962 and 1964, in which he used the cocktail therapy approach to control rejection, and almost immediately his success rate began to grow. "By the first week of September, 1963," Starzl wrote in a 1978 article, "when an international meeting was convened at the National Research Council to consider the past and future of renal transplantation, our Colorado series of kidney recipients was up to twenty-seven . . . I remember the surprise, if not incredulity, that greeted our report of a very high survival rate (twenty of twenty-seven patients were alive)."

Starzl's classic textbook, *Experiences in Renal Transplantation*, published the following year, reported the results of the application of double-drug therapy with sixty-four patients receiving kidney transplants, at that time the largest study group of transplant patients ever, and provided the necessary documentation to justify past and future research and experimentation. With the proper regimen of immunosuppressant medication, Starzl had concluded, "rejection was a highly controllable and reversible process." This significant point had never before been established.

At the same time, Starzl realized that even though his double-drug therapy was an important step, it was far from the ultimate answer. For although many of the original sixty-four patients for his landmark kidney study remained alive for many years, their experience indicated that the side effects from the drugs were quite harmful. The combination of azathioprine and steroids made an extremely powerful and jarring impact on the body, not unlike dropping a hand grenade into the immune system. The body is laid open to many dangerous infections, including bone marrow toxicity, anemia, and a general retardation of growth potential. Steroids and azathioprine will also retard the healing of the wound from surgery— again making the body susceptible indefinitely to infection.

The side effects from high-dose steroids alone were even more destructive than from azathioprine, and much more difficult to control, as Denton Cooley discovered in Houston, when he employed double-drug therapy for his heart recipients. Because such massive doses were required, patients suffered terribly, as reported by the journalist Thomas Thompson, whose book, *Hearts*, captures many of the details of the transplant era in Texas in 1968–69.

"With the first large doses of cortisone [steroids], the typical transplant patient became positively euphoric," writes Thompson. "But a week later, many became depressed, and for brief periods, psychotic. Some had total withdrawal, lying mute, catatonic in their beds, staring out at a blank unknown that only they could see. Others burst into tears for no apparent reason. One sobbed so hysterically, that his wife and child began to cry as well, and tranquilizers had to be administered to all. Some were unable to eat. Others had memory lapses. Alice [nurse in charge] handed one patient his toothbrush and he looked at it with such total bewilderment that she had to demonstrate what he was supposed to do with it. Some could not move their limbs. Some could not sleep, others *would* not sleep. To close the eyes was to die, in the mind of one transplant.

"Disorientation, confusion, and memory lapses seldom lasted more than a few days, although all could return with altered dosages of cortisone. But there was another side effect that no one liked. Their faces swelled up like balloons. 'If I were in a crowd of 20,000 people in Madison Square Garden, I could spot a transplant,' said one doctor. 'Their faces began to haunt me.' "

Facial puffiness, even 'balloon-like' didn't begin to accurately describe the distortion and disfigurement that could be caused by steroids.

"One transplant suffered the horror of having his face chewed away by herpes virus. His body resistance was so lowered by the immunosuppressive drugs that the disease ran rampant. Whenever he fell fitfully asleep, Alice would creep silently into his room and bathe the black scabs with peroxide and try to remove them. The patient had been a splendid-looking man, but could no longer even bear to look at himself in the mirror. She worked the longest on his nose. By the time he died, Alice had done her work: there were no more black scabs, not even on his nose. In his last hours, as he lay in terminal failure, Alice urged him to keep trying, to fight for more life. 'I'll try one more day,' he gasped, 'but then I'll give up.' Fifteen minutes later, he was dead."

Although, double drug therapy represented significant progress—while they suffered a great deal, transplant patients were living longer than ever before—it was clearly only an interim answer, and not the final solution to the puzzle of rejection. This realization was reflected in Thomas Starzl's ongoing experimentation in his laboratory at Denver, adapting an animal's immune system to create a potion for use in a human, called ALS (anti-lymphocyte serum).

To create ALS, Starzl would inject human white cells (which contained T lymphocytes) into an animal, usually a horse, and over a two- or three-week time period, the horse's immune system would begin to recognize the white cells as foreign— and would consequently make antibodies to destroy them. At this point, blood would be drawn from the horse, and "separated" in a centrifuge, a device that spins test tubes at high speeds. When "spun," red cells settle at the bottom, while a straw-colored plasma (the white cells) float at the top. This plasma, the "serum," ALS, was subsequently injected into a person who was rejecting, the idea being that the antibodies made by the horse to kill the invading human cells would then destroy the T lymphocytes attacking the transplanted heart.

ALS was another important step in this seemingly neverending sequence—antibodies did combat rejection and improve survival rates—but it also produced a reverse effect. Just as the horse would make antibodies to fight human cells because it recognized it was foreign, the patient's immune system would invariably recognize that the serum from that horse was foreign and make its own antibodies against it. There were a great many side effects as well, most especially "serum sickness," which caused nausea, fever, swelling, joint pain, kidney problems. Later, a more purified version of ALS, called ALG (anti-lymphocyte globulin), and ATG (anti-thymocyte globulin), in which the serum is made from the thymus (an organ above the heart that helps to develop the immune system) alleviated some of the more destructive effects, so that the medication, although painful for patients, was tolerable.

Starzl also extended his cocktail creativity to a triple-drug regimen in which steroids, azathioprine, and ALG were combined. ALS (and ALG and ALT), incidentally, had been used before with animals. Thomas Starzl's significant contribution was to adapt it and develop it clinically, proving it could work in humans. No one had had the knowledge or the courage to do that before.

Nor had anyone learned how to detect rejection early enough to maximize the effect of the medication that Starzl was helping to develop. The earlier that rejection is treated, the more effective the immunosuppressant that is being employed. By the time Louis Fierro and Everett Thomas and other cardiac patients returned, sick and depressed to the hospital, their rejection was too far advanced to respond to treatment. They died.

To solve the problem of rejection recognition, Philip Caves, a young Scottish surgeon serving a fellowship at Stanford under Shumway in 1973, developed an endomyocardial (the innermost layer of the heart muscle) biopsy technique, a mild and relatively safe invasive procedure, allowing patients to be monitored regularly for the earliest signs of rejection. This is accomplished by threading a catheter through a vein at the patient's neck and following the vein to reach the heart. A small piece of the heart, about the size of a grain of rice, is then retrieved with a tweezer-like instrument, and subsequently examined under the microscope for evidence of encroaching T cells.

"The heart biopsy quickly became the 'gold standard' for diagnosing rejection," according to Dr. Bruce Reitz, Professor of Surgery at Johns Hopkins University School of Medicine in Baltimore, Maryland, and Cardiac Surgeon-in-Charge at the Johns Hopkins Hospital. "Before the biopsy was available, we looked at the EKG [electrocardiogram], listened to the patient's heart sounds, and looked at the blood pressure. These are pretty 'soft' findings, and the heart has to be really hurting in order to show signs of rejection in this type of examination.

However, if you have an actual piece of muscle, you can detect rejection at a very early stage. That's the real advantage of a biopsy. We take a piece of muscle about two millimeters in diameter. Some of the patients accuse us of giving them a new heart, and then taking it away, millimeter by millimeter," said Reitz. "But it is a small price for them to pay."

The results of Caves's efforts, combined with Starzl's "triple drug" therapy were noted immediately in Shumway's work. Shumway reported five-year survival rates, from 1968–74 of 25 percent, and from 1974 (after Caves developed the biopsy) to 1980 of nearly 60 percent. Because the liver is such a complicated organ, with so little understood about it, the biopsy technique was not too helpful in determining rejection in liver transplant patients, however. In fact, through the entire decade of the 1970s, while Shumway at Stanford had been able to continue his cardiac transplant work and nurse nearly half of his patients back to some semblance of health, Thomas Starzl in Colorado, Shumway's lone liver transplant counterpart, had been experiencing a disconcerting and unending lack of success.

Chapter 3

THE CRUSADER

The man is an enigma. He is a person who has an energy quotient that is so far off the scale of most humans that it is almost unbelievable. If you really want to write a book, find out what makes him tick. I wouldn't know how to begin, but that's probably not for a journalist to do, that's for Sigmund Freud II.

—Keith Reemstma, M.D., Chairman, Department of Surgery, Columbia University College of Physicians and Surgeons

Thomas Earl Starzl, born and raised in Le Mars, Iowa, the "corn and hog capital of the world," as proclaimed in a sign at the edge of town, simultaneously earned his Ph.D. in neurophysiology and his M.D. at Northwestern University in Chicago in 1952. Over the next four years, he served as a surgical intern, fellow, and resident at Johns Hopkins University in Baltimore. In 1958, he became Chief Resident at the University of Miami Medical School, before serving a final residency in thoracic surgery at the Veteran's Administration (VA) Hospital in Chicago. In 1961, back at Northwestern, he accepted an appointment as an assistant professor of surgery. It was at that time that Starzl, in his characteristically scientific and methodical fashion, set out to choose his life's work.

"I went to the library to try to think of some subject or topic which might support a lifetime of effort. I wasn't really looking for a cheap shot, and so I finally decided upon two possibilities. One of them was transplantation, which in 1958 was said to be hopeless by no less an authority than F. MacFarlane Burnet, who was to share the Nobel Prize with Sir Peter Medawar. The other possibility was to work in oncology, but it was being said in those days that the cure for cancer—just as it is today—was right around the corner. And so I decided to work in transplantation."

He subsequently joined the University of Colorado Medical School in Denver as an assistant professor, where he remained for nearly twenty years, rising rapidly through the ranks to become chairman of the Department of Surgery. In 1981, he accepted a professorship at the University of Pittsburgh School of Medicine, with its clinical affiliates Presbyterian-University Hospital (Presby) and Children's Hospital. First in Denver and then in Pittsburgh, Starzl honored his full-fledged commitment to transplantation with unwavering dedication—despite the many inevitable sacrifices in his personal life.

Starzl sleeps many nights in a wrinkled, flannel-lined sleeping bag in the aisle on chartered airplanes (on organ procurement runs) or under the round wooden conference table in his office (between surgeries). He is known as one of the world's true eccentrics—a notion verified by the clerks at the nearby Mr. Donut shop, who report that Starzl will frequently appear, wrinkled and unshaven, day or night, in his blue scrubs and battered, blood-stained running shoes for a quick donut fix. He will scan the cases of jelly and custard-filled, and cinnamon or apple or cherry toppings, with the same experienced eye that has helped make miracles on a surgical field, and he will select the ugliest, the most misshapen derelict of a donut in the store to devour. His favorite restaurant is a local campus hangout called "the O," (the Original Hot Dog Shop), where he consumes great quantities of french fries, swimming in rivers of melted cheese.

Up until 1982, when he experienced a sudden pain in his chest after a marathon forty-eight-hour period of surgery and cigarettes, Starzl was a three-pack a day smoker. He quit on the spot, and as a temporary diversion, adopted Pacman, which he found to be "positively arresting." Pacman was a way of relaxing while simultaneously keeping his adrenalin pumping, burning some of his enormous energy. "But I had to quit that, too," Starzl says. "It was ruining my hands." His fingers are impeccable: long, slender, delicate, perfectly manicured—beautiful, with one exception. The little finger of his left hand is slightly misshapen and paralyzed, a side effect of a hepatitis infection he received working in the laboratory.

Starzl's reputation as a volatile and unyielding taskmaster is legion in surgical circles. People come to study with him and work under him with a mixture of excitement and dread, says Dr. Oscar Bronsther, a surgical fellow (surgeons who have already completed surgical residencies) in Pittsburgh for six months in 1984–85, today director of the liver transplant program at the University of San Diego. "You will work substantially harder and longer in Pittsburgh—seventy-two to eighty-four-hour nonstop shifts—than in any other position before or after." Working with Starzl on a day-to-day basis was not only arduous, but potentially volatile. "He can be in a foul mood and lash out at the world. You gotta always watch your backside a little bit."

In addition to his obsession for work and his ability to drive others far past any boundary of sweat and labor they had ever before achieved, Starzl's phenomenal memory is also legendary among his colleagues, patients, and staff. He can recall the first and last names of each and every transplant patient he has encountered, the names of relatives (wife, parents, etc.), the date of transplant, the size, blood type of the transplanted organ, and any special problem related to the surgery or the postoperative care, with startling precision.

Starzl not only recalls the people on whom he has performed transplant surgery, but he displays an uncanny recognition of the organs he has taken out of them. He will look at a slide and say, "This is Julie Rodriguez's liver; I transplanted her in Denver in 1973." He will grab another slide. "We took this liver out of Terry Avery in November 1984." How could he remember two livers out of hundreds? "How could I ever forget?"

Starzl's memory is necessarily and sometimes irritatingly selective, however. "He will often not acknowledge me when I walk by him in the hall," says liver transplant social worker

Donna Rinaldo. "But whenever he needs something, he instantly knows who I am and how to find me."

There is no question that Thomas Starzl uses people for his own ends and without a moment's hesitation, says Robert Gordon, a surgeon who coordinates the kidney transplant program under Starzl's direction. "He is looking, always, for answers. And he looks at every facet, he wants every fact; he'll go around and ask everybody about some problem, and it looks as though he's going around behind your back to ask that guy, and that guy, and that guy. But this is how he works; he simply wants to know what everybody thinks so he can make a decision. He knows that everybody interprets situations in the way that sheds the best light on themselves. So he listens to everybody; he weighs all the angles. That's the way he works; he's ruthless in that regard. But it is the kind of intellectual ruthlessness that you have to have to be successful."

Gordon first joined Starzl in Denver and then followed him to Pittsburgh, along with Starzl's closest associate, Dr. Shunsaburo (Shun) Iwatsuki of Japan. "I had been planning to stay in America to study transplantation only a year," says Iwatsuki, "but after I saw first hand Starzl's work, I realized it would be wrong to go back. I wanted to be a part of what Starzl was doing." Dr. Byers (Bud) Shaw, the first surgical fellow under Starzl in Pittsburgh in 1981, says that he, on the other hand, at first did *not* want to be a part of what Thomas Starzl was doing, at least as it pertained to liver transplantation.

Shaw's interest in transplantation was first aroused while working as a surgical resident, part of a three-year program in the kidney transplant unit at the University of Utah. "I started looking around at transplant fellowships, and about that time there was a medical student from Denver that came in—I was taking him on a tour of the hospital—and he asked me what I was interested in, and I said transplantation, and he asked me where I would go, and I said that I didn't know. I mentioned four or five places, and he said, 'Why don't you go to Denver?' I said, 'You gotta be crazy, I wouldn't go to

Denver and work for Starzl. I've heard all kinds of things about him. The guy is the toughest taskmaster alive. Besides, liver transplants, that's all he wants to do. That's the biggest joke ever played on the medical community.'

"I thought it was ridiculous, liver transplantation. All I had heard was that most people died. I mean, 25 percent survival rate after a year . . . what a joke! I had heard all of these horror stories of people lying around miserable and yellow [from jaundice] for weeks and weeks and finally dying, and I thought, 'That's got to be the craziest thing I ever heard of.' But then, it was funny. I looked around at all the other [kidney] transplant programs, and I met the people who were in charge of them, people who had made a name for themselves in transplantation—and they were kind of sitting back, enjoying their successes, not looking further into the future. The more I thought about it, the more I realized that if I really wanted to get involved in transplantation in a big way, that probably going and working with Starzl was the most important step."

Even after he had been accepted as a transplant fellow in Pittsburgh, the idea of liver transplantation did not particularly appeal to him. "When I came to Pittsburgh, first thing I told Starzl was that I really wasn't interested in liver transplants; I came here to learn about kidney and pancreas transplants. I distinctly remember telling him, first of all, that I would like to *see* liver transplants, but I really don't think I was capable of ever learning how to do them; and secondly, I thought that liver transplantation must be one of those exotic things that really wasn't practical to offer to a large number of people. But then I began feeling better after seeing my first couple of liver transplants, seeing the patients able to sit up in bed after that long operation, and I can remember one day on rounds, saying something to Starzl, like 'This operation is for real; this really works!'

"It was something very special to come in here and watch what Starzl did, the whole procedure. People, fatally ill just weeks before, woke up after surgery, went home. I couldn't believe it. I figured that I'd be taking care of all these deathly ill patients who'd sit around for a month and then die." Shaw's speculations and observations about liver transplantation, made in the early 1980s, perhaps may have been a bit exaggerated for the time, but not too terribly naive.

From the very beginning, liver transplantation had represented considerably more difficulty than the challenge posed by kidney or cardiac transplantation, although Starzl points out that even in the very early 1960s, it was "inevitable" that sooner or later "transplantation of the liver would be performed. Optimism was high because of the success of double-drug immunosuppression" and the assumption "that the same therapy would be applicable for other organs." Also, through a five-year period beginning in 1958, Starzl and his associates had conducted hundreds of experimental liver transplant procedures in dogs. The time arrived for the therapy to be attempted in a human subject.

On March 1, 1963, Thomas Starzl, like Murray before him and Barnard later, made medical history by transplanting the liver of a three-year-old boy who had died during brain surgery into another boy of the same age, who had been dying of liver disease. Unlike Murray and Barnard, however, there was no joy, not the least measure of satisfaction either for the surgeon or the patient's family, for the child bled to death even before the procedure was concluded. Two months later, Starzl tried again, transplanting the liver from a patient who had died of an inoperable brain tumor into a forty-seven-year-old janitor, with liver cancer. This man lived twenty-two days, although "he was in remarkably good condition postoperatively" and might have had the opportunity to survive if infection had not set in. Starzl transplanted livers three more times during that year, with his recipients living six, seven, and twenty-three days respectively. Returning to the laboratory for further research, he did not attempt another liver transplant in a human until November 1966.

After studying the results of his work, Starzl concluded that the poor quality of the transplanted livers (the organs he had used had been damaged during the death of the donors), combined with the massive blood loss caused by the radical nature of the surgery, were immediately responsible for the deaths of not only his first five patients, but of more than half of the first twenty-five patients on whom he attempted these procedures from 1963 to 1969. Five of those first twenty-five actually survived more than a year. The situation improved through the decade of the seventies, but not nearly in such a steady and positive manner as with Shumway's experiences in heart transplantation. Not only were infection, blood loss, and organ quality important factors, but rejection still loomed as the primary nemesis. Starzl's one-year survival rates leveled out at approximately 35 percent, and nothing he could do, including use of the biopsy or the introduction of triple-drug (with ALG) regimen, seemed to make much difference. The barrage of ridicule and criticism Starzl suffered at the hands of the scientific-medical community at that time was unending.

The problem, said Starzl, was "that there was little public understanding" of the progress that had been achieved. "Early in 1964, there appeared an editorial in the *Annals of Internal Medicine* written by the editor, condemning these attempts at what he considered human experimentation. I don't even remember the title of the article, except that in it was contained the flash word 'cannibalization,' as well as references to possible violations of ethical codes."

Dr. Lawrence Hunsinger, president of the American Council on Transplantation, and a kidney specialist who studied at Harvard under John Merrill, observes that such comments must be put into the proper context. "You have to understand what the world was like back then," he explained. "Tom Starzl got into liver transplantation when it was a thing that only a madman would do, and he plugged away at it, kept going, despite all obstacles."

Hunsinger compares Starzl's work with livers twenty years ago to the isolated incident of the "Baby Fae" transplant, which occurred in 1984, when a surgeon from Loma Linda, California, transplanted a baboon's heart into an infant child, who died soon after. The negative criticism from the medical community, combined with the angry accusations from religious and animal rights groups, highlighted and exaggerated by the national media, were devastating. "Would the person who, having done the first Baby Fae, go ahead and do the next Baby Fae? And then a third and a fourth, and keep on going, indefinitely?* That's comparable to what Starzl was doing in a very real way. You are doing a procedure that doesn't work; you are cutting out people's livers, and they are dying in the wards. It takes a certain amount of 'chutzpah' to keep pushing at it, when you are not meeting a great amount of success, and people are criticizing you from every direction."

Starzl, however, claims that he "didn't think much about the criticism. I don't want to overdramatize that aspect [pressure from criticism]. I didn't honestly pay any attention because I knew perfectly well that I was right, and I knew there were some people who agreed with me, people who were quite creative and intelligent in their own way, and so I paid a lot of attention to them. I never felt like I was exactly alone in the whole thing."

Indeed, this is one of the secrets of Starzl's success, says Bud Shaw, today Director of Liver Transplantation at the University of Nebraska in Omaha—Starzl's absolute refusal to accept defeat, a word that simply doesn't seem to be a part of his vocabulary. "When somebody tells him 'no,' he responds by just taking another route around the situation and going ahead anyway; he doesn't take 'no' for an answer. And he doesn't really care too much about the opinions of other people. Most of us are concerned over whether other people think we're doing the right thing, but I don't know that he's ever relied on what anybody else thinks. When he decides something, he has a very deep conviction that he's right and everybody who doesn't agree with him is wrong. I think that's what it takes to be an innovator or a pioneer in anything."

It also takes courage, the courage to face nearly insurmountable odds and continue fighting, says Denton Cooley who, to this day, remains disturbed with Norman Shumway's criticism of him and his heart transplant work in the late 1960s. Cooley stresses that many people have also been very critical of Norman Shumway, who has often been accused of enhanc-

---

* To date, another *xenograft*, a transplant between one species to another, has not been attempted again anywhere in the world, and this is more than three years since the Baby Fae debacle.

ing his statistics by being extremely selective in the patients he has accepted for transplantation—not taking chances with those patients who are most desperately ill. Says Cooley of his own surgical team: "We don't worry so much about the statistics. We are trying to do good for the largest number of people. We take patients who are at the point of death. I believe that that is an obligation we have."

Starzl concurs. "People liked to take potshots at that 35 percent to 40 percent one-year survival rate [in 1975]," he said in his soft, reedy voice. "But I always asked myself, 'Thirty-five to 40 percent? Yes, but it was compared to what?' That's the answer. I always had the idea that it was more dignified to go down swinging if you knew that there was some dividend, whether it be 40 percent or not, other than letting people bleed out in some back room of a hospital. That didn't make any sense. Any moralists who were approaching me about the sub-optimal results got nothing but agreement from me on that score, but I didn't see it as genuine grounds for criticism because at least we were trying.

"I think that the patients and the families always felt as I did about transplantation because I was never sued or even threatened. Usually, if we failed, they would say, 'Well at least we tried. We didn't have to have that awful sense of having let our baby die and not doing anything, especially now that we know that it works.' That's their perception of it. And I think they are right in retrospect, and I knew at that time that I was right.

"It stands to reason that if you are succeeding one in three times and failure to take action results in failure three out of three times, then you are already comparing a chance, although not a perfect chance, with no chance at all. We showed in Colorado that if you were admitted as a candidate for a liver transplant and didn't get one [a transplant] that within three or six months, you were dead. *You always died.* So the poor results were, in my mind, always being compared with no results whatsoever. Now, I don't think that was a distorted position at all."

C h a p t e r 4

THE MAKING OF A MIRACLE

In the end, the key that unlocked the riddle of the immune system did not emerge in Starzl's laboratory in Denver, at Shumway's facilities at Stanford, or anywhere else such a discovery might have been expected. The answer was literally "unearthed" in 1969 in an isolated highland plateau in southern Norway known as the Hardanger Vidda. This vast and untouched primeval landscape, carpeted with mosses, lichens, and treeless grasslands, dotted with crystal blue lakes, rolling hills, and gigantic glacial boulders, is where a microbiologist from Sandoz, Ltd., a pharmaceutical firm based in Basel, Switzerland, dug up a soil sample to bring back to company laboratories.

Like many other pharmaceutical firms, Sandoz is always searching for microbes (bacteria cells) that might produce chemicals with antibiotic activity, and employees traveling on vacation or on business are encouraged to gather and submit soil for screening even, if possible, from the ocean floor. The microbiologist visiting the Hardanger might have discovered arrowheads, traps, and other tools deposited by primitive hunters who inhabited this land 7,000 years before, but instead, he returned to Switzerland with a soil sample that, when analyzed, contained an amino acid (an organic compound) heretofore undiscovered in any other form of life.

At the outset, the substance, which was called "cyclosporine," did not show much promise as an antibiotic, but it did contain some unique properties that particularly intrigued a thirty-five-year-old Swiss scientist at Sandoz, Jean-François Borel. Educated at the University of Wisconsin, as well as in England and in Zurich, where he received his Ph.D. in immunogenetics (the study of genetics by use of immune responses), Borel subjected cyclosporine to a second set of tests that led to the discovery that this substance had the power to suppress the immune system in an unprecedented way.

Whereas azathioprine and prednisone wipe out most types of immune cells, thus stripping patients of any protection from a slew of infections, cyclosporine seemed to work primarily on killer T lymphocytes—those that especially detect and attack foreign invaders, like transplanted organs or tissue. Borel's studies demonstrated that cyclosporine had the potential of permitting the immune system to protect the body from infection while fending off—not destroying—the T cells that normally attacked donor organs. He could not then and does not now completely understand how or why cyclosporine worked the way it did, but what was important to Borel was that, for whatever reason, it did seem to be impressively effective.

It was not important, however, to Sandoz executives—or at least not important enough. Borel's superiors agreed that cyclosporine's properties were unique—potentially fascinating, in fact, but was it potentially profitable? That was the question to answer. It had taken three years for Borel's tests to reveal the results he had presented, but even in 1972, the field of organ transplantation was still at its barest beginnings. The prospects for a drug that could control the immune system were negligible, especially when weighed against the amount of time and money necessary for proper research and development. Including further testing, marketing, advertising, packaging, and (most especially) investing in the design and manufacture of equipment and machinery for mass-producing it, Sandoz estimated a $30 to $40 million expenditure for cyclosporine over a period of ten years.

Drugs such as cyclosporine cannot be manufactured in the

traditional manner, rather they must be nurtured, cultivated, and fermented. The long and arduous process began with quantities of soil from the Hardanger Vidda being transported to Switzerland, where it would be broken down and isolated. Coincidentally, back in 1969, in approximately the same month the soil sample had been sent from the Hardanger to Basel, a second soil sample was also submitted by another vacationing microbiologist, who had been visiting the state of Wisconsin. Tests revealed that this soil sample also contained the mysterious and heretofore undiscovered amino acid, cyclosporine. Since that time, cyclosporine has been isolated in soil samples sent from other parts of the United States, but the crucial difference between the soil from Wisconsin and that from Norway had to do with where in the soil the cyclosporine was detected. In Wisconsin, said Borel, it was in the "surface culture" whereas in the Hardanger it was in the "shaking culture," or in other words, deep in the ground. One could dig deep for large quantities of the soil, rather than dragging and scraping the landscape.

Technically, cyclosporine lay in fungi that grew in the Hardanger soil, not in the soil itself, and the next step in producing the drug was to isolate the fungi, replant it, and then cultivate it so that a maximum yield could be grown in the smallest possible area. The fungi then had to be fermented, and subsequently broken down into its purest possible form, a process that, from beginning to end, could (without the specially designed machinery) only be completed by hand. "Back then, considering production costs, an ounce of cyclosporine was worth hundreds of times its equal weight in gold," said Borel. "So, you could not really fault Sandoz for their reluctance. I didn't blame them at all."

Borel did not blame his employers, but he also did not easily give in to them. He lobbied for his drug, and he protested, until he was eventually able to persuade management to permit him to pursue his research into cyclosporine on a limited basis. "I would have done it all on my own time had they declined," Borel said. Further tests in mice over the next three years not only demonstrated the amazing effectiveness of cyclosporine against T lymphocytes, but also its gentleness. There were very few serious side effects evident in the research so far conducted, a crucial point considering the fact that the terrible side effects from azathioprine and prednisone were the primary stumbling blocks toward further expansion of organ transplantation, the field in which cyclosporine would potentially cause a miraculous transformation. In November 1976, Borel traveled to London where he had agreed to present a paper that touched upon his work with cyclosporine.

Dr. David White, an immunologist and a junior associate of Sir Roy Calne, the surgeon who had first used azathioprine clinically in kidney transplant recipients, went to the meeting of the British Society of Immunologists that day—the day that might be described as the "second coming" of cyclosporine—because he too had been thrust into a new and fortunate situation. His superior at Cambridge University had suddenly resigned his position as director of the department in a dispute over promotion and White, at only thirty-two years of age, "fell into the job."

Borel's paper, according to White, "was essentially a review of the many immunosuppressive agents that he had worked with in the lab over the years, and in his talk, he concentrated on one rather peculiar immunosuppressive agent called cyclosporine." Listening quietly in the audience, White was intrigued, although he did not know why specifically. Just instinct. There was really nothing truly significant in what Borel was saying. Many experimental products with mysterious ingredients and thought-stimulating properties come and go in the field of immunology without a ripple. With the exception of Borel's limited work in mice, this stuff had never been subjected to real clinical study. But there was something about cyclosporine, and Borel's enthusiasm, that sparked White's curiosity. And although he did not make himself or his suspicions known at the time, he immediately returned to his office in Cambridge and wrote to Jean Borel. "I said, 'You send me some of this stuff, because I think it might be of value in transplantation. And so, Jean Borel sent me two grams to do some test-tube work. And we did some test-tube work," which, as Borel had known years before, indicated that cyclosporine had major potential as an immunosuppressant in organ transplantation.

"One of my duties [in his new position] is to direct the researches of a number of foreign visitors that we have in our department," says White, "and one of those visitors was working in the lab doing heart transplants in rats. Sounds pretty grandiose, but actually it is a very simple surgical technique. You just put the heart onto any convenient artery and vein. You don't actually take out the rat's own heart; it's just an extra one. And we took [used] this drug to see if it would stop these animals—the rats—from rejecting."

Initially, "we made some super mistakes," said White, beginning with an overwhelmingly large dose, a quantity, White discovered later, about twenty times the maximum amount actually necessary to contain rejection. Also, "Jean Borel had given the dose down the mouth, and I was convinced that we should do it by intramuscular injection."

Back in 1972, Borel had been stymied about the way in which cyclosporine should be administered. For the second set of tests, which had revealed the immunosuppressive effect, cyclosporine had been injected into mice. But, Borel recalls, "at the time I said that when you have a drug which people will have to take everyday," in significant quantities and for the rest of their lives "it is no use to inject it; try to give it orally and see if it is absorbed [into the bloodstream]. It was a rule that you give such a drug three or four more times higher orally than if you give it IV (intravenous) because a person will not absorb 100 percent. So we did that, gave it to mice orally and," said Borel, laughing, "we completely failed to reproduce the result. We did it a third time, and the third time also we failed." Finally, Borel "enhanced the dose at least ten times more" than had been injected, "until we produced the same results with oral activity."

Borel was having similar difficulties in his tests using human volunteers, who were given doses in powdered form in a gelatin package. The drug would pass directly through the digestive tract and never make an impact on the bloodstream. Thus, David White, in early 1977, after first receiving the drug, became certain that it would be more effective and efficient to inject it—at least for experimental purposes. And to do that, White explained, the substance, which came to him in a white powder, had to be dissolved.

White began by dissolving the cyclosporine with alcohol (most other liquids would not reduce it) "and to make a long story short, we killed an awful lot of rats." The alcohol, White explained, combined with the intensity of the cyclosporine being injected directly into the bloodstream tended to "poison" or "paralyze them." For this initial round of experiments, "we got a lot of toxic problems, partly from the alcohol, partly from injecting the drug, but what we *didn't get* was any rejection. So, despite the difficulties, I was keen to go on.

"At that stage, Jean Borel actually came and visited me and brought another five grams of cyclosporine to continue our tests, because I had mentioned to him over the telephone that we were quite encouraged—the rats had not rejected their hearts, although there had been a lot of other problems. And so Jean Borel and I then met for the first time and discussed the problems we were having, and he suggested that the drug might be better dissolved in a lipid [something greasy—fatty acids, etc.], rather than in alcohol, and made a number of suggestions." He also convinced White to give cyclosporine orally.

"I was sitting at the bench in the laboratory one day sometime later trying to dissolve this thing in every kind of lipid that you have seen," said White. "I had a Greek surgeon colleague who was very keen on Greek cooking, which has to be done in Greek olive oil. You can't actually buy Greek olive oil in Cambridge, but there is a Greek restaurant that has it imported in great big drums, and my colleague had an arrangement. He used to go and take a bottle, it was a whiskey bottle, down to the restaurant to actually fill it up with olive oil. And he came into the lab that day, wanting to know when he could get started with the next set of experiments— when was I going to get this stuff suitably dissolved?—with a bottle of Greek olive oil in his hand. 'Oh,' I said, 'you know, I'll bet it will dissolve in olive oil.' So we took Greek olive oil, and it dissolved like a dream. And that's how we started working. And I should say that it is dissolved in olive oil to this day."

Significantly reducing the dosage and giving it to rats, orally, with oil, rather than alcohol, produced such astoundingly good results in the laboratory that when White presented the product of their research efforts to Calne for his approval, "the Professor looked at them and said, 'I don't believe you. Go and do it again.'

"We went away and repeated them again. In fact, what we did was to drop the dose right off until we could actually get rejection, because we were finding that [with cyclosporine] the animals were never rejecting. We actually had to get some rejection to convince the Professor that we really had an immunosuppressive worth looking at.

"I had to write to Jean Borel to get enough cyclosporine—five grams is enough to do some rat experiments, but if you are actually going to do dogs, you are talking many more grams than that. Jean Borel wrote back and said, 'Oh, Sandoz has dropped cyclosporine. They don't think it is worth proceeding with, but we'll send you what we've got,' which was fifty grams, which was then what we thought was most of the world's supply.

"This was August, 1977," said White, "and everyone was away on a holiday. I'm not a surgeon, so it was rather strange for me to actually find myself assisting the Professor in the surgery, holding the strings and things. We did those experiments, and it became immediately clear from the results of the first six dogs, that this was a very, very powerful immunosuppressant. We were getting quite prolonged survivals before we ran out of the drug. When it became quite clear, I rang up Jean Borel and said, 'This is a winner. You've got to get us some more drug.' "

Jean Borel explained that his cupboards were dry. But he said, "Why don't you come over to Basel and tell us what you've been doing and see if we can convince the money men that it is worth going for?"

Meanwhile, Borel had been fighting for the life of his precious drug since Sandoz had made its decision to suspend development. "The marketing people thought it [cyclosporine] was impractical because the first [sales] estimates that were done were based on the selling points of azathioprine," said Borel, "and I went to the marketing people and I said 'Look, you're nuts! You have to add to azathioprine all of the other drugs, like steroids, used for transplantation, and then you have to at least multiply that number by four, because things [transplantation] will increase as soon as cyclosporine becomes available. That computation gave a number that was something like 50 million Swiss francs, which was about $30 million a year volume, and by that number, you may think of developing a drug; it becomes worthwhile." With that figure in mind, the Sandoz people were anxious to hear what David White and Roy Calne had to say.

"I presented the data on cyclosporine," said White, "because we had done a lot more studies in the lab by this time, and Roy gave, as only he can, a kind of general exposé of transplantation, what transplantation was about, because people from Sandoz were just not in that field at all. He said something about the dog experiments and tried to put them in context. Then the Sandoz people adjourned into big rooms with big cigars and mahogany tables, and small calculators," said White, lowering his voice and raising his brows, "and after a while, they came back and said, (in a German accent), 'Ah, ve put our high-risk money into cyclosporines.'

"I should say," White commented, "that it has paid off for them a millionfold. And it was an interesting experience, in a way, actually having to sell a pharmaceutical company its own drug. To their credit, they accepted what we said, and they made it for us initially at great expense, because it was being made virtually on the bench [by hand], many kilos of cyclosporine."

Says Borel: "Sandoz realized that from an image or public relations point of view, it would be beneficial to develop cyclosporine, and of course, they were astonished by the results of Calne's and White's work. Also, Sandoz had a firm near Innsbruck, Austria, which is one of the largest manufacturers of penicillin [made also from a living substance—bacteria] in the world, and they took over the cyclosporine job. They had surprisingly quick success in figuring the methods of up-scaling the production." Today, cyclosporine is fermented in vats that are five stories high.

Although people might criticize Sandoz for its hesitancy and its calculated businesslike approach to pharmacology, it is important to understand that scientists and surgeons can be equally calculating. They too recognize the need to profit from their investment of time, energy, and sheer brain power, and they can be as political and as competitive as any large corporation—often more so. These are the rules of the game, as played by all scientists—Cooley, Shumway, Starzl, Barnard, as well as White and Calne.

"Coming back in the plane," White recalls, "Roy said, 'Now what we've got to do is, we've got to publish this stuff quickly, so that we can get precedents.'" In the world of medicine and science, researchers cannot plunge whimsically into animal or human experimentation: they must show reason, a "precedent" to proceed with their work. Thus, they must "publish" the results of their labors in one of the many medical journals, to be noted by the scientific community. But when you are on the verge of an earth-shattering discovery, you want to make sure that no one steals your ideas—or your thunder—as happened to Shumway and Lower in 1967. Not only had they opened their laboratories to Barnard, but they had published the entire transplant procedure, step by step, with illustrations, in a number of major journals. "You want to publish," said White "where not too many people can see it."

As they flew from Basel to London, and then jumped the train for the one-hour ride back to Cambridge, White and Calne decided to "go public" with their work with cyclosporine and dogs in an obscure "research-communications system, which is one of these computer-run journals, where you publish on a single sheet, while the longer paper is essentially stored in a computerized retrieval system." Anybody who wanted to read the Calne-White paper could read it—but it wouldn't be easy to find.

It wasn't as if White and Calne wanted to forever conceal their work, but as in all professions and walks of life, timing in the world of medicine is crucial. Every two years, the entire global transplant community, some 2,000 to 3,000 strong, counting surgeons, immunologists, nephrologists, etc., gather for the International Transplantation Congress. In 1984, it was held in the United States in Minneapolis, sponsored by the University of Minnesota's transplant program, and in 1986 it convened in Helsinki, Finland. That year, 1978, it was scheduled for Rome.

"The professor's profound ambition," said White, "was to actually get it [cyclosporine] into patients before that meeting, at the end of August. We were then in January 1978—so we had absolute mayhem over the succeeding months. We tested it in rabbits, in pigs, in dogs, in rats, in monkeys. Our abstracts went off in April. I then submitted for oral presentation to the British Transplantation Society meeting in June the bare bones of what was going on in our laboratory, simply so that we would have had the courtesy of telling the English transplant community what was going on before telling everybody else. So the word began to get around."

And the word was incredible. Calne's and White's experiments had revealed "stupendous" results in all of the animals tested. They were convinced, as was Jean Borel five years before, that cyclosporine could change the course of the entire field of immunosuppression. And in the early summer of 1978, White and Calne were ready to attempt to use cyclosporine in humans. "Actually, the first person ever to take cyclosporine was Jean Borel," White recalled, "He took it not in olive oil, but he dissolved it in the equivalent, he tells me, of a liter and half of wine. So having actually taken the drug, he was then too drunk to do the experiment [blood test]. He just lay there and giggled.

"The first patient we actually transplanted with cyclosporine as the immunosuppressive was a young man who got a kidney in July 1978," said White. "Nothing happened." That is to say that nothing "terrible" happened, as might have happened with double-drug or triple-drug therapy. "The inevitable rejection response was effectively controlled by the medication, and the destructive side effects so prevalent with azathioprine, prednisone, or ALG were nonexistent." White shrugged nonchalantly, as if it had been a foregone conclusion.

As David White looks out the window from his laboratory at Addenbrooke's Hospital at Cambridge, where no less than nine Nobel laureates in medicine currently work and reside (he calls Addenbrooke's the "Nobel laureate-infested ivory tower of all ivory towers"), he recreates with both joy and discomfort the details of that day in Rome when he and Roy Calne introduced cyclosporine to the leaders of the world of transplantation.

It started in the afternoon, and their paper was scheduled for presentation on the first day of the Congress. Although everyone who was anybody in transplantation knew through the grapevine about White's and Calne's amazing success with this mysterious miracle, nobody had actually bothered to notify their Italian hosts, and so they had been put in the smallest and stuffiest of the five conference rooms being used. "There we all were," said White, "I suppose, about two and a half thousand people, trying to get into this room, designed for about 350. And I was first speaker, and they kept pouring in and pouring in, and of course, when people see crowds trying to get into the room, everybody else wants to go in and see what's going on. So there was a good deal of commotion.

"I remember having to stand there. I always get nervous when I have to talk, even after fifteen years. My hands still sweat, you know? And this was a particularly important paper. So I had to stand there and wait. I'll never forget, Sir Peter Medawar, who was in a wheelchair [because of a crippling stroke], was lifted up and passed over the heads of all these people crowding in, with him sitting straight up in the wheelchair, and they put him right down in front. And all these people, out of respect, parted to make room for him. I gave a very technical paper on the immunology of cyclosporine. And then Roy gave the stuff that everybody had come to hear: the dog experiments and our [human] clinical experience that we tracked."

White enjoys telling about the dramatic and amusing way in which Calne began his presentation. As it turned out, Jean Borel had hoarded a second stash of cyclosporine, which he was doling out to another group of medical scientists, two

British colleagues, who were following a slightly different trail of research than Calne and White, but which had resulted in similarly positive, although not nearly as useful and well-documented indications. In fact, they had made the announcement of their success with cyclosporine months before Calne and White had elected to go public.

"They had given a press conference on this drug," said White. "Unfortunately—I wasn't there, so I don't know what specifically happened—but the only publication that actually took up the story was what we would describe as a 'tit and bum' magazine called *Reveille*. And the next day, they had this huge big headline. It was a front page. 'Miracle Drug for No Hope Patients.' But the gorgeous bit about it," White chuckled, "was that right next to the article, there appeared a naked lady, and the headline, 'High Flying Donna.' It was a stitch!"

Subsequently, when Roy Calne stepped up to the podium in Rome in late August 1978 to unveil the results of their work with cyclosporine, he began his presentation with a large color slide of *Reveille*'s front-page report, featuring "High Flying Donna."

C h a p t e r 5

THE SAGA CONTINUES

"After Rome," said Jean Borel, "I had everybody at my door begging for an audience, in order to get some of this cyclosporine stuff." The Swiss and the French were especially put out at him for giving cyclosporine to the British for testing, and subsequently to the Americans.

They said, 'You know, we have dogs in our country, too, for the cyclosporine?'

"And I said, 'Yes, but your dogs did not want to eat it.' "

Borel explained that he had many times offered cyclosporine to scientists from both countries before sending it off to White and Calne, "but they would not take it until there was clinical proof that it was effective, and the English and Americans were the only people willing to do the clinical work. So I gave them the drug."

It was not, however, easy sledding either for Borel or cyclosporine from that point. In fact, a potential "catastrophe" then occurred, said Jean Borel. "That was the publication of the paper by Calne in the *Lancet* [a prestigious British medical journal] in 1979 outlining his experiences with his first thirty-four cyclosporine patients." Calne and White had been forced to conclude, based upon a much more extended review of kidney transplant patients receiving cyclosporine—more thorough than the results presented in Rome—that the drug was nephrotoxic (poisonous to kidneys) and that it had induced lymphoma (growth of tumors). "He had three patients with lymphoma," said Borel, "and of course everybody thought that this beautiful dream, this cyclosporine, was finished now; the joke was over.

"It is important to remember that the approach for immuno-suppression at that time was to use the highest possible level, just avoiding the toxicity." That was how azathioprine and prednisone were administered. Calne did the same with cy-closporine, and that had been his nearly "catastrophic" mis-take. When he decreased the dosage for his patients, the lymphoma was eliminated and the nephrotoxicity was sig-nificantly reduced. In the years since cyclosporine was intro-duced, however, the damage that it can do to the kidneys has remained a serious, although not necessarily an insurmount-able danger.

On a more manageable level, scientists have learned that cyclosporine can cause other side effects: hot flashes or sweat-ing; numbness or tingling of the hands and feet and mouth; sinus drainage ("runny" nose); overgrowth of gums, some-times associated with soreness, swelling, and redness. More physically apparent is a constant and uncontrollable shaking of the hands and feet, similar to the trembling of someone with a very slight case of palsy. Cyclosporine also causes an increase in hair growth, most especially on the arms, legs, and face, a situation that women find especially annoying and embarrassing. But most serious indeed is the fact that cyclosporine exerts a great deal of strain on the transplant recipient's kidneys—whether the patient be a heart, liver, or kidney transplant recipient. During the first post-transplant year, most patients suffer a harsh reduction of kidney function caused by cyclosporine. Although the reduction seems to stabi-lize at about 20 percent, many surgeons have recently begun to wean patients on a combination of azathioprine, steroids, and cyclosporine, adapting specific immunosuppressive for-mulas for each individual, thus maximizing effectiveness while minimizing side effects.

In 1979, Jean Borel presented cyclosporine to Thomas Starzl in Colorado for testing—one of only two American surgeons Borel was initially willing to trust with such an important and delicate responsibility; the other was transplant pioneer

Francis Moore at "the Brigham." Starzl was convinced that although cyclosporine had great potential, Calne was not utilizing it to its utmost advantage. "Although there was some good news in Calne's work, there was also some bad news that really disqualified the drug for widespread use," said Starzl. "The bad news was that 40 percent of their patients died, and none of their kidney recipients had normal kidney function." Some of these results were due to overdosing, but there were other factors to consider, as well.

Cyclosporine was also given a trial at the Royal Free Hospital in London. Both the Royal Free, which combined it with azathioprine, and the Brigham trials, which utilized cyclosporine alone, as had Calne, failed. The results were not appreciably better than for traditional prednisone-azathioprine cocktail therapy without cyclosporine. "So of the first four trials of cyclosporine in humans," said Starzl, "one was interesting [Calne's], two failed, and the fourth one was ours at Colorado. If it hadn't been for the Colorado trial, that drug would have been scrapped. Calne was recommending that the drug be used by itself, that it was not to be combined with anything."

But Starzl took a page from his own successful past in the world of organ transplantation and, as he had done with azathioprine fifteen years before, added a small amount of steroids. "Then we 'racked off' [transplanted] about twenty-five or thirty kidneys, and we were enormously impressed with it. We reported it [published a paper] in the summer of 1980, about eight months after Calne's report." Starzl's clinical trials in Denver yielded a 79 percent one-year survival rate. The following year, a randomized trial comparing cyclosporine-steroid therapy with therapy by azathioprine and prednisone was carried out, said Starzl, revealing a one-year survival rate in the cyclosporine-prednisone group of 90 percent versus the expected 50 percent in the azathioprine-prednisone group. "So we had these tremendous results and [after arriving in Pittsburgh] we took it right into livers."

Prior to 1980, the reported five-year survival rate for 170 liver transplant recipients, was 18.2 percent. But then, using cyclosporine and steroids, the projected five-year survival rate, based on 244 patients, had risen to 68 percent. In 1983, when the Food and Drug Administration (FDA) approved cyclosporine for use in all transplant centers on all transplant patients (Starzl and Moore had been required to obtain temporary FDA approval for their experimental trials), it was stipulated that the drug could only be used *with steroids.*

Shumway at Stanford had received the drug for experimental trials in cardiac transplantation in 1980, not long after Starzl had received it in Colorado. By following Starzl's lead, combining it with a moderate amount of steroids, the Stanford people were literally ecstatic with the results—so much so that the persistent and insistent Norman Shumway thought that now, with cyclosporine, perhaps once again it was time to give heart-lung transplantation—that is, the heart and both lungs, *en bloc,* another shot.

Shumway and Lower had experimented with heart-lung transplants in dogs in 1960 and 1961, but the animals didn't survive during the postoperative period. According to Bruce Reitz, "Usually they would wake up, but their breathing would be very slow and deep, totally different from the way a dog normally breathes. But Shumway had it in his mind that if we continued doing this operation in dogs, it would eventually be successful. So every couple of years he would mention to somebody working in the lab, 'Why don't you see if we can't get somewhere on this heart-lung thing?' Most of us had done it once or twice, but no matter how hard you tried, you couldn't get a dog to survive more than four hours or so.

"I started looking back through the literature at the things that had been done before in the way of heart-lung transplantation. There were a few papers, all reporting the same disappointing results as had Shumway. "But there was one article that apparently hadn't gotten much attention when it came out in the early 1970s by Dr. Aldo Castenada at Minnesota, who had done some heart-lung transplants in baboons." Castenada had removed a heart-lung bloc and then put the heart and lungs right back in the same animal. "There were some technical failures, but there were also about a half a dozen animals who woke up, breathed normally, and survived. This was right there in the literature, but no one had paid much attention to it because, I guess, the feeling was that heart-lung transplants just weren't possible. But it just suddenly seemed very clear to me right away."

The problem, Reitz concluded, was how the animals breathed. "There are stretch receptors or nerves in the lungs in dogs which seem to be very important. But if you cut the nerves that go to the lungs in man [which is what happens in a heart-lung transplant], it doesn't matter. Man [and primates] controls respiration almost entirely from the brain." With this in mind, Reitz went a step further than had Castenada by transplanting heart-lung blocs from one monkey to another rather than returning the organs to the same primate. "And the monkeys would survive," said Reitz, "a fact which made Shumway so excited that he would just come back to the laboratory each day and look at those animals and jump up and down."

At the beginning, Reitz's transplanted primates would only remain healthy for seven to ten days. "They would get a lot of infections and eventually die." Then cyclosporine came into the picture. "That's when we really got excited because these animals looked healthy and they kept going. When we finally did the first heart-lung transplant in a human, one monkey was a year and a half old."

When Thomas Starzl, Denton Cooley, and Norman Shumway had first resolved to pioneer the transplant frontier, there were few administrative and governmental regulations prohibiting experimentation; these men could proceed on instinct and the power of faith. The situation had considerably modified for the second generation of transplant pioneers, beginning at Stanford with Bruce Reitz. Approval for experimental therapy was required from ethics and research boards within the university—and from the federal government through the National Institutes of Health (NIH), which in 1980, after about a six-month wait, approved Reitz's proposal for six heart-lung transplants in humans.

By this time, Reitz had interviewed many patients dying from heart and lung disease and had selected the person whom he felt would be best suited: Mary Gohlke, a forty-three-year-old wife, mother, and advertising executive, suffering from primary pulmonary hypertension (PPH), an obscure lung disease that eventually destroys the heart. Not only was Gohlke spunky, honest, and straightforward about her feelings, but size was in her favor. At 5'2" and just a little more than 100 pounds, her body frame could accept a heart-lung bloc from a woman, or a teenager of either sex.

By early fall 1980, Reitz and Mary Gohlke had become friends and partners in this courageous venture, and although they were ready and willing to take the plunge, one roadblock remained. Initially, no one had thought of including heart-lung transplantation in the original application to the FDA for experimental use of cyclosporine because, at the time, heart-lung transplantation was inconceivable. And yet, it became clear that if Mary Gohlke had any chance of remaining alive after surgery, it would be because of cyclosporine. Consequently, Stanford had had to re-apply, and now, despite Mary Gohlke's tenuous grasp on life, the FDA was taking its time passing judgment.

Reitz was impatient, but he felt helpless in the face of the federal government. Mary Gohlke was also helpless—physically—more than anything else. She was bed-bound, and had been for months, experiencing difficulty breathing and suffering from repeated blackouts. She knew deep within her that one day she would lose consciousness, and never open her eyes again. In her 1985 autobiography, *I'll Take Tomorrow,* she describes what happened the day she resolved to wait no longer—that it was time to fight in order to live. She had been talking with Reitz on the telephone from her home in Mesa, Arizona.

"How long do you think it's going to be [for FDA approval]?" she asked.

"Mary, I hate to tell you this. I feel bad about it, but I think it's going to be at least another five to ten weeks."

"I don't think I've got ten weeks. I'm afraid I don't even have five weeks."

"All I can tell you is, hang in there. We're going to get this done," Bruce said.

Later that day, she picked up the phone and called her boss, the editor of the *Mesa Tribune,* and told him that if he knew anyone, anywhere, in an influential governmental position, to please pull some strings—help before it was too late. Max Jennings flipped through his Rolodex and phoned Senator Dennis DeConcini's office. Less than two days passed before Bruce Reitz was again on the phone to Mary Gohlke, this time asking if she was finally ready to come to Stanford. "We've got the approval," he informed her.

The surgery took place on March 9, 1981, with Reitz assisted by his mentor, Norman Shumway, and it was long and arduous, nearly eight hours, but relatively uneventful. Few details of that historic operation have remained with Reitz over time; surgeons involved in these marathon procedures are somehow able to put themselves in a kind of trance-like state, oblivious to all outside stimuli. What he remembers most was how tired he was after the surgery; he had stayed in the hospital two nights straight before putting an end to his sleeplessness.

Within six months, Mary Gohlke returned to Mesa and her family, and eventually went back to work part-time; she wrote her autobiography with Max Jennings, dedicated to Reitz, with a forward by Norman Shumway. More than five years after her historic transplant, Mary Gohlke caught a cold, which eventually turned into pneumonia. She died in her sleep. Today, there are still only a few centers (compared to those doing heart transplants) throughout the world willing to attempt this difficult and highly dangerous procedure, which results in about a 50 percent one-year survival rate.

But Reitz is obviously pleased, not only because he has been the surgeon who made heart-lung transplantation a reality and gave hope to hundreds of potential recipients around the world, but also because he has been able to witness the entire "transplant business" becoming an integral part of the world of medicine. "Used to be you would go to a meeting and give a paper and then stand there looking foolish for there was no discussion."

Now, five years later, Jean Borel has dedicated his life to the drug that helped make Thomas Starzl, Bruce Reitz, and Norman Shumway modern medical heroes, and as his research continues, more valuable and important mysteries of cyclosporine are being uncovered. Within those mysteries, Borel and his colleagues are discovering that cyclosporine's incredible therapeutic umbrella casts shadows of hope and relief in many directions other than organ transplantation.

Scientists have been experimenting with the use of cyclosporine in treating uveitus, an autoimmune disease that can result in blindness. Cyclosporine has been encouraging in newly diagnosed juvenile-onset diabetes patients, and half of those treated have stopped using insulin, at least temporarily. Cyclosporine has shown indications of being useful in curing disorders analogous to rheumatoid arthritis and multiple sclerosis. It has been effective in eliminating psoriasis, and there are some scientists who envision cyclosporine as an element that will help unravel the puzzle of AIDS.

Borel cautions that all of this experimentation is in the very early animal-study stages, at about where he found himself in 1972; nothing can be assumed or even hoped for at this point in the game. Besides, he emphasizes, with cyclosporine's obvious and potentially dangerous nephrotoxicity, the cure could be considerably more harmful than the disease itself. But the seeds he alone planted so deeply with remarkable determination and persistence are beginning to root and blossom in a myriad of revolutionary directions.

PART II

THE DONOR

Chapter 6

RICHIE BECKER

Soon after the accident, Sharon and Dick Becker of Huntersville, a tiny suburban community a few miles from Charlotte, North Carolina, counted up all of the keys to Sharon's flashy white Mazda RX-7 two-seater sports car. There was one key extra, one key they had never seen before—the key their son Richie had used that Wednesday, April 30, 1985.

The Mazda had been Richie's dream car—the one he hoped his parents would present to him on his sixteenth birthday. But Sharon had recently become pregnant, and the Beckers had decided to sell the car and buy a station wagon. Richie was extremely disappointed, but he seemed to understand and accept the practicality of his parents' decision.

The previous Sunday, Richie had labored with his dad, polishing the wire wheels of the Mazda with a toothbrush. Later, as a special treat, Dick had permitted Richie to drive the car from the street into the garage. After all, with the car on the market, this was a rare and final opportunity for Richie to experience the sports car firsthand, or so Dick thought. Perhaps this privilege had sparked Richie's uncharacteristic actions later that week, perhaps not. No one will ever know. There are but a few bare fragments of detail remaining of Richie's final half hour of life.

From all that the Beckers can piece together, Richie had arrived home from school as usual, at about 3 P.M. He dumped his books on the kitchen counter and ran upstairs to change clothes. Sharon and Dick were both at work—Sharon, an agent for an insurance broker, Dick, a designer of electronic security systems.

"Why he got into the car is something about which we can only speculate," said Sharon, a tiny, pretty brunette with a thick, lilting Carolinian drawl. "He and his girlfriend had had a fight that day in school and he told her then, 'Well, I'm coming to see you after school. I'll be there this afternoon.' "

Richie left the house within a few minutes, got into the car using his mysterious key, and pulled out of the driveway. On the desk in his room, alongside a photo of himself leaning proudly against the hood of his beloved sports car, was a book open to a page providing a series of directions and illustrations. It was an automobile driver's manual.

"The accident happened about three miles from the house on a curvy little road," said Dick. "He was following a school bus and showing off, just generally showing off, and got involved in one of those curves, couldn't negotiate it. The police estimated that he was traveling at approximately 70 m.p.h., when he lost control of the car and slammed sideways into a magnolia tree."

The driver's side of the car was nearly untouched, but Richie's head went through the windshield on the passenger side.

Early the following morning, a doctor at Charlotte Memorial Hospital and Medical Center told Dick and Sharon Becker that their son Richie would never again regain consciousness. The term that the doctor used to describe Richie's condition, "brain dead," is defined by the American Bar Association for all legal purposes as "the irreversible cessation of total brain function."

In describing the importance of the concept of brain death, which is law in forty-four states, Denton Cooley has observed that "civilization as we know it today has lasted 3,000 to 4,000 years, and during that time, we have never defined when life begins and when it ends—both ends of the spectrum. We are still arguing about the former, in relation to abortion, but on 'the other end' we have finally worked out a reasonable answer. At one time, we thought that when the heart stopped, that was death. But it is not when the heart stops. It's when the brain stops. That's when people die. Life exists in the brain. That's where your soul and your mind reside. Your heart, your liver—are just servants to the brain. Think of a brain as a master of the household. The master dies, and these servant-organs keep doing meaningless tasks. But those servants actually ought to be employed by some other master, who needs another servant."

It isn't death that is so terribly difficult to accept, said Dick Becker—not even the death of a fifteen-year-old son— but that very idea described by Cooley, *brain death*, because it is such an invisible concept. The majority of organ transplant donors are victims of deaths that are neurological in origin, meaning that the brain incurs damage, but the vital parts of the body maintain the ability to function normally, such as in the case of Richie. It was nearly midnight when Dick was finally permitted to see Richie for the first time in the Intensive Care Unit (ICU), and despite what the doctors had told him about the hopelessness of Richie's condition, Dick was momentarily relieved. "He had a couple of bruises on his face and a bandaged thumb." Dick shook his head, shrugged and sighed. "Gosh, nothing seemed to be wrong with him. What was all the big fuss? I told the nurse, 'Well let's get him up and get him on home.' I figured everything would be back to normal tomorrow."

Richie looked healthy—to his parents, he was indestructible, a kid with a lifetime yet to live—but his appearance was seriously misleading, for he was in no way being supported by his own resources. Every vital function was connected to a corresponding machine, a process initiated the moment the ambulance had brought him to Charlotte Memorial.

He had been immediately intubated—a plastic endotracheal tube was inserted partway down his throat into the trachea to open his airways—and ventilated, meaning that the tube was connected to an electronic ventilator that would force a prescribed measure of oxygen into his system. As Dick lingered in the tiny curtained cubicle in the ICU, he could see Richie's heart beating strongly, the boy's chest rising and falling twelve times each minute to the perfectly paced thump-clunk sound of the ventilator, which sustained his breathing. Richie was being fed intravenously a solution of glucose and saline through a plastic tube connected to a plastic bag extending from an IV pole above his bed, while a similar apparatus, called a Foley catheter and Foley bag, below the bed, helped him pass urine. Despite the monitors and the machinery, said Dick, "it just looked like he was in a peaceful sleep."

If there was anything more difficult at that time in their lives than personally coming to understand and accept brain death, said Sharon Becker, it was the task of attempting to communicate the concept to other people, especially Richie's classmates, unfamiliar with the frightening reality that brain death brings. "The day after the accident, the phone kept ringing off the hook," Sharon recalled. "It was kids from school, and they kept saying, 'I've heard the horriblest thing, that Richie is dead.'

"I would listen, and I would say, 'No, not exactly, he's still on the respirator.'

" 'Oh, thank God.'

" 'Wait a minute. You don't understand. Richie is clinically brain dead.'

" 'Well, just so long as there's hope.' "

Sharon still cries when she talks about her stepson: "Having to explain brain death to the children and to all of the others who inquired, that the respirator was actually breathing for Richie, and that there was just no hope he would ever come out of it on his own, I think was the hardest part of all. I guess I said it often enough, so that sooner or later I myself came to accept it."

At some point the morning after the accident, one of the doctors attending Richie Becker had picked up the phone and dialed Sandy Bromberg, a member of the organ procurement team at Charlotte Memorial, itself a major kidney transplant center, with plans in the works to begin a heart transplant program within the next few months. Bromberg, a registered nurse (RN), was told that tests would soon be initiated confirming Richie Becker's brain death, and that it would now be appropriate to broach the subject of organ donation to the family.

Organ donation in the United States has always been conducted on a voluntary basis—a concept often referred to as "encouraged voluntarism," meaning that a certain systematic and legal framework has been established that maximizes the opportunity for individuals or their next of kin to donate organs and tissue. The framework for this policy took shape on July 30, 1968, when the National Conference of Commissioners on Uniform State Laws approved the Uniform Anatomical Gift Act (UAGA), which served as a model for states to utilize in adopting legislation that would encourage organ and tissue donation. The UAGA, which goes into effect at the time that death is pronounced, called for assigning the right to individuals to donate organs by means of written directives such as donor cards. It also gave the right to families to make donations where the deceased had not expressed an opinion. The UAGA was subsequently adopted (with some variation) in all fifty states and the District of Columbia during the 1970s.

Transplant experts estimate that organ transplantation could potentially extend life and quality of life today to hundreds of thousands of people, but the finite amount of resources available, most especially donor organs, severely limits the potential scope of transplant therapy. Because of the dearth of organs, only the very sick and dying are accepted as candidates for transplantation. And even then, approximately 30 percent of all adults and perhaps 40 percent of infants and young children accepted as candidates for extrarenal transplantation at approximately 200 organ transplant centers across the United States will die while waiting for a donor.

It would be comforting if all death could potentially lead to a second chance at life through transplantation for people who are terminally ill, but unfortunately, only about 1 percent or 25,000 of the 2.5 million people who die each year in this country die under circumstances suitable to become candidates for organ donation. What is even more unfortunate is that only about 15 percent of the possible 25,000 actually become donors.

There are many prerequisites, beginning with age and the general state of health of the dead person. Chronological age is less important than physiological age, and as transplant technology continues to evolve, surgeons are constantly testing and subsequently expanding the age boundaries, but generally, an organ donor should be between the ages of birth and fifty-five years for livers, heart, or heart-lung, and between twelve months and sixty years to qualify for kidney donation. There are no age limits for bone, tissue, and cornea donation.

People within the prescribed limits would not qualify if they have a history of disease or trauma involving organs considered for donation. They would not qualify if they suffered from diabetes, hypertension, cardiovascular or peripheral vascular disease, or malignancies (cancer) other than brain tumors, untreated fungal, bacterial, or viral infection. They would not qualify for heart or heart-lung transplantation if they were heavy smokers, or for liver, kidney, and pancreas transplantation if they were drug or alcohol abusers. Overall and ironically, the ideal organ donor should be, except for the isolated and singular cause of death, in relatively good health.

Many people in the United States mistakenly believe that they are potential organ donors because they have signed organ donor cards, or because they have checked the specially allotted spaces on drivers' licenses provided by some states. But though these are binding documents, surgeons, nurses, and other qualified personnel, citing both legal (fear of malpractice suits) and ethical considerations, will always seek consent from the next of kin. Under the UAGA, authoritative priority is designated as follows: (1) spouse, (2) adult son or daughter, (3) either parent, (4) adult brother or sister, (5) guardian, (6) any other authorized person.

As defined by the UAGA, consent may be given in person through a witnessed signature on the consent form, by telegram, or by phone. When possible, a telephone consent should be taped, with two witnesses listening to the proceedings, and each caller identifying themselves. As a precautionary measure to the transplant team, the tape, along with a transcription, should be entered into the donor's permanent file. If family members are under the influence of alcohol, drugs, in shock, or under sedation, it is necessary to wait for consent until a time when the priority next of kin is alert and aware of the critical nature of the process.

Expenses incurred as a result of donor evaluation, maintenance, and retrieval are automatically assumed by the transplant agency, which is reimbursed by the federal government under Medicare and/or the recipient's insurance carrier. The donor family must pay charges resulting from the patient's diagnosis and treatment related to the primary illness and for the disposition of the body after organ removal. Under no circumstances will the family receive remuneration for the gift of donation. Although the donor family retains the legal right to determine which organs will be donated (in fact, each specific organ must be individually listed on the consent form), any stipulation regarding race, location, or origin of the prospective recipient is discouraged. Ethical and practical considerations make it standard operating procedure to refuse organs if any member of the immediate family objects to donation.

Are families opposed to donating their loved ones' organs for transplantation? Not according to a recent Gallup Poll, which indicated that 80 percent of the families asked to donate organs of a brain-dead spouse or sibling would comply. Ironically, the scarcity of donor organs begins with hospital personnel—most especially the attending physician—reluctant to broach the subject to grieving families. There are many reasons for this reluctance, beginning with the fact that some physicians, especially in rural areas, remain generally uninformed about the advanced state of transplant technology, continuing to believe that it is a pipe dream, far removed from medical reality. But even in cases where doctors and nurses have the best intentions in relation to transplantation, emergency medical crews can get so involved in the lifesaving process (cardiac massage, etc.) that, when and if the patient is lost, they forget to maintain life support systems, especially the ventilator, so that normal circulation can be continued, thus maintaining the prospective donor's viability.

A much more serious and widespread problem is not one of education or reflex, however, but of ego. Many physicians will not allow themselves to think about organ donation because of what it represents to them, personally: "Which is failure," according to Donald Denny, former Director of the Pittsburgh Transplant Foundation, the organ procurement organization that services the western Pennsylvania area, most notably Children's Hospital of Pittsburgh, Presbyterian-University Hospital and the University of Pittsburgh School of Medicine. "An inability to have applied their years of training and experience, and to have saved the life of one of their patients."

Indeed, confirms Dr. Felix Rapaport, Director of Transplantation Service, State University of New York at Stony Brook, "physicians apparently do not want to face the failure implicit in the death of their patient; they do not want to further burden a grieving family by making the request for donation; they are aware of taboos in some religions about organ donation; and they may fear legal recrimination in what has become a highly litigious society."

Also, most physicians are not particularly good communicators, says Denny. They are not taught in medical school or in any part of their internship or residency how to talk to the people they treat. This inability to communicate combined with their reluctance to accept defeat make it "difficult enough to confront a family face-to-face and to tell them that a loved one is dying, let alone turn around and ask them for the heart, liver, and lungs."

To lift the burden from physicians, usually it is the procurement coordinator who broaches the subject of organ donation. Procurement coordinators have been described as the unsung heroes of transplantation, the conduit through which the system flows, for it is their responsibility to stimulate interest in organ donation, to locate the potential organ donor, to meet with the grieving families, to obtain consent, to determine whether donor organs are viable for transplanting into another human being, and finally to link that donor with the transplant surgeon. The procurement coordinator is responsible for the entire process—including transportation and organ preservation—from the time the donor is identified to the moment the organ is to be implanted into the recipient.

Denny, aged fifty, received his master's degree in social work from the University of Pennsylvania and subsequently took a job in his field in Philadelphia, until one day while scanning the newspaper "help-wanted" section, he spotted an ad from the local Society of Transplant Surgeons seeking someone to approach families of potential kidney donors. At this time, 1975, transplantation of extrarenal organs was not yet being widely practiced. He applied and got the job, and four years later was recruited to Pittsburgh. When the transplant program in Pittsburgh began to mushroom, Denny offered a coordinator's position to a young paramedic, Brian Broznick, who had helped him retrieve and transport kidneys. Since then, the Pittsburgh Transplant Foundation has added many additional coordinators and technical assistants.

Denny, Broznick, and Sandy Bromberg are among the 600 members of NATCO, the North American Transplant Coordinators Organization, which has divided the United States and Canada into 115 territories to serve each transplant center. Through frequent phone calls, direct mail flyers, and personal visits, coordinators attempt to inform and educate hospital personnel, primarily nurses, about organ donation and the benefits of transplantation. Each coordinator will make a goodwill visit to the Intensive Care Units of the hospitals (119 in the Pittsburgh area) in their procurement territory once or twice a year.

Beginning in September 1982 and continuing through mid-1987, Pittsburgh maintained 24-ALERT, the talking computer system, which matches extrarenal organ donors with potential recipients. Accessed by telephone, with a capability of handling four incoming calls simultaneously, the system allows an organ procurement coordinator in one part of the country with a possible donor to enter donor information (weight, blood type, age, organ available, etc.). In return, the computer immediately provides the caller with recipient matching information by means of synthesized human speech. If more than one recipient is available for an organ, the computer identifies the patient(s) who are most urgently in need of transplantation through a series of "Status" designations.

A hard-copy (printout) computer system, United Network for Organ Sharing (UNOS), operated by the South East Organ Procurement Foundation (SEOPF) similarly linked all kidney transplant centers throughout the United States and Canada. Although both systems function adequately, organ procurement coordinators have long been united in their belief that a centrally controlled national organ sharing network, linking all transplant centers for all donor organs, would be more efficient and more equitable. In the summer of 1986, following a two-year feasibility study by the National Organ Transplant Task Force, a group appointed by President Reagan, the Department of Health and Human Services allocated $400,000 for the establishment of a procurement network, which went into operation on October 1, 1987, under the UNOS banner.

Although organ donation in the United States has always been conducted on a voluntary basis, there are seventeen countries, including France, Sweden, Greece, and Israel, in which a "presumed consent" system has been instituted, meaning that a brain-dead patient is automatically an organ-donor candidate unless he or she has previously objected in writing. The supply of organs in countries using "presumed consent" has increased, but not nearly as dramatically as had been predicted when the system was introduced.

Most surgeons and coordinators in the United States do not support "presumed consent" because they are certain that it would never be accepted by the very democratic and independent American public. They reason that any attempt to introduce "presumed consent" might create a backlash that would decrease rather than enhance donations. (Actually, for those rare situations in which family members cannot be located or consulted, there are ten states, including Ohio, Texas, and Florida, where a limited "presumed consent" system permits medical examiners and coroners to donate tissues or organs of the deceased.)

Many states, with Oregon and New York leading the way, have sidestepped the situation by introducing a compromise system that restricts the freedom of hospitals and health care providers rather than potential donors. Under "required request," a system devised by Dr. Arthur L. Caplan, formerly of the Hastings Institute, today Director of the Center for Biomedical Ethics at the University of Minnesota, someone on the hospital staff—physician, nurse, or administrator—must offer the option of organ and tissue donation to families of patients declared dead by using brain death or other criteria.

One year after the 1985 implementation of "required request," Oregon reported a 30 percent increase in donation of vascularized organs, a 300 percent increase in skin donation, a 200 percent increase in cornea donation. Based upon these figures, nearly three dozen other states passed legislation for required request over the next two years. Interestingly enough, it was not the initial scarcity of donor organs that eventually triggered the New York legislature into action, but the effects of the mandatory seat belt law, which saved so many lives that it significantly exacerbated the shortage of organs for transplant.

The original state-adopted required request laws often threatened no recourse if hospitals did not comply, but with the establishment of the national organ distribution network, the U.S. Department of Health and Human Services agreed to deny Medicare or Medicaid reimbursement (programs benefitting the elderly and the poor) to hospitals which do not belong to the network and/or do not establish "written protocols for the identification of potential organ donors." In 1987 nearly all of the nation's 7,000 private or public hospitals participated in Medicare or Medicaid.

Many of the same people who favor "presumed consent" have also endorsed the possibility of expanding the search for live donors. Despite the staunch objections from Thomas Starzl and other prestigious transplant surgeons, some seventy-five U.S. transplant centers perform *living-related* kidney transplants as standard practice. Most experts object to *unrelated* living donors because they fear that such an action would immediately trigger a situation in which organs become a commodity for buying and selling. Such an act has been illegal in the United States since a proposal by one Virginia physician to create and operate an organ and tissue brokering service elicited such a strong negative reaction within the transplant community that a special section in the 1984 National Transplant Act was passed into law, making dealing in live organs punishable by imprisonment or up to a $10,000 fine. A similar law is also in effect today in Europe.

Arthur Caplan outlined the ethical arguments presented during congressional testimony by the transplant and bioethical communities in the successful prohibition of a market in organs and tissues. In addition to the inherent danger to the donor associated with the procedure, there was the very persuasive argument that a market in organs would create the "ghoulish spectacle of desperately ill and, as a result, vulnerable patients bidding furiously against one another for invaluable biological materials."

The action of Western nations in forbidding a commerce in donor organs and tissue has had very little effect on many third world and some oriental countries, however. Organ brokering is a perfectly acceptable profession in Taiwan, Indonesia, Pakistan, Korea, and other countries where poverty makes people desperate for dollars. In Brazil, people will often sidestep the local organ broker and place advertisements, offering kidneys or cornea for sale in the newspaper. Such transactions have generated as much as $100,000 in Tokyo, and as little as $1,500 in Bombay, where cultural traditions prohibit the use of brain-dead donors for transplantation. Many advertisers in South American newspapers employ the old-fashioned hard-sell techniques of American used car salesmen: "Kidney or cornea. Any time, any place. Must sell. Best offer." Kidney and cornea donation is also often viewed as a sign of rehabilitation for prisoners applying for parole in the Philippines.

The third world is not so far removed from the Western world, however. Kidneys purchased on the streets of Mexico City or Manila have ended up in England or the United States for transplantation. This does not happen because of greed or dishonesty on the part of the American or British medical establishment, but more so because of its trusting nature and its willingness to help people who are gravely ill.

A citizen of Saudi Arabia, Kuwait, or any country where transplantation is prohibited by religion or law might arrive at a kidney transplant center in the United States with a man or woman who claims to be a "nephew" or "cousin," and who explains, usually through an interpreter, that because of emotional or humanitarian reasons, he has decided to donate one of his healthy kidneys to his "uncle." Through the help of a professional broker who will match blood and tissue, it is relatively easy to "buy" a donor similar enough to pass the general tests conducted by American hospitals to verify a possible relationship, especially one as elusive as "cousin." In a Pulitzer Prize winning report entitled "Selling the Gift" and focusing on profiteering in kidneys, the *Pittsburgh Press* told of one wealthy Indian warehouse owner who forced more than 100 of his employees to undergo blood and tissue matching tests in order to find a suitable donor for his ailing wife. The person selected to donate was rewarded with a trip to England, where his kidney was removed—and the opportunity to keep his job.

Importing of foreign organ donors by potential foreign recipients will always be a problem, according to Dr. Hans Solinger, a transplant surgeon at the University of Wisconsin Medical Center in Madison, who told the *Pittsburgh Press* that he mistakenly transplanted a kidney from a paid foreign donor into a foreign recipient. (The patient confessed after the surgery.) "If I get a Wisconsin dairy farmer with his wife of thirty-five years in here, and she wants to give him a kidney, I can go to a whole town full of people who go to church with them, watch them milk their cows, and know that they are really married. I can't do that with a foreign national," Solinger was quoted.

Solinger and other surgeons insist that it would be unfair and incorrect to heap the blame for the scarcity of donor organs wholly upon the shoulders of the medical community, either because of their lack of responsibility or their fear of showing weakness or admitting failure—especially considering the results of a 1985 Gallup Poll of 1,500 people, eighteen or older, sponsored by the American Council on Transplantation. The poll concluded that Americans overwhelmingly believe in organ donation, that they feel it is the proper and generous thing to do—*as long as the liver, hearts, kidneys, and pancreases being donated are someone else's.*

Gallup reported that 74 percent of the adult Americans polled said that it was not wrong "to prolong life through the use of human organ transplants." Sixty-seven percent of the respondents used the words "loving" and "generous" when asked how to best describe a donor. Would they approve of transplantation of a loved one's organs? Assuming that the relative had indicated a desire beforehand, 71 percent said yes. Nearly half of the people polled indicated their willingness to donate their children's organs in case of accidental death. But how many of those 1,500 people were likely to donate their own organs? Says Gallup: Just 27 percent.

The contrasting figures perhaps suggest that although it is difficult to deal with the tragic loss of a loved one, it is considerably more difficult for the average man on the street to come to grips with his own mortality. Indeed, 18 percent of the respondents, choosing from a list of nine possible reasons for declining their own organ donation, replied: "I don't like to think about dying." Other answers included the squeamish 16 percent who "don't like the idea of somebody cutting me up after I die" and the religious 12 percent who "want my body intact for the resurrection or for a healthy afterlife."

Brian Broznick says that during the half dozen years he has worked full-time as an organ procurement coordinator, he has received very little resistance on religious grounds, with the exception of the Christian Scientists, who reject all medical cures, preferring to believe that the body will heal itself. "For a considerable time we had trouble obtaining consent from Orthodox Jews, but public statements from many highly respected rabbis endorsing donation and transplantation have improved the situation significantly." In Israel, where a liver transplant program was introduced by Dr. Igol Kam, a surgeon trained for three years by Thomas Starzl in Pittsburgh, the ultra-orthodox Jews continue to oppose donation and transplantation, defending the sanctity of the human body.

Experience indicates that location, race, and nationality of the donor and family also make a difference as to willingness to donate. In western Pennsylvania, for example, an area known for its transplant activity, families asked to donate organs will respond at a rate above the eight of ten national average, as reported by Gallup, but in New York, only half the families approached will consent to donation. Denny and Broznick attribute the poor rate of donation in New York, especially Manhattan, to the hostile atmosphere caused by high crime in the city, and the large and generally less-educated population. Denny says that people of Latin or Middle Eastern backgrounds are less likely to be willing to donate organs primarily because of superstition and lack of medical sophistication.

Broznick estimates that only 20 percent of the blacks (whether the coordinator is black or white doesn't seem to matter) approached agree to donate. "I've had black people say to me, 'Oh, if you're going to give these kidneys to white folks, we're not going to donate.' " (Broznick points out that, ironically, the vast majority of the people on dialysis are black.) Similarly, have white people refused to give organs to black people? "Twice in my experience. I told both families if that's the way they felt about it, they shouldn't donate." Broznick says that there is some difference in tissue type in the kidneys of blacks and whites, but not enough to make an impact on the selection of transplant recipients.

Of course, there is no way to guarantee who would receive an organ being donated, and no way for the donor to trace the recipient after the donation is completed. Because of the many kidney transplant programs around the country and because so many kidneys are transplanted annually (about 8,000), there is a good chance that a kidney will be given to a recipient in the immediate area of the hospital, but extrarenal organs, most especially livers and heart-lungs, might end up anywhere in the United States or Canada simply because there are so few centers capable of attempting these delicate operations. Procurement agencies will supply some general information to either the recipient or the donor family: the sex, age, the location of the donor or the recipient surgery, but no more. This information is held in the strictest confidence.

Foreign nationals traveling to the United States for transplantation have also become a significant issue, even if they are not accompanied by a "cousin" to facilitate donation. In July 1985 the *Pittsburgh Press* triggered an ongoing controversy by publishing a large front-page story that revealed, in part, that 28 percent of the kidneys transplanted by Thomas Starzl's surgical team at Presbyterian-University Hospital over a fourteen-month period in 1984–1985 were transplanted "into patients from foreign countries, primarily Saudi Arabia. In most cases, there were U.S. citizens waiting who would have benefitted from the specific kidney available." This was in violation of "hospital policy," the *Press* said.

The *Press* listed a number of examples of "foreign citizens— especially Saudi Arabians—[given] preference over Americans for kidney transplants," including a "member of the Royal Saudi family," (a princess) and the "daughter of the King of Qatar."

In addition to statements from Starzl and other Presbyterian surgeons, the viewpoint of Don Denny, Presbyterian's procurement head, was prominently covered in the *Press*'s story. He focused upon the potential ramifications of transplanting so many foreign nationals. "I am concerned that the numbers of foreign national transplants may create an appearance of favoritism which will negatively affect the willingness of Americans to donate," he was quoted. He recommended that "protocols and policies" be established to clarify some of these ethical concerns, and stressed that the decisions that were needed were beyond the province and authority of medical professionals.

Denny also broached the subject of political pressure, which, he claimed, can sometimes play a role in who receives donor organs, a contention confirmed in the *Washington Post* by reporter Howard Kurtz, who described "a new form of political patronage, in which obtaining the support of a state legislator, member of Congress, or even the president can spell the difference between life and death for those who need a costly organ transplant."

Such decisions, one congressman told Kurtz, often depend

upon political clout. "It's which patient has gotten to someone who can influence the state Medicaid program . . . or whether the president or some congressman decides to give you visibility." Kurtz quoted another official, "weary of the constant pressures from Capital Hill," who "said that some members of Congress act like 'ambulance chasers,' and are all too eager to exploit these situations for publicity."

There are no indications that President Reagan's involvement in the transplant world has been motivated by purely political gain, but his efforts, although extremely helpful to some patients, have been quite unfair to many others. Early in his administration, Reagan appointed a staff assistant, Michael Batten,* as a special White House transplant liaison, and over the years Batten has responded to personal appeals for assistance from hundreds of desperate patients throughout the United States. The problems have been nearly always financial—conflicts over coverage between insurance carriers and/or state medical assistance bureaus and patients requiring transplants. Batten could not allocate money, but by personally "inquiring" into the situation, he was able to exert the considerable weight and influence that only the White House could muster.

Despite the fact that Batten has saved many lives, his efforts have also triggered serious questions concerning a subtle but important form of discrimination. One might ask: What about the many hundreds of patients dying from heart or liver disease who may not have money to pay for the procedure, but who also might have never heard of Michael Batten and would not know how to contact him? What about the people too proud or too intimidated to ask the White House or anyone else for special treatment? What about the people who cannot write articulate letters or sound irate and/or desperate over the telephone? Does the very existence of Michael Batten's position as transplant liaison, combined with President Reagan's tendency to publicly and individually respond to isolated instances of personal tragedy, constitute unfair treatment to

---

*With the influx of the Bush administration, Batten's tenure at the White House ended.

the vast majority of the people who are unwilling or unable to access the media or draw attention to themselves? On TV, or for his Saturday afternoon radio broadcast, Reagan has frequently made personal appeals for organ donors for dying children, but when was the last time he spoke out on behalf of an adult? Wouldn't the thirty-five-year-old father or mother of three children be as important, or perhaps even more important to save than a child of eight?

Brian Broznick and most other organ procurement coordinators around the country point out that Reagan's efforts, as generous and well-meaning as they may be, are often detrimental to the organ allocation system as well as to the credibility of the program. "Special media events (press conferences, etc.) mislead people into believing that the child on whom the press is focusing is the only child waiting for an organ when there are probably 100 just like this kid, and three or four just as sick. People will be led to believe that once the child is transplanted, the need for donor organs is then less severe."

Broznick, Starzl, and Chief of Surgery Henry T. Bahnson deny having to confront any overt political pressure on the determination of who will be selected for transplantation, and they insist that the *Pittsburgh Press*'s stories, although valid to a certain extent in detail, were extremely unfair, unbalanced, and one-sided. They do not deny that many foreigners were given kidneys prior to Americans during the period in question, but in most cases, there were reasons for their actions.

At the outset, they say, it was never any secret that foreign nationals, many from the Middle East, came to Thomas Starzl for liver or kidney transplantation. The *Press* itself had featured stories focusing upon the economic activity wealthy Arab families had generated, especially at hotels, where the Saudis would occupy not rooms or suites, but entire floors. But there were many other patients from many other countries being treated by Starzl's transplant team. In Pittsburgh from March 1981 through December 1985, Starzl had transplanted livers into 518 patients, 60 of whom were from countries outside of the United States, including Peru, Germany, Finland, and Canada. During that period, more livers were transplanted into Israelis than into patients from all other Arab countries combined.

The *Press* made no mention of these statistics in this story, nor did it fully explain the circumstances under which so many foreigners, especially Arabs, ended up in Pittsburgh for transplant. Obviously, liver transplantation was rare, with only a few centers in the world capable of such challenging surgery, which is why Thomas Starzl would often find mothers and fathers with dying children arriving uninvited from Ireland, Argentina, even England, where the second largest liver transplant center was located, pleading for help.

Kidney transplantation is not so new, however, and although lengthy and relatively difficult, today it is considered routine surgery in most countries, with the exception of Arabic countries, where, up until recently, religious beliefs prohibited cadaveric transplantation. Because there are approximately two American patients waiting on dialysis for each kidney that becomes available, most of the largest U.S. kidney transplant centers had recently adopted policies denying or limiting the transplantation of foreigners. Starzl, however, had transplanted a number of foreigners at Denver, and he continued to accept foreign kidney patients after arriving in Pittsburgh in 1981. The Saudi government provides all of its citizens with preferred medical treatment wherever it is available.

The "policy" the *Press* had accused Starzl of violating, had been recommended by a colleague, who had become concerned that the many foreigners attracted to Pittsburgh by Starzl might somehow give the wrong impression to potential donor families, thereby reducing the number of kidneys available for transplant. In 1983, a letter was circulated stating that foreign nationals would not receive kidney transplants unless every effort had been made to make the kidney available to an American. The letter had been initialed by Daniel Stickler, then the President of Presbyterian, but Starzl had refused to agree to it. Many foreigners had already been accepted into the program, he explained, and foreigners were continuing to be accepted. To put them on the bottom of the list would mean that they could never receive kidneys; they could die waiting.

There were a number of other complicating issues, but if one was to boil it down for Starzl and other members of his transplant team, an important and overriding principle was at stake here having to do with the Hippocratic Oath and the tradition of sharing lifesaving therapy, especially with the underprivileged. As surgeon Robert Gordon stated: "I want to practice medicine, not discrimination."

Chief of Surgery Bahnson, who reviewed each of the thirty-five kidney transplant cases questioned by the *Press*, says that "there were a few little things in that whole episode [the *Press*'s reports] that we, if we had to do it over again, would have done a little differently in retrospect," but primarily he stands behind the decisions made by his surgical services. Bahnson says that on many occasions foreigners did receive kidneys prior to Americans who had been waiting for transplant longer, as the *Press* had reported. But there were explanations, extenuating circumstances, in nearly every situation.

For example, in two cases, Starzl and/or Gordon had determined that the foreign patient would die without immediate transplant, and in two other cases (a Syrian and an Egyptian), their governments had decided to withdraw financial support and force the people to return home (and perhaps eventually to die) if they were not transplanted immediately. One patient had previously been transplanted in Denver by Starzl and another patient was a child; it is policy to give priority to former patients and to children. In two other instances, the Americans on the list had been too ill for surgery, and the kidneys were given to the back-up patients standing by, who happened to be Arabs. One of the two Americans, a woman, had had a heart attack on the way to the OR and died, at which point the Arab was summoned.

"There is no question that in some cases foreigners got special treatment, but it was because they *didn't* have money," said Robert Gordon, "not because they did. The newspaper portrayed it as the hospital making big bucks off Arab oil sheiks, so they are giving them preference for the kidneys. That's not why people got special treatment. They got special treatment for medical reasons or for financial reasons which were the exact opposite of what the newspaper portrayed."

Gordon and Bahnson did not agree with Starzl's decisions in each instance, nor was Starzl's rationale always supportable. For example, Starzl partially justified transplanting an Italian woman because she was the daughter of the chairman of the Department of Medicine at a prestigious university. He gave another kidney to the mother of a religious leader who was working toward changing the cadaveric donor law in his home country. But in these and in many of the remaining cases, the situations were extraordinarily complicated, and perhaps that is why the *Press* did not attempt to explain the intricacies and variations in each and every instance to its readers.

In his zeal to defend himself, however, Starzl also made things worse than they might have been. Once, he agreed to a two-hour, off-the-record, tape-recorded conversation with Andrew Schneider, one of the reporters responsible for the series, and a few days later, he discussed the conversation with a reporter from a rival paper that, in essence, violated the off-the-record agreement. Schneider, in response, wrote a long and damaging accounting of the behind-the-scenes issues involving foreign nationals at Presbyterian, based upon the tape-recorded conversation.

At one embarrassing and unfortunate point in this interview, published in the *Press*, Starzl confided to Schneider that some of the kidneys transplanted into foreign nationals were "bottom of the barrel" organs. Later Starzl said that the kidneys given to the wife of the financial adviser to the King of Saudi Arabia were crumbs. "They were crumbs. They were crumbs," he said, meaning that they were bruised or subjected to unusually long storage times. Starzl was attempting to illustrate that he had taken these substandard organs— kidneys that would not have been transplanted into American citizens—and because of his experience and surgical skill made them usable. He had transplanted them into the foreigners on Presbyterian's waiting list.

Starzl's confusion and frustration with the relentless reporting of transplant revelations by the *Press* kept him perplexed for many weeks, and provided an interesting insight into his character. As much as he tried, he couldn't seem to understand the newspaper's motivation for its pursuit of him. He realized that he was wrong on a certain bureaucratic level, but he seemed to justify his actions as necessary, in light of his obsession to save lives through transplantation. The bottom line was that he had made those "crumb" kidneys—kidneys that ordinarily would have been discarded—work for foreign nationals who might otherwise have not received a transplant, or whose transplant might have denied an American a kidney. And as far as Thomas Starzl was concerned, a successful transplant superseded or neutralized practically all other considerations. Nothing was more important than transplantation.

"What else does that newspaper want?" he asked. "You know how we work. We pull a name from the list—the sickest kids. I don't even know who they are, what color, or where they come from. Sandee (his senior coordinator) tells me who's the sickest and that's who we do.

"We brought a heart in last weekend for a very beautiful woman here. It came from a fifteen-year-old girl from Venezuela, who was only in this country for twenty-four hours. Her parents didn't worry about who got the organ, or from what country the donor was. They just wanted to help somebody. I think that's payment for some of the other foreign nationals we do."

Just as people feel differently about the nationality of both donor and recipient, so too are there definite preferences concerning the donation of different organs, according to Brian Broznick. The pancreas, kidneys and even the liver are more readily donated, but the heart will sometimes be omitted because it is considered by some to be "the essence of life." Broznick says that many families are reluctant to sign away a loved one's skin, bone, and tissue because they are afraid that the body will be mutilated and unsightly for burial. This is untrue. The body is restored from wherever bone is taken, and skin, removed at a thickness of approximately 10 to 15 one-thousandths of an inch, similar to a mild, peeling sunburn, is taken from areas normally concealed, and transplanted to victims of fire and chemical burns. (Even after the removal of larger organs, the donor's appearance is restored for burial.)

More than 23,000 people received cornea transplants in 1985, while bone, the second most transplanted tissue today, second only to blood, has a myriad of uses, including restoration or replacement for bone cancer and other degenerative bone diseases, back and spinal problems, and congenital defects of the face and head. Some bones are kept intact for replacement, and others are ground up into "cancellous" (spongy tissue) for repair and restoration of existing bone. Tissue recovered from a brain-dead donor also includes cartilage, tendons, joints, ligaments, nerves, blood vessels, and in cases in which the heart cannot be transplanted, often the heart valves. Skin and cornea are stored in freezers, and while cornea will remain viable for only up to six months, skin will keep indefinitely.

"Sometimes you have skin in your freezers for six months or a year and all of a sudden there's a major industrial accident and there's all these burn victims," said Broznick, "and you wipe out all of your skin overnight. That's the kind of thing you try to stockpile, so when the need comes up, you have it available." Bone has an indefinite storage life because it is cryogenically frozen—freeze-dried like coffee, and then vaccuum packed. "Just add water and mix."

The primary reasons people are reluctant to donate their own organs, however, according to Gallup, have to do with what would happen to them *before they died,* rather than after. Twenty-three percent responded by admitting their fear that surgeons "might do something to me before I am really dead," and 21 percent said: "I'm afraid that the doctors might hasten my death if they needed my organs." Sandy Bromberg's colleague, RN Mike Callahan, a former army medic, once dedicated hours answering questions and explaining organ donation to one family "only to have a neighbor lady come in and say that the young boy [brain dead] would feel the pain" as the doctors cut the organs away. The mother did not believe the neighbor, "but she couldn't get the thought out of her mind, and eventually decided not to donate."

Surprisingly, these naive ideas are shared by some ICU

nurses and other health professionals involved in the organ donor process. Writing in the *New England Journal of Medicine*, a group of eight psychologists, nurses, and surgeons from Case Western Reserve University School of Medicine contend that the process of maintaining organs for transplantation, which necessitates treating dead patients as if they were alive, is as disturbing to some health professionals as it is to the general public. Underlying this disturbance "are concerns that organ donors are not dead, despite a declaration of brain death, and that the organ recovery process itself is somehow disrespectful and may indeed kill the donor."

The authors also highlight more subtle reasons health professionals, primarily nurses, refuse to cooperate with organ donation, beginning with the lack of a special term or category to describe dead patients whose organs and systems continue to function. They are not "corpses" in the traditional sense, and although they are dead, they do not resemble other dead patients, who would not be on life support systems, but on their way to the morgue. "When the patient is admitted to the operating room [for organ removal], the recorded diagnosis is 'beating heart cadaver'—a term that is offensive to most people." The lack of an accepted term for "taking of the organ" is also troublesome. "Harvest" is most common, but in Pittsburgh "retrieval" is used, according to Denny, ever since an angry surgeon told him not to treat one of his patients "as though he were a cash crop."

There is an interesting message in the final item in the Gallup Poll, concerning this "glitch" in what is otherwise a very well-planned system of donation: Sixty-two percent, *more than double the 27 percent very likely to donate their own organs*, added that they wouldn't mind if, upon death, their organs were donated, even if they hadn't initially given their permission—a revelation that rather abruptly leads the discussion of organ donation back to the original starting point: the physician.

Doctors are not only reluctant to bring up the subject of organ donation, but worse, are initially remiss in their responsibility to the family in explaining the meaning of the term "brain death." In a 1984 survey conducted at hospitals with more than 200 beds, it was discovered that nearly 90 percent of the neurosurgeons responding, 80 percent of the hospital administrators, and 60 percent of the nurses believed that the brain-death criteria was generally accepted by the medical community. One-third of the medical professionals responding, however, maintained that brain death remained a complicated and difficult concept to communicate to potential donor families.

"Some doctors," says Denny, "prefer to let the patient deteriorate on the ventilator until the heart runs down, as it inevitably will. That makes it extremely difficult on the family. They haven't been told that their relative is dead. They've been told 'he's hopeless.' This prolongs the agony of the family and the patient." Doctors often take another course of action to protect themselves from pain and embarrassment by asking the families if *they* want to disconnect the ventilator, as if the official expiration of their loved one is in the family's hands. This is not true. "The patient is dead, connected or disconnected. Why put that burden on them?"

And no family who thinks that their father or daughter is still alive will want to discuss organ donation. "It brings up all sorts of negative images—someone hovering around waiting for him to die, or worse, hastening his death. Families must understand that brain death *precedes* donation."

If the concept of brain death is confusing to the parents of brain-dead children, it is often totally frustrating to the parents of anencephalic (a condition in which the brain and spinal cord have completely failed to develop) children. In September 1986, the *New York Times* reported the experience of a twenty-six-year-old Canadian woman, five months pregnant with twins, who was informed that one of her infants would be anencephalic, and thus would die at birth or very soon thereafter. Because Canadian transplant centers are not at this time equipped to operate on newborns, the woman's physician attempted to arrange for organ donation in the United States. To simplify matters, the woman volunteered to deliver her babies at a major U.S. transplant center.

Unfortunately and necessarily, the woman's offer was turned down. Because the brain stems of infants suffering from anencephaly are still functioning at birth, they do not fulfill the prevailing legal definition of brain death. Consequently, the parents of this Canadian child, along with the parents of approximately 3,500 anencephalic children born in the United States annually, have been denied the opportunity of donating the organs of children who have no possible hope for survival beyond a few hours or days. This is especially tragic because the demand for infant donors is undoubtedly most acute. The *Times* interviewed one official at the Loma Linda University Medical Center near Riverside, California, who observed that the hospital was forced by law to turn down two or three anencephalic children offered by parents as organ donors each month, while fifteen infants who had been accepted into Loma Linda's transplant program died in 1985 awaiting new hearts. Anencephalics have been used as donors in western Europe and Japan in recent years, however. A small group of California legislators are attempting to change the law in their state.

As mentioned in a previous chapter, Loma Linda was also the sight of a spectacular attempt to identify and demonstrate the feasibility of another alternate source of pediatric donor organs when, on October 15, 1984, the heart of a baboon was transplanted by Dr. Leonard Bailey into a fifteen-day-old girl called "Baby Fae." Transplants fall into three distinct categories. There are *homografts*, transplants of the same species (human-to-human, dog-to-dog), *heterografts*, which link closely related species, such as dog-to-wolf. Up until Baby Fae, the idea of an *xenograft*, transplants between distantly related species, specifically, animal-to-man, had not been publicly explored.

Most of the surgeons at Children's and Presbyterian-University Hospitals in Pittsburgh were cautious, but in no way opposed to the possibility of animal to human transplantation. "My initial reaction was repulsion," said visiting Australian surgeon Stephen Lynch. "But when you sit down and think about it logically, it is not so bizarre. Many of the heart valves put into people these days have been man-made from pig valve cuffs. Pig skin is used in severely burned patients, and that's a transplant—pig skin onto the original skin. That was the original transplant, long ago—a skin graft." Cows have also played an important role in extending human life. Patches are taken from a cow's pericardial sac (the membrane surrounding the heart), and utilized to repair human heart valves, and cow tendons and bones are actually used to replace those damaged in humans. The "catgut" once used in surgical procedures comes from the intestines of sheep.

Actually, the concept of animal to human transplants should not be surprising to anyone involved in the world of transplantation in any significant way. On about a half dozen occasions between 1906 and 1923, kidneys were removed from a pig, goat, lamb, or primate, and transferred to patients who were terminally ill. Interest quickly waned because all of these patients died, but in 1963 and 1964, Dr. Keith Reemstma, today at Columbia-Presbyterian Hospital in New York, but then at Tulane University in New Orleans, attempted a dozen xenografts over the course of eighteen months—chimpanzees' kidneys into humans—and was able to extend the lives of two patients for more than two months.

At about the same time, Dr. James Hardy, Chairman of the Department of Surgery, University of Mississippi School of Medicine, performed a surgical feat of stunning magnitude, according to the journalist Thomas Thompson, who recorded Hardy's recollection of that experience in his book, *Hearts*.

"On January 23, 1964—how well I remember—a man named Boyd Rush from Laurel, Mississippi, a man who had had heart trouble for years, was brought into our hospital in shock. We examined him and told his family that there was nothing that could be done for him surgically—but that there was a possibility of a cardiac transplant. We explained that there was a neurological case in the hospital, with the patient near death, and that if death did occur, then we could perhaps use the heart. But if death did not occur, then would they agree to the heart of a suitable primate? They were less enthusiastic about a 'suitable primate,' but they finally agreed." According to Hardy, the medical community was also very squeamish. "Even the cardiologist, who had earlier agreed, stood outside the surgery doors wringing his hands and saying, 'I don't know, I just don't know.' I said, 'Look, when you're going to jump, you're going to jump.' "

Despite all doubt, Hardy and his team proceeded. "We put in the chimp's heart and it started up right away. It beat regularly for a while, but it only lasted two hours because the patient was in terminal shock. He was too sick to accept anything."

Soon after the Baby Fae transplant, at a regular monthly University of Pittsburgh Medical School forum called "Ethics for Lunch," in which faculty members discuss their particular area of specialization, Starzl, in his typical brief, direct, and thorough manner, highlighted the history and brought some perspective to the present and future potential of animal to human transplantation. Based upon Reemstma's work in 1964 at Tulane, Starzl said, "I used two chimp liver donors for children in the sixties, for whom we did not find a human donor. One of those two children died because of an infection, but the death had nothing to do with the liver. And one of Reemstma's kidney transplants from a chimp to a human," Starzl added, "was to a woman who lived almost normally, out of the hospital, for almost a year.

"The situation is very awful and frustrating," Starzl pointed out. "Every week that goes by, one of these children waiting for transplantation here will die. This has been a continuous source of anxiety for all of us." He estimated that approximately 100 children were currently awaiting livers, at least a half dozen under six months of age, "with very little prospect or hope."

"So why not use chimps?" a student asked.

"The chimp is an endangered species," Starzl answered. "And there is the potential ethical problem of essentially 'executing' a living thing capable of rather high and integrated intelligence. That is a problem that would trouble everyone."

One who has long been troubled by the use of chimpanzees in medical research is the anthropologist Jane Goodall, author of *The Chimpanzees of Gombe*, who points out that there are numerous behavioral, psychological, and emotional similarities between humans and chimps, "resemblances so striking that they raise a serious ethical question: are we justified in using an animal so close to us—an animal moreover that is highly endangered in its African forest home—as a human substitute in medical experimentation?"

Goodall is primarily concerned with the fate of chimpanzees, but Starzl warned of the "potential outcry" from all different sorts of animal protection groups similar to those that had immediately set up pickets at Loma Linda in 1984 and loudly criticized Bailey's actions. "And then," said Starzl, "there is also the problem about where one would get a supply of chimpanzees" to do transplants.

RN Frank McSteen, director of the animal laboratory at the University of Pittsburgh, pointed out that the choice of using a dog, pig, or other laboratory animal in transplant clinical experimentation is often dependent upon economics. "From the time a dog comes into our holding facility and until he reaches us, we will spend $250. A pig is a lot less expensive than a dog—about one-fifth. A rhesus monkey, who has been quarantined, inoculated, born in this country, labhoused, you are talking a cost of $700. If you want a baboon— $1,200. A chimpanzee, however, is out of the ballpark."

Starzl estimated that there were probably no more than thirty chimps in the United States for all investigators in the whole country to use. "The great competitors would be for use in research in hepatitis and AIDS. Finally there is the pure raw question of expense. Right now it costs about $10,000 to purchase a chimp."

Brian Broznick, who approaches approximately 100 families a year, points out that the idea of using animal organs is beyond the scope of imagination of most ordinary people, who usually have trouble enough grasping the normal issues of life, death, and transplantation, beginning with the intricacies of brain death—a primary challenge.

"I want them to feel absolutely, positively comfortable that their loved one is dead. That there is no hope for this person. There's no miracle cure coming down the road. Nobody is going to come in and bless the patient, and then the patient will get up and walk. That's not going to happen. I want them to feel comfortable about that first, and then we'll talk about organ donation. I'm not there to convince them of something. I am not going to twist their arm. If they say 'no,' that's fine; that's their decision. I tell them that up front."

Jo Burton, a former ward sister (nurse), now an organ procurement coordinator at Addenbrooke's Hospital at Cambridge, believes that it is essential to "get the family to talk about the person who has just died, and I think it is very, very important to mention the word, 'death.' I ask them, 'When so and so was alive, did he talk about organ donation?' The idea is to help them look at that individual's wishes. The most important thing is to try to be informal about it, and I know sometimes I've sat on the floor when there hasn't been a chair, just give them a cup of coffee and let them talk."

Burton and Broznick agree that organ procurement coordinators—despite the country in which they work—are primarily facilitators. Says Broznick: "Although I am supposed to find organs for the people who are waiting, I see my job more as a person who is a mediator [between the system and the family] for that family to give that gift; I am part of the process that allows them to derive something positive out of something that has been tragic and senseless for them."

He is, however, critical of fellow coordinators and hospital public relations departments who in literature and public statements lead people to believe that "a part of their loved one will live on through organ donation. That's their liver, not the person they knew. It's one part of the body. The heart is nothing but a pump. That part of the body that made that person a loving person, a caring person, and a knowledgeable person is the brain, and that's gone."

Dick and Sharon Becker only vaguely recall the conversation that took place between the coordinator at Charlotte Memorial, Sandy Bromberg, and their family in the waiting room adjacent to the ICU, but both parents agree, counter to Broznick's objection, that the idea that a part of Richie would be able to live on in other people was a primary motivating factor in their decision to donate. "We are all put on this earth to accomplish one thing or another," said Dick, "that's what I truly believe. And perhaps, you never know, this was Richie's purpose—to give life to others. We do know that Richie would have wanted us to donate; Richie was a truly generous and compassionate young man, and our decision was ultimately based upon our strong sense that this is what he would have wanted, had he himself been given the choice."

Dick's parents are deceased, but his two brothers had flown in immediately, the day after the accident on May 1. When the subject of organ donation was broached, the entire family participated in the decision. "What was especially important to us was the fact that Sandy [Bromberg] never exerted the least bit of pressure. She made it clear over and over again that what happened to Richie was completely under our control." Before deciding in her own mind, Sharon consulted with their minister. "I wanted to be sure that the donor program would not interfere with Richie going to heaven." Dick and Sharon subsequently signed the consent form, authorizing donation.

Methods used by coordinators to approach families of potential organ donors vary, depending both upon the situation and the personality of the coordinator, as well as the type of people with whom they might be dealing. Bromberg, who has been a coordinator since 1984, says that she hardly ever knows what she will say to the grieving family in advance. "I let my instincts guide me when I walk through the door. You can tell right away whether they want to talk with you, and whether they will be receptive, inquisitive, or even hostile."

Only a very few coordinators report that the families they approached have gotten openly threatening: "The biggest problem is that these families are actively grieving and you are interrupting this grief," says Bob Duckworth, formerly a procurement coordinator in Pittsburgh, now Director of Organ Procurement for the University of Nebraska at Omaha. "But it can't be helped. The patient is breathing and his blood is circulating only because of life support systems, and our job is to determine whether he or she is a viable donor, and then we must get the family's permission. This all has to happen immediately, within hours. We can't wait until the family feels better about the situation. Believe me, it is uncomfortable to go into a room with people sobbing and broken down, but it is part of our job to do it. I've never had anyone get mad at me or try to beat me up; that has not happened, although I realize full well it might just happen in the future."

Broznick, Denny, and the other coordinators who approach and counsel families of prospective donors, soon discover that the absolute agony of the experience is inescapable—for everyone involved. The family members with whom Broznick comes into contact are often so shocked by the suddenness of the death, so bleary eyed from constant crying and from lack of sleep, that they cannot always pay attention to what he is trying to say, and he will have to repeat ideas and explanations again and again. Although they are usually interested, they frequently cannot express their feelings about organ donation or articulate questions for which they want answers. Not only do Denny and Broznick exhibit an extraordinary capacity for patience in such situations, but they are somehow also able to maintain a distance and a compassionate yet businesslike approach.

One mother's desperate need to maintain a connection with her son through organ donation was particularly painful and heart-wrenching. The boy was only a year or two older than Richie Becker, and he had been riding his motorcycle on the highway near his hometown, about an hour from Pittsburgh, when he was sideswiped by a pickup truck. Doctors in the local hospital emergency room rushed the young man to Presbyterian. ICU nurses in large transplant centers are not at all surprised to see procurement coordinators like Broznick suddenly appear under such circumstances. They refer to the many tragic motorcycle accident victims they are forced to treat as "donor-cycles."

At 4 A.M. the young man was lying, intubated, in the ICU with a couple of dozen big black stitches zigzagging up both of his arms. His legs were also skinned and cut, but like Richie, his face was just slightly bruised. The attending physician, who had already explained brain death to the mother and father, introduced and identified Broznick to the parents when he arrived. Broznick offered his condolences, then asked politely if they could spare a moment so that he could talk with them. The parents agreed, but first concealed themselves behind the curtain that circled the young man's bed.

"I needed to say goodbye to my boy," the mother said to Broznick, as he ushered the parents into the tiny closet-like room. She was a tall, slender woman with a drawn and wrinkled face, gray at the cheeks, and red around the eyes. "Funny, I just said goodbye to him a couple of hours ago. I said I'd see him in the morning."

Broznick nodded politely, but did not respond. He waited until they settled themselves into the two chairs, then he sat down behind the desk and hunched forward.

"I'm here to tell you about organ donation, but I don't want you to feel any obligation to respond in any way. I just wanted to tell you a few things and answer any questions you might have." Broznick spoke quietly, in a voice that was flat, without expression. He paused, waiting in the silence of the tiny cramped room, listening to the muffled activity of the hospital outside. "I know that the doctor has explained much of this to you, but do you have any questions?"

"Why don't you start telling me things, and then if I think of something, I'll ask it." The mother's voice was raspy from cigarettes, and she was somewhat belligerent, not at Broznick, or the doctor, or anyone else particularly.

Broznick began to explain, but even before he reached the end of his first sentence, the mother interrupted: "Will I be able to meet the people who get my son's organs?"

Broznick shook his head, and looked down at the desk. "Absolutely not." Then he paused, studied his fingernails, as if he was actually reconsidering the woman's request. "I'm sorry," he said, "but we find that people get too involved, too attached.

"But I won't," the woman said. "You can count on it."

"But it's human nature," Broznick said, "no matter how hard you try."

"I've seen it on television, parents meeting children who have received their own children's organs."

"The news media will sometimes track down donors and recipients when the evidence is obvious . . . articles in other newspapers, police reports, and things like that . . ."

"So why not us?"

"But we will never cooperate. It might happen, but it won't happen through any help from us."

"Please."

"I'm sorry."

The mother paused, bit on the tips of her fingers. "I see, all right," she finally said.

"Actually," Broznick continued, "you have two distinct choices. Your son is legally dead. You can turn off the ventilator and take him home, or . . ." he pointed with his ballpoint pen down at the standard organ donation consent form on the desk, "or you can give his heart, liver, pancreas—whatever you choose—to organ donation." He paused again, waiting while the woman looked over the consent form. "Maybe you want to take some time and discuss it. Take all the time you need."

To this point, the father had been sitting silently, squeezing his wife's hand intermittently, staring straight ahead. Now he looked at Brian, cleared his throat. "We've already discussed it."

"And what have you decided?"

The man turned slowly toward his wife. She too was looking straight ahead, in an exhausted stupor of grief. It wasn't as if the decision was difficult to make—it had obviously already been made. What was so hard was letting go, finding the energy to form the words that would forever relinquish her child to the mysteries of medical science. "He was a good boy," she sighed, "and his body should also do good. We'll give the organs."

C h a p t e r 7

DEALING WITH DEATH

According to Ginny Smith, a writer who worked as a secretary and statistician at the Pittsburgh Transplant Foundation, most organ procurement coordinators protect themselves from the bizarre and haunting reality of the job by employing language that masks the true nature of their work. "We didn't talk much about death," she wrote in a column in a local newspaper. "The terminology we used avoided that word. The coordinator who is with a grieving family is 'on a donor.' A patient in an intensive care unit sliding into brain death is a 'referral.' Until brain death is declared and the organs recovered, the coordinator is 'working a donor.' Transplant surgeons anxious for a donation tell us they're 'strong' and call often to ask if 'anything's going on.'

"Besides calls and letters and visits from health professionals and media representatives, the Transplant Foundation hears from individuals anxious to make a buck. How much, they want to know, will the foundation pay for an organ? (Nothing.) Some ask for advice on how to commit suicide so as to leave organs intact for transplantation."

With the perspective of a five-day, forty-hour per week schedule for nearly a year, observing the procurement team in action, Ginny Smith says that most of the coordinators she knew in Pittsburgh "lock their feelings inside themselves, refusing to discuss the tragedy or how it might have personally affected them." Coordinators, she observes, become "emotional time bombs, dangerously close to going off."

Over lunch or at leisurely moments in the office, Denny, Broznick, and Duckworth release some of this pressure by telling grisly stories about surgery and joking incessantly about death. They are a very independent and close-knit breed, maintaining an almost monk-like isolation from the surgeons and from patients waiting for an organ. One of the most pressured coordinators in the field, RN Marguarite Brown, the only organ procurement coordinator at Stanford, the second largest cardiac transplant center in the United States in volume of transplants performed (Pittsburgh is larger), readily admits to the difficulty of working with people balanced temporarily on that precarious borderline called "brain death."

"As a nurse, first of all, it is difficult to work with the dead constantly and to know that they will not get better, that the only thing I can do is make sure their organs are recovered. There is not going to be that opportunity to change that person's [the donor] outcome. It is also very hard not to keep focusing on the donor, and get caught up in the details of his death, how he committed suicide or what brought about the traffic accident."

Brown says that she appreciates the responsibility as the only procurement coordinator at Stanford—she is on immediate call, twenty-four hours a day, seven days a week—but she lacks a support system, a reality that complicates her ability to deal with her emotions. This aloneness, combined with the intimacy with which she interacts daily with death, is an ever-present and nagging reminder of her own fragile vulnerability.

"Constantly knowing that every time you pick up the phone you are going to be hearing about somebody else who met with an unexpected death, starts me thinking about how we are lulled into the sense that we will live forever. You come to realize that you are no different than the people who have had that accident. It could likely happen to you, someone in your family; it is very difficult to escape being confronted with that kind of thought."

Most people are unaware of the unrelenting demands of

the job, says Brown; it is the epitome of the hurry up and wait kind of existence. Wait until someone dies; wait until they are pronounced brain dead; wait until the family agrees to donate; and then suddenly, no matter where you are or what you are doing, the phone will ring, and you will be given six hours or twelve hours to arrange for transportation, coordinate a surgical team, and travel perhaps a thousand miles or more to retrieve an organ.

"I make plans," says Brown, "but I just sometimes don't keep them. It gets to be a difficult kind of life, but I wouldn't be doing it if it wasn't something I thought was pretty important, and I wouldn't be doing it if the work wasn't a fairly large part of my life. Right now it is, but I don't know that it will stay that way. I'm not sure how much longer I can do it."

On the other hand, she says, "I think to myself, could I stand it if I wasn't doing it anymore? You get to be a crisis junkie. Just last night, we flew off to Albuquerque, New Mexico, for a heart, and coming back we couldn't get into the air after the retrieval because of a series of snow squalls. Then, when the snow let up, the airport maintenance crew plowed out the lights on the runway. So it was a struggle. But that kind of drama, that kind of excitement, that kind of 'living on the edge,' makes coming home, doing the laundry, and going to Safeway every morning for cat food, very dull. It gets to the point where you find that that 'normal' part of your life is less than satisfying, and you can't wait until the beeper goes off again."

Jo Burton's fellow procurement coordinator at Cambridge, Celia Wight, expresses similar feelings. "You walk into the office and you don't know what is going to happen. You might have a whole day planned, and it will, in fact, end up being totally different, and I suppose it must suit my type and other coordinators' types of personality to enjoy that sort of working life or working environment."

Says Burton: "We had about a week when there were no calls, and we really didn't know what to do with ourselves. There were little things to be done, very minor things, but we both found it very difficult because we are used to being under pressure. I think I'm addicted to stress."

That's the "Catch 22" dilemma of being a donor procurement coordinator, says Brown: "Yes, I'd like to take more time off, but then if the time that I take off means that I miss one of those moments, which is what I am doing the job for anyway, it is like you miss the 'icing on the cake.' I came home last night after the crazy trip to Albuquerque and it was pretty hard to unwind from a night like that—plus you know that back at the hospital, everything is still going on. The recipient was still on the table [being transplanted], but when I came back with the heart, that was the end of my job. Then at home, I couldn't help but think about it. I'm always thinking about the off-chance that, just in case something goes wrong, the phone might ring and they will tell me they need me again."

In Pittsburgh, the procurement coordinators will only infrequently meet the candidates—the patients waiting for organs to be transplanted into them. But in Stanford, in addition to working as a liaison with the media and with ICU nurses in many hospitals, Marguarite Brown will often communicate with patients and families waiting for a heart or heart-lung (Stanford does not transplant livers or kidneys).

"They very much want to know the person who is responsible for the donor procurement, want to know how it is done, and what they could do to make it better. They don't apply pressure, but it is very hard for me to deal with their frustration, to relieve some of the anger and bitterness that some of them feel because they are waiting so long for a donor. They think that nobody out there—the public—cares about them. I try to turn it around and ask them, 'Before you were ill or before your wife was ill, how often had you thought about being an organ donor? The answer usually is, 'Never.'

"They need to realize that it is not a malicious thing on the part of the public, but it is something caused by a lack of education, something that will be improved with time, but time is just something that these people do not have. It's pretty hard to tell them that, because you'll say, 'Things will get better by a certain time'—maybe 'next year'—but they know and I know that they don't have next year. They only have now."

It is unlikely that Brown or any procurement coordinator will have contact with the donor, *before* they become a donor, but that summer, around the same time of Richie Becker's accident, Don Denny had had a conversation about organ donation with a woman who strongly suspected that she would become an organ donor within the next few days.

The woman, who had been in a local hospital for more than a week with a deteriorating brain tumor, had phoned the Pittsburgh Transplant Foundation, explained her situation, and was promised that a donor card would be delivered the following day. For some reason, the card did not arrive, and at 11:45 P.M., she once again phoned the Foundation. Don Denny's beeper went off at home.

The woman said that she was going into surgery early the next morning, that her prognosis was not good, and that she wanted to make certain that her organs would be used to help other people. Denny said that her husband could sign on her behalf if she were to die, and that she should inform him of her wishes. "She had obviously taken the time to think things out, the life and death issues that people usually ignore," Denny said, when he was informed that the woman had not made it through surgery.

When he arrived at the hospital to see the woman's husband and to obtain his permission for organ donation, Denny was informed that the family had departed, having given the neurologist permission to disconnect the ventilator whenever he thought it appropriate. They did not plan to return. Denny was surprised and discouraged, and though a cursory examination indicated that the woman's organs might be too far gone to be used for transplantation, he elected to proceed with the tests that would determine the woman's suitability, anyway.

As to the tests, Brian Broznick explains: "We all have kind of a standardized protocol in this regard. There are certain tests that we always run, like hepatitis and blood cultures, urine cultures, AIDS screening, screening for venereal diseases. That's a standard thing we do on every donor we come across, whether it is a kidney donor or tissue donor or cornea donor or whatever.

"One of the other big factors we examine is social history. What kind of life did this patient live? If you get a seventeen- or eighteen-year-old person that shoots themselves, you have to worry about why. Were they on drugs? What was going on in their life to cause suicide? You want to gently talk to that family to try to find out what kind of lifestyle this person led. That can be a very important factor. Was the person a homosexual? Was the person very promiscuous? It just gives you a better indication about how much you should really push to dig into this person's past. There are also essential questions concerning how the person died. Could there have been some trauma during a collision in an auto accident, for example, that might have injured an organ? If necessary, we'll bring in a specialist for a consult.

"We always have to be real careful. I remember a case that a donor had rabies and it wasn't discovered until after one of the corneas were transplanted, and the recipient then developed rabies himself. The last thing you want to do is to give somebody who is going to die without this organ something that is going to kill them anyway."

As the necessary tests were being conducted, Denny sat down at a desk in the head nurse's office and began attempting to contact the woman's family to explain the situation. No one answered the phone at her home, nor could he reach the other relatives for whom the hospital had numbers. He sat there repeatedly dialing the few phone numbers available to him, until eventually, he connected.

Although a taped phone conversation would have been acceptable, it is always preferable to obtain direct signatures from the donor family. "What I need is to have you sign the form in person, sir," he said to the husband. "No, we would have to have you sign beforehand [before taking a organ] to know that we had your consent." The husband agreed to meet Denny at a point halfway between the hospital and his home.

"It must not seem real to you," said Denny, as the two men finally faced one another.

The husband was a black man in his early thirties, a Baptist minister. "What a difference a day makes," he answered politely.

"I can't get over that I talked to her," said Denny. "She seemed like such a nice person, a thinking person, a good person."

"She called you at midnight?" said the husband.

"Eleven forty-five from the ICU nurse's station. Last thing I said to her—and I thought later that it was such a stupid thing—is 'good luck.' I guess that's not too encouraging." Denny paused, then said very softly, "She seemed to have had everything thought through."

The husband nodded, said that they had three children. "We all knew what might happen. She prepared us well."

Upon returning to the hospital, after examining the results of the tests he had ordered, Denny was forced to conclude that, with the exception of the corneas, the woman's organs were no longer viable for donation. Too much time had passed and too much damage had been incurred during surgery. "It happens quite often," Denny said.

Before leaving, Denny walked around the ICU, thanking the nurses, residents, and the attending physicians for all of their help and cooperation. Although this was a major metropolitan medical facility, they did not refer many prospective donors to the Foundation, and he wanted to be certain to show his appreciation for their efforts on this occasion. Denny's last stop was to visit once more with the woman who had phoned him. She was still ventilated, breathing regularly and normally, at five-second intervals, looking as if she were immersed in a deep and peaceful sleep.

She was a heavyset black woman with short hair and a large patch of light skin, partially bandaged at her scalp, where she had been shaved for surgery. The fact that she was brain dead, and connected to life support machinery, in no way diminished the strength of character in her face, bloated and bruised from surgery and medication. Denny reached out, patted her a couple of times heartily but tenderly on the shoulder, humming a kind of strange wordless mumbled prayer. It was a meaningful and memorable gesture in that lonely, shadowed room.

Donald Denny resigned as director of the Transplant Foundation a few days before Christmas, 1985. He was replaced by Brian Broznick.

Because of the many tests they had conducted, the physicians in the ICU at Charlotte Memorial knew that Richie Becker was brain dead, but certain additional procedures were required for official certification. The process began early on May 2.

A physician first conducted an in-depth examination, probing—unsuccessfully—for any sign of normal circulatory or neurological function. Richie showed no response to painful stimuli—needles, etc.—applied to his head and face. He exhibited no spontaneous movements, no pupillary reaction, no corneal or gag reflexes, no response to ice water in the ear canal. His eyes appeared frozen in their sockets when his head was turned.

Two technicians wheeled in a bulky electroencephalograph, taping ten electrodes to his skull, waiting and watching for thirty minutes, searching the depths of his brain for the barest indication of any electrical activity. Nothing was visible. Another physician conducted a second in-depth examination, subsequently supporting the conclusions of the first physician's examination.

Meanwhile, Mike Callahan, Bromberg's associate coordinator at Charlotte Memorial, accessed (telephoned) 24-ALERT to ascertain what transplant centers across the United States were listing a need for donors of Richie's size and blood type. Based upon the information it provided him, Callahan then phoned Pittsburgh, alerting them to the possibility of a "multiple" donor, meaning the heart or the heart-lungs *and* liver, as well as the kidneys. Pittsburgh was listing an urgent need for a liver, and a serious need for a heart-lung bloc. If and when the donor was "confirmed," meaning that the brain death of Richie Becker was officially established within hospital protocol so that a death certificate could be signed, Callahan would recontact Pittsburgh, thus triggering the transplant team into action. The plan was to offer Pittsburgh the liver and heart-lung bloc, while Charlotte Memorial would keep the kidneys for transplant themselves. The Beckers had not donated corneas, skin, tissue, and bones.

Hours before, Dick and Sharon Becker had said their good-byes to Richie and returned home to finalize arrangements for Richie's funeral, scheduled for May 4. There was no doubt in anyone's mind that Richie was forever gone.

The stage was now set for the final test of brain death. The results of all other examinations and conclusions would mean nothing without this crucial determination: Could Richie Becker sustain himself without help from the mechanical ventilator? If he were able to breathe, and thus sustain his own life cycle, he might, under law, have to remain there, in a state of extended vegetation, similar to the famous case of Karen Ann Quinlan, who existed in this manner in a New Jersey hospital for more than ten years before passing away.

The ventilator was disconnected from the tube in Richie Becker's airway, and a small and silent cadre of physicians, nurses, and technicians clustered around the young man, waiting and searching for the barest hint of life. Within three minutes the search was finally over, for the doctors could then legally sign the young man's death certificate. Richie was immediately re-intubated, to continue the crucial oxygenation of his organs, while Callahan rushed back to his office to contact Pittsburgh.

Brian Broznick told Callahan that a five-person surgical team would leave Pittsburgh within three hours, by 5 P.M., and that their estimated time of arrival in Charlotte was 6:38 P.M. Callahan said that he would have an ambulance waiting at the airport to speed them to Charlotte Memorial, and that operating room personnel would be ready to assist them the moment the surgeons were gowned and scrubbed.

PART III

PITTSBURGH

Chapter 8

THE COURT OF LAST RESORT

The University of Pittsburgh's School of Medicine towers over Oakland, the cultural center of the city, etched into one of the steepest hills in this city of hills—Cardiac Hill—so named because of the heightening heart rate of students and faculty who slough off the campus bus and attempt to climb it. With the exception of Pitt Stadium, where the Pitt Panthers play a rugged and always wild brand of football on Saturday afternoons, Cardiac Hill is crammed with sprawling, architecturally indistinctive medical edifices. From top to bottom, there is the Veteran's Administration Hospital ("the VA"), where nursing students medical interns, and residents receive much of their training; Western Psychiatric Institute and Clinic ("Western Psych"), of worldwide prominence for its research into sleep disorders and tranquilizing medications; the School of Public Health, where a comprehensive, federally financed five-year study into the causes and possible cures of AIDS is now taking place; Montefiore Hospital, a private institution loosely affiliated with the university; and the School of Nursing.

The School of Medicine is headquartered at Scaife Hall, situated in the middle of the hillside, in which the libraries, laboratories, classrooms, lecture halls, and faculty offices are all located. Scaife is the nucleus of the medical center, connected by a ribbon of elaborate tunnels and bridges to the major clinical facilities, which, although independent organizations, have been closely allied with the university for many years. These include Eye and Ear Hospital, a small and specialized institution, as well as Presbyterian-University Hospital and Children's Hospital. In western Pennsylvania, Presbyterian and Children's are premier health care institutions, with a number of high profile programs, but in the challenging, complicated, and evolving world of organ transplantation, the University of Pittsburgh, Children's Hospital and Presbyterian-University combined, are internationally unequaled.

In Pittsburgh, the largest organ transplant center in the world, there is a liver transplant every day, a kidney transplant every second day, a heart transplant every third day, a heart-lung transplant every fifteen days. In all, there is an organ transplant in Pittsburgh every twelve hours, 365 days of the year. More hearts, heart-lungs, and livers were transplanted in Pittsburgh in 1986 than were transplanted in the entire world five years before. In many respects, this phenomenal progress—the quantum leap from dream to reality—is the real miracle of organ transplantation.

It is the numbers, even more than the expertise behind the numbers, that draws so many sick and dying people (nearly 2,000 in 1987) from across the United States and dozens of foreign countries, to Pittsburgh for evaluation for transplantation. "Evaluation" can be defined as a test or series of tests to determine if the patient qualifies for transplantation. During evaluation, the transplant team will confirm the referring physician's diagnosis—usually a gastroenterologist for those with liver disease, and a cardiologist for patients suffering with heart disease—and investigate the possibility of alternate therapy. Can a patient be kept alive, and can the quality of their lifestyles be maintained in pharmacological or surgical ways other than transplant? If so, for how long? There are economic and psychosocial aspects that will also enter into the evaluation, but the critical questions are initially and primarily clinical, while the answers rest upon the frightening reality of the transplant experience. It is a sad cliché but true all the same that in a transplant, the surgeon literally takes the patient's heart (or liver) into his hands, and once the organ is taken out of the body, it cannot be returned. No machine today exists similar to dialysis, that will artificially and safely simulate the critical function of extrarenal organs over an extended period of time.

This is why transplant surgeons in Pittsburgh and elsewhere search tirelessly during the transplant evaluation for reasons to avoid or delay what they do best: Not only because the shortage of organs necessarily makes extrarenal transplantation a scarce and selective opportunity, but also because there is no turning back once the procedure begins. Surgeons know that one of every five cardiac patients, one out of every three-and-a-half liver transplant patients, one out of every two heart-lung patients rolled into the operating room for transplant surgery will not be alive within a year from the moment scalpel breaks skin. More than one-third of the remaining survivors will not live out the next two years. On the other hand, they realize that most of the people who come to see them will die eventually from their disease. So, whether to operate or not to operate isn't a matter of yes or no as much as it is a determination of when.

The transplant patients who come to Pittsburgh for evaluation are often tugging the surgeon in a somewhat opposite direction. They are not anxious to continue living indefinitely in an impaired manner, especially compared to quality of life before their sicknesses became acute, and in light of the fact that their disease will gradually incapacitate and destroy them; they want help now—no matter what the consequences. If they are going to die anyway, they reason, why not go for "the big fix" and get it over with? Indeed, the patients would not have traveled hundreds or thousands of miles to Pittsburgh to be poked, prodded, tested, interrogated, and frequently humiliated if they had not been told by many physicians beforehand and did not know deep down inside that transplantation was their only chance. The stakes during the evaluation are elementary and frighteningly clear. If they are not transplanted, they will soon die, and if they are not accepted for transplantation in Pittsburgh, then they will probably not be accepted anywhere else in the world. Because of Pittsburgh's size and international reputation, Pittsburgh can afford to take great and unorthodox risks that few other centers would dare

attempt. When patients come to Pittsburgh for transplant evaluation, they are inevitably and unequivocally committing
themselves to the court of last resort.

Even after her sickness had been diagnosed as Primary Pulmonary Hypertension (PPH), a constriction of the blood vessels
of the lungs which leads ultimately—fatally—to the destruction of the heart, forty-year-old Winifred (Winkle) Fulk continued teaching at her local junior high school in Kansas City,
Missouri, from September 1983 through June 1984. "All the
while, I could feel myself getting weaker, 'under the weather,'
having more difficulty with my breathing. But I didn't give
the future much thought." Despite the fact that PPH had
no known cause—or cure—"I refused to consider the possibility that it would not work out."

Writing in the medical journal, *Heart Transplantation*, senior social worker Virginia C. O'Brien of Papworth Hospital
near Cambridge, one of England's three cardiac transplant
centers, explains that the ability of terminally ill patients to
continue working helps them maintain in their lives an aura
of normalcy, while delaying acceptance of reality. O'Brien, a
transplant social worker since the inception of the Papworth
program in 1979, and one of the very few social workers currently writing about the special challenges posed by transplant
candidates and recipients, reported that her patients gradually
grew hostile as their illness became more debilitating. Winkle
remembers exactly when her hostility became evident and
to whom it was directed. "I was in the hospital because of a
negative reaction to some of the medications the cardiologist
was prescribing for me, and one day, he came in, sat down
in a chair, and he said, 'Well, here it is.' He had all his records—
my records—in front of him."

The cardiologist briefly reviewed the disease process of PPH,
which causes the muscle in the walls of the pulmonary arteries
to become increasingly inelastic or inflexible. The pulmonary
arteries, which carry deoxygenated blood from the right ventricle of the heart to the lungs for oxygenation must be flexible
to stretch, or expand, as the right ventricle pumps, he told
her. Inelasticity of these arteries forces the pulmonary pressure

to rise severely (hypertension), leading to a significant back pressure. As the disease progresses and the pressure escalates (at that point, it was two-to-three times above normal), she would suffer from congestive heart failure (CHF). It is because there is no known cure for PPH, and because she would suffer from CHF, the doctor concluded, that the lungs *and* the heart would be destroyed.

Winkle, who received a Ph.D. in physiology at Iowa State University, where she had met her husband, Dave, had been presented with this information many times before, and she understood the scientific realities perfectly. But her cardiologist had observed that she was not coming to grips with the practical realities of the situation, for he was direct and brutal:

" 'We had hoped last year that you, your condition, would have leveled off,' he told me," said Winkle. " 'But you haven't. What you've done is gone downhill to the point where there's absolutely nothing I can do for you.' Then he closed up his book and his files and walked out." He estimated, said Winkle, that she had less than another year to live.

Winkle watched as the physician exited the room, his white lab coat flapping behind him. She will never forget the frightening silence, the aloneness, he left in his wake. "I was so upset! I cried. But I was also mad because he gave up. He was a doctor and he gave up. He was not looking at the literature anymore. This was it. This is what I had, PPH, and as far as he was concerned . . ." She paused, and her eyes glistened at the memory. Her voice, normally somewhat gravelly in texture, grew thick and hoarse. "As far as he was concerned," she repeated, " 'tough bananas.' "

Ironically, she now admits, even her anger did not dissuade her from continuing to resist the inevitable for a few months longer. She proceeded with her life, as if she could go on in this manner indefinitely.

"But my bubble burst," said Winkle, "when I went to my family doctor in August to get my teaching health form OK'd. I handed it to him, and he took it and he ripped it up, right in front of me, and he said to me, 'You've got to be kidding. There's no way you can teach.' And that just crushed me. I had already called the school, arranged for special classes and special treatment—I was sure I could do it. I certainly did not want to sit home and feel sorry for myself. But he felt that that would be less stress, sitting home. So," said Winkle, "I sat home."

Along with the psychological pressures during this stage, says O'Brien, are profound social changes that affect the entire family, including: "The inability to work; the loss of earnings; the loss of status and a reversal of roles . . ." As Winkle's condition deteriorated, her husband Dave, a Ph.D. grain management specialist for the U.S. Department of Agriculture, began to assume responsibility for much of the housework and cooking. And then, Winkle's mother, who had been living alone on the family farm near Davenport, Iowa, moved in with the Fulks for an extended visit.

As the disease continued to eat away at her, Winkle could not walk downstairs to the basement to help clean her childrens' newly remodeled rooms. Normally robust and athletic—an avid gardener, horseback rider, championship bowler—she now found physical activity impossible; breathing was hard enough. She spent most of her time in bed—she slept twelve to fourteen hours—or on the couch, watching TV. Without an oxygen bottle at her bedside, which she pulled along with her when she moved about the house, she would not have been able to draw a breath. She could move from the bedroom to the living room once or twice a day on her own steam, but if she wanted to go to the supermarket or to church, or to sit out in the afternoon sun, her husband or her mother or one of her children would have to push her in a wheelchair, a situation that she considered intolerable— not only because it was physically exhausting, but more importantly because it was unbearably embarrassing.

This dependency, especially parental dependency, is one of the low points in the entire transplant experience. As Mary Burge, a heart transplant social worker at Stanford University Medical Center observes: "It is difficult enough when a teenager becomes very sick; you have all kinds of tension. The teenager has just been trying to get away from the parents and now he is forced once again to be more dependent. But an adult patient who, after years and years of independence from the parent, is once again forced to live as a dependent of the parent, is worse. That seems like a very difficult relationship."

It was during this long and protracted period of decreased activity and energy that she began to accept her diagnosis— not necessarily her prognosis—and to attempt to seek out ways of possibly extending her life. With the guidance of a family friend, a physician, she read medical journals, newspaper articles (Dave would make endless trips to the library)— anything available about PPH. One article focused on the Stanford University Medical Center, where the first six heart-lung operations had been attempted.

Winkle learned that heart transplant pioneer, Dr. Norman Shumway, and his young associate, Dr. Bruce Reitz, had performed nearly two dozen heart-lung transplants since 1981— more than any other facility in the world at that time—and that about fifty such procedures had been attempted worldwide. The diseases, in addition to the more obvious lung disorders, such as emphysema, that might lead to heart-lung transplantation, included PPH. Although only half of those patients on whom Reitz and Shumway operated lived a full year and only 35 percent remained alive by 1984, there was one shining hope: Reitz's and Shumway's very first case, a forty-five-year-old mother of three from Phoenix, Arizona, Mary Gohlke who, like Winkle, suffered from PPH, was, at that time, healthy enough to have returned full-time to her job as a newspaper executive.

The knowledge that someone like Mary Gohlke existed was a great elixir to Winkle's depression. She realized now that the doctors who had told her that she would die unless some miraculous cure suddenly materialized, might be wrong. The odds were stacked against her, but Mary Gohlke was alive, so there was a chance that Winkle could also survive. Immediately, she wrote Drs. Shumway and Reitz, but unfortunately, Stanford could not accept her because they felt that her overall condition was much too weakened at that point. In contrast to its reputation as the consummate cardiac transplant center, Stanford has always been a relatively conservative institution.

Even if they would have accepted her, however, Winkle would have had to move to Stanford to wait for a donor organ(s) to materialize (Stanford insists that all transplant patients be located within an hour's drive of the hospital), and that—relocate—Winkle categorically refused to do. If she were going to die a slow death with shortness of breath and exhaustion and heart failure, it would be in her own house and in her own bed, and not in some furnished apartment in a strange and friendless city.

Stanford did suggest an alternative possibility. They were doing some heart-lung transplant work in Pittsburgh; in fact, they were doing a lot of it, more than Stanford these days. And because Drs. Robert Hardesty and Bartley Griffith were young, and at that time their heart-lung transplant program was new, Pittsburgh was accepting the most difficult cases as candidates into the program. Most of Pittsburgh's initial fifteen to twenty heart-lung transplant patients had sought help at Stanford first.

Administrators and social workers at Presbyterian-University Hospital report that many patients who eventually arrive in Pittsburgh for evaluation for transplantation are there due to their own personal research and their own persistence. Numerous physicians either refuse to accept or remain unaware of the increasing success of transplantation. Those physicians who do value the potential of transplantation are often stymied by the difficulty in knowing where the best transplant centers are to be found. Ever since the FDA had approved the use of cyclosporine in 1983, transplant centers have appeared with increasing frequency, but often with little justification. Most surgeons are simply not experienced or skillful enough to face the varied and unpredictable challenges of surgery and the immunosuppressant follow-up. In addition to lacking qualified personnel, most hospitals do not have the facilities or support services (specialized social workers, ICU staff, etc.) to justify a transplant program.

According to the 1986 report of the federal Task Force in Organ Transplantation, nearly half of the approximately 70 heart and 35 liver transplant centers in the United States and one-third of the 180 kidney transplant programs could easily be eliminated without a reduction in the number of patients who are transplanted in the United States. The Task Force has presented a thirteen-point set of guidelines for transplant programs, which include the establishment of a minimum number of transplants a year, based upon current donor organ supply and patient demand: twelve for hearts, fifteen for livers, and fifty for kidneys. The Task Force also recommended that regional centers for transplantation be established where personnel and facilities could be more efficiently combined, and that these centers should be located at teaching hospitals affiliated with major universities, where significant research and development are more likely to occur.

"The Bob and Bart Show," as some of the patients glibly refer to the Hardesty-Griffith heart transplant team, was responsible for 51 of the 434 heart transplants performed worldwide in 1984 when Winkle Fulk first came to Pittsburgh, more than any other institution. Of the first twenty heart-lung patients transplanted over three years in Pittsburgh—a number second only to Stanford's twenty-three—there were nine survivors. Pittsburgh has transplanted patients with a number of different lung disorders, but the therapy has been most successful on patients with PPH, a disease that, for some reason, strikes mostly women. As of December 1984, only sixty such procedures had ever been attempted. Two years later, Hardesty and Griffith would more than double Pittsburgh's number of heart and heart-lung transplants, far exceeding Stanford as the leading cardiac transplant institution, while slightly improving the one- and three-year survival rates in both categories.

There are three ways of being evaluated for cardiac transplantation in Pittsburgh, according to heart transplant coordinator, Ann Lee, a nurse practitioner (a nurse with an advanced degree and enhanced diagnostic skills). First, if the referring physician has not conducted the necessary tests (or if the tests have not been conducted recently), the patient will be admitted to the hospital for a few days to confirm the physician's diagnosis. This might happen once every ten times. Second, "which is not a very desirable way, but maybe the easiest way for us to make a decision, is when you are on 'death's door,' and you are being transferred here as an emergency." This situation is relevant only to heart transplant candidates, says Lee, because for "heart-lungs, there is very rarely an emergency 'death's door' situation because we could never ever get a donor in time to save them." Lee estimates that approximately "25 percent to 30 percent of the patients coming in for heart transplants are emergency situations." She points out, however, that "the survival rates between those who came for prior evaluation and the 'death's door' categories, assuming the availability of donor organs, were relatively the same."

The third and most frequent variation of evaluation is for candidates who have already been thoroughly examined and diagnosed by knowledgeable and qualified cardiologists, and who know or at least suspect that transplantation is a strong future possibility. Thorough medical workups are consequently unnecessary (these people have sent records in advance), but blood tests are initially taken upon their arrival, and interviews are conducted between the patient and surgeons. "For the heart-lung transplant, we will also do a chest X-ray, to look at the size of the lungs," says Lee. "Dr. Griffith also measures the torso, the chest around, and he will measure down from the clavicle [collarbone] to the 4th or 5th intercostal [between the ribs] space, which gives him a real good idea of the size and depth of the lungs." A chest X-ray is not usually necessary for a heart transplant candidate, however. The surgeons rely on height, weight, and body type to determine if a particular organ will fit.

Hardesty's and Griffith's approach to the entire transplant process, beginning with evaluation, has a soft and humanistic edge, for they are men who, according to one ICU nurse, "are not afraid to let their feelings hang out once in a while." This willingness to show vulnerability by taking a personal interest in their patients was particularly important and memorable to Winkle Fulk during her very brief outpatient evaluation in Pittsburgh in August 1984 with the man who was to become her surgeon, Bartley Griffith. As in many cases with patients with heart and lung diagnoses, Winkle Fulk's disease and prognosis were clear-cut and well documented, and Griffith had talked on the telephone to Winkle's cardiologist prior to her visit to Pittsburgh.

"Right away he asked me how many children I had," said Winkle of the moment she first met Griffith. "And then Dr. Hardesty poked his head in the room, and he only stayed a minute, but he also asked me how many children I had. Which impressed me because they were concerned that we were a family." The evaluation took place in Falk Clinic, which is located on the very bottom of Cardiac Hill, also connected to Children's and Presbyterian by tunnels, bridges, and passageways, where most of the evaluations for both the cardiac and the liver transplant teams take place. Falk Clinic, which has been newly modernized in a "high-tech" decor, is also the headquarters for the Pittsburgh Cancer Institute and the Benedum Geriatric Center, institutions of rapidly emerging national prominence.

"They consulted for a while by themselves and I got very nervous because I was afraid that we would not be accepted. I knew that they did not accept everybody. I did not know what the criteria was, so I really did not know what to say to him to try to convince him to take me. I just told him what I could do and what I couldn't do, gave him a bit of my family background. I remember being extremely surprised at how young Griffith was—thirty-six years old and performing a surgery that only a few others had ever attempted—and handsome."

Griffith is tall, slender, and athletic-looking, and he still moves with the fluidity and grace of the young and skillful varsity soccer star he once was. ("He was a guy who hated to lose," a friend and former teammate commented, "always gracious in defeat, but always mad as hell at himself for allowing it to happen.") Griffith is also handsome, as Winkle Fulk observed, but his forehead is deeply lined with worry and, because of the marathon pace at which he works, he often seems on the verge of being completely overcome by weariness. Although equally hard-driving and dedicated, Hardesty is considerably less obsessive about his work. He is a man who knows his limits. In describing her boss, Ann Lee has said, "Bob is as steady as a rock ever gets."

Consulting briefly, Hardesty and Griffith quickly agreed that Winkle Fulk was a good candidate, first of all because at the rate of her deterioration since diagnosis, she would undoubtedly be dead within a year, and second because, considering her condition, Winkle was comparatively healthy and strong, one of those patients "most likely to survive" the surgical ordeal. The fact that she had PPH was another plus, a disease with which they had had some positive experience. Seventy-five percent of their long-term survivors have had PPH. At 127 pounds, Winkle was also somewhat heavier than most of the other women on the waiting list. They had probably been as heavy as Winkle when healthy, but they had dwindled since becoming ill down to anywhere from 90 to 110. So this was a final plus—less competition in her weight range, when and if a donor were to become available.

After a while, Griffith returned to the examination room in which the Fulks were sitting "and praying," and he was smiling: "OK, we'll accept you on our list." And although they had talked for only fifteen minutes at the most, Winkle remained in her wheelchair long after they had shaken hands and said goodbye, and sobbed with relief.

Because his disease had been diagnosed early enough, and because he had been able to quickly make contact with an experienced and knowledgeable transplant center, Frank Rowe, a thirty-five-year-old industrial psychologist from Philadelphia, who also suffered from PPH, had actually been accepted into the Stanford program without having to submit to the ordeal of the evaluation. The Stanford surgeons had examined all of Rowe's test results and X-rays and thoroughly discussed his case with his cardiologist in Philadelphia before issuing a terse mimeographed letter inviting him to relocate to Stanford to wait for the availability of a donor organ. And although Rowe had taken leave from his position at Philadelphia Electric Company and rented out the large old house in which his family had lived for the past two years (Joyce Rowe had grown up in this house) with the intention of moving to California, he had decided to come to Pittsburgh—much closer to home—for evaluation.

In contrast to Winkle Fulk, Frank Rowe had not attempted to deny the existence of the disease that threatened his life: In fact, he had foreshadowed the possibility of his diagnosis. A couple of weeks before Thanksgiving 1983, during a routine checkup, a company physician had recognized an unusual inelasticity in Rowe's pulmonary arteries and referred him to a cardiologist for a more thorough examination. But before seeing the cardiologist, Rowe spent the weekend in the library, investigating the possible consequences of his symptoms.

"Frank is a very scientific person," said Joyce, "very methodical, medically inclined. He keeps a copy of *Gray's Anatomy* by his bedside for pleasure reading. I'm not joking," she adds, laughingly. There was little pleasure in Rowe's research at this point, however. "He came home with a whole list of possible diseases and problems," said Joyce, "the worst of which was Primary Pulmonary Hypertension. At the time, I told him, 'Yeah, I know, it sounds terrible, but it's not going to be that. You're young, healthy, and you know, except for this shortness of breath, there's nothing wrong with you.' "

He was hospitalized the following Monday for a cardiac catheterization, a painful process in which a tiny plastic tube is passed into the heart through a blood vessel. Samples of blood are withdrawn, while blood pressure and cardiac output (the amount of blood the heart pumps) are measured. Later, the cardiologist walked into his room. "I was flat on my back and pretty miserable, but he was straightforward, which I appreciated," said Rowe. Tall and Germanic, with thick brown hair always combed neatly to the side and a slightly hooked nose that is too large for his face, Rowe has a smooth distinctive voice, and an aura of self-importance that makes it seem as if he is always lecturing to a large audience, even when speaking in privacy about the most intimate of subjects. "He [the cardiologist] looked me straight in the eye and told me I would not live to see my children graduate from high school," Rowe said. "I spent the whole night looking out the window at the clock face on the side of the *Philadelphia Inquirer* Building. I watched every tick of that clock. The next two weeks we spent a lot of time yelling, 'Why me? What's going on here?' We were filled with desperation—fear, anger, and confusion."

Rowe explained to Bartley Griffith that he had been accepted by Stanford, but that he did not want to travel so far unless it was absolutely necessary. So there he was in Pittsburgh, and from Rowe's prejudiced point of view, it would seem as if he were perfect, "a blue chip candidate," he told Griffith, "the kind of patient of which good statistics are made.

"Griffith told me that he doesn't like to expose people to the catastrophic ordeal of transplantation until it is clearly the only alternative," Rowe reported, after his evaluation one autumn afternoon in 1984. "He's not so sure that I won't be able to live with reasonably the same symptoms for another year before the transplant becomes imperative. He's concerned. He does not want to take a guy in reasonably good health and subject him to the risk of killing him on the table."

In retrospect, Frank and Joyce Rowe realize that they probably should have remained in Philadelphia for another year and held on to their jobs (Joyce was the office manager of a dental clinic), but "procrastination" was not a word that invaded Frank Rowe's vocabulary very often. Rowe's favorite word was "opportunity," which he said symbolized the philosophy by which he lived. He categorically and unwaveringly believed that life consisted of a series of windows of potential opportunity. The fact that he had another year before the disease would begin to seriously impinge upon his life presented for Rowe an opportunity to fight to increase his chances for survival. He would do this by dedicating himself to the concept of organ donation, and to spending quality time with his wife and family. So when Griffith questioned the wisdom of putting him on the transplant list so early, Rowe was ready to jockey for position. He had prepared himself with answers.

"I understand," said Rowe. "I hear what you are saying as far as my potential for staying active for a while. But as far as I am concerned, I've been damn near dead since last November when I was first diagnosed. There's an awful lot of things I cannot do. I can't go running around with the kids. I can't pick up the kids. That's not life. Yes, I may die on the table, but I think there's a low probability in that." Rowe told Griffith that he could feel himself deteriorating day by day: "If I don't get this thing done by next year, I'll be in real bad shape." What did Griffith say about his chances of surviving the operation? "Two words: 'No guarantees.' He said, 'I think you are a better than average candidate, and I'm convinced that you don't want to die.' He said that it might be realistic that I could get three or four years after the surgery, if I got through surgery, but that he couldn't guarantee that I would see my six-year-old or my eight-year-old graduate from high school." At that time, there were too few heart-lung transplant survivors on whom to base a long-range prognosis. "I told him that what I wanted to do is to buy time for the scientists to learn more. I told him that in my point of view my case would be an excellent opportunity for them to get a patient who has the potential for some post-surgical longevity to commit a team of their doctors to study and analyze me.

"I said to Griffith, 'I have all the confidence that it is all going to work, and life is going to get somewhat better. It may not be perfect, but it is going to be somewhat better, and I am willing to take that risk.' " Rowe told Griffith that he was going to turn this tragedy into a grand opportunity. "I am going to grab the brass ring. We're going to win. I'm not going to let myself die. I'm going to fight like hell after the surgery. They're going to have to hold me down. I can taste it. I'm so damn anxious to get out there and win, I can't wait."

Griffith agreed to accept Frank Rowe into the program as a low priority (Status 3 on the NATCO scale) candidate, but despite what Rowe and other patients might think, Griffith's decision probably had little to do with Rowe's enthusiasm and resolve. "Everyone who comes to Pittsburgh has the same story to tell," says Griffith. " 'Doc, I'm going to make it. I'm the one. I'm not going to fail you.' But you know from the beginning it's [the transplant] going to fail at least 20 percent of the time in the first year for hearts [and 50 percent for heart-lungs], no matter how strong-willed and determined they are."

Griffith warned Rowe then that it would probably be an

extremely long wait, since he was in much better condition than most of the other men and women on the list. Waiting is a fact of life that many transplant candidates initially refuse to think about. They seem to prepare themselves for future happiness the moment the transplant becomes the vaguest possibility. "For the first time since their illness, they can contemplate a future in good health," says Virginia O'Brien. "This leads them to ignore all obstacles."

"So often," says Dr. Robert Hardesty, "the patients don't listen. You tell them the facts. They say they understand completely, but then later, you find out they haven't heard a word. I once told a husband and a wife that we were going to try a certain procedure on their child, but that I didn't think it would be successful, that there wasn't much hope. We talked about some other things for a while—practical matters such as when and where the operation would take place. But the message was clear. We were in trouble. And then when they were ready to leave the office, the wife turned to me and said, 'So you think everything will be alright?'"

Chapter 9

SLOWLY DYING

When she first began feeling ill, U.S. Army Specialist Fourth Class Rebecca Treat had not exhibited the more obvious symptoms of liver disease—yellowness in the eyes and skin (jaundice), a severely distended belly, constant itching, vomiting of blood—but what had motivated her to go on sick call at Fort Campbell, Kentucky, where she had been stationed, was a general feeling of tiredness and a sudden swelling of her legs. Rebecca had always been broad shouldered and muscular, but never fat. Almost overnight, she told the doctor at the base hospital that morning, she had gained over twenty pounds.

"He knew what was wrong right away," said Rebecca, "but before he said anything, he sent me to have some blood tests done. It was confirmed in about twenty minutes that I had Chronic/Active Hepatitis, Non-A, Non-B. But I didn't know exactly what that meant—I mean to me, to my husband, to our future—until I was sent, airlifted, to Fort Gordon, Georgia, for a liver biopsy."

Rebecca's memory of most of the events that preceded transplantation is rather clouded, but the details of that day, that very frightening moment, when her prognosis was explained, are crystal clear. "This was a Sunday morning, nice and sunny and hot and beautiful; they have a lot of fine trees on the base," said Rebecca. "I was in a room by myself, and my husband [Michael] and I were waiting there together. We had been waiting for them to release me, but they wanted to talk to me first."

The doctor sat down beside her bed, and then he cleared his throat and his face got kind of white. "He said that if there was anything that I had ever wanted to do in my life that I should do it within the next six months because I was going to become very ill. When he said that, I thought, 'Well, I could die.'" But she, like Winkle, steadfastly refused to allow that thought to linger.

"I immediately started to make jokes about it," she said. "I was just joking the whole time the doctor was talking to me. I kidded about touring Europe, hiking in Alaska, or some of the other stuff I wanted to accomplish in my life. From that point on, I never really took it seriously because I just couldn't believe that that was going to happen; I'm young, and it was such a shock. How could I be dying? I had never been sick before a day in my life."

Patients who are suddenly, rather than gradually affected with a fatal illness, particularly those who are younger, such as Rebecca Treat, twenty-one, have little time to make the necessary mental adjustments. This is especially the case for people suffering from hepatitis, a virus that rapidly infects the entire body.

Although not necessarily the most fatal, hepatitis is certainly the most prevalent of all liver diseases, with more than a million cases reported in the United States annually. Some hepatitis can be traced to substances such as alcohol, chemicals, and drugs, but more often than not hepatitis is caused by several highly contagious viruses: Hepatitis A is spread through contaminated water and food and excreted in the feces. Hepatitis B is usually transmitted through blood transfusion, kissing, or sexual contact, puncturing of the skin with contaminated instruments (for tattooing, ear-piercing, even acupuncture), or from mother to child, during pregnancy. Obviously, hepatitis will flourish in institutional settings such as colleges, hospitals, or the military.

Very little is known about the third category of hepatitis, that from which Rebecca Treat suffered, which, says senior liver transplant coordinator Sandee (Alexandra) Staschak, is diagnosed "through a process of exclusion. If you do a thorough examination, and you discover it is not A and not B, but you are convinced it is hepatitis, then you have your answer."

Both B and Non-A, Non-B strains of hepatitis could lead to cirrhosis, a condition in which damaged liver cells are replaced with scar tissue, thus impairing the liver's ability to function normally as the body's refinery. Staschak emphasizes the important distinction between the liver and the kidneys. "As a refinery, the liver breaks down blood cells, protein, and sugars into smaller chemical structures, whereas the kidneys serve as the body's filter; it filters out the toxins." There are many different conditions of cirrhosis, some so rare that they are barely footnotes in medical textbooks—*hemochromatosis* (abnormal handling of the body of iron), *Wilson's Disease* (abnormal handling of copper), *glycogen storage diseases* (inability to properly utilize sugars)—to name a few. But overall, cirrhosis is deadly. Behind heart disease, stroke, and cancer, liver disease is the fourth largest killer in the United States, responsible for more than 50,000 fatalities annually. Sixty percent of all people dying from liver disease die of some type of cirrhosis.

In retrospect, Rebecca suspects that her initial denial of the possibility of her death had a great deal to do with her new husband, who had been a very ambitious and steadfast suitor. When Rebecca had put in for a transfer to Alaska, Michael, whom she had been dating for only a few months, had immediately proposed, and she subsequently had agreed to withdraw her request—and to marry him. "And then, suddenly, we were told that I might not live too much longer. Well, we couldn't conceive of it; we wouldn't talk about it. Sometimes my husband and I would just sit and cry, and he would hold me and I would say, 'I'm going to die, I'm going to die.' We could not come to terms with it."

"People are often angry when somebody is going to die or when somebody's illness is disrupting their life," says Reverend Leslie Reimer, an ordained Episcopal minister, who serves as a full-time chaplain, addressing the special needs of transplant patients at Presbyterian and Children's. "But they are usually too guilty to admit to that. They don't want to say,

'I hate you because I can't be at work,' or 'I hate you because we have to live in Pittsburgh for six months.' So they clam up and stew inside."

The situation between Rebecca and her husband temporarily stabilized, but the medication that was helping Rebecca maintain some semblance of normalcy became less effective as her symptoms grew more prevalent. She became jaundiced and her body itched incessantly.

Jaundice is caused by the overabundance of bilirubin, an orangish-red pigment in bile, which is an essential component of the digestive system. When the liver, the body's filter, is damaged, bilirubin builds up, causing the skin to turn a deep yellow (greenish in severe cases) and act as a toxin. Normally there is .3 mg of bilirubin per 100 cc of the body's blood, but the bilirubin count in patients with liver disease can, at its extreme, reach 50 or 60. An excessive amount of bilirubin in the blood is an irritant that causes constant itching, extremely annoying to adults, but agonizing to children, especially those too young to help themselves. "The itching made me a little nervous," Rebecca Treat recalls, "but I was acting pretty crazy anyway. I would run around like a chicken with nowhere to go, then suddenly I would get amazingly exhausted. Nothing made sense to me sometimes; I couldn't remember things."

Ammonia is a waste product of the digestive tract, normally processed in the liver. The toxic combination of excess ammonia, combined with high bilirubin, usually causes one of two opposite extremes of behavior: hyperactivity and disorientation, or a decreased level of consciousness. People with high bilirubin and ammonia counts can be very lethargic, and a different person with a similar bilirubin can thrash wildly, out of touch with reality. At different times, a person with a high bilirubin count, along with high levels of ammonia, can exhibit both "crazy" behaviors.

Not only can liver patients be distinguished by their yellow color, but also by their shape. A damaged liver destroys appetite and disables the digestive tract, thus causing a gradual loss of overall body weight. Depending upon the severity of their cases, people suffering from end-stage liver disease have narrow shoulders, pinched faces, collapsed chests, because of the lack of protein over a prolonged period. Some will shrink to half of their normal size. These same people will often have severely distended bellies (ascites) or swollen legs (edema), both resulting from excess accumulation of fluids, as a result of obstruction of normal circulation.

By the end of December, Rebecca was so run down, she could hardly lift herself out of bed. "I was sleeping through most of the day, and I guess I finally realized that the situation was serious, just as serious as the doctor at Fort Gordon had assured me it was." When she had been initially examined at Fort Gordon, her physician had offered to contact Dr. Thomas E. Starzl on her behalf. At the time, Rebecca had been reluctant, but at that point she re-contacted the doctor, who was able to arrange for an evaluation in Pittsburgh.

Rebecca Treat's decision to attempt to become a candidate for liver transplantation in Pittsburgh, might possibly have been her last clearly succinct and rational act for many months. From that point on, she began to lose more and more of her memory; her concept of reality rapidly diminished. She knows that she went to Pittsburgh January 12, 1985, and that she remained there for nine days. Rebecca knows that all of this happened while she was in Pittsburgh that January, but she cannot recollect any of it, except for the steep hillside that surrounded the hospital, and the bitter mid-winter cold. The solitary image that remains with her from that moment in time was climbing out of a taxi, dashing to the nearest doorway—the Western Psychiatric Institute and Clinic—and hiding "for the longest time." She could see the Presby building across the street and around the corner. "I just couldn't work up the courage to face the cold outside."

Gastroenterologist David H. Van Thiel, who supervises most of the medical evaluations conducted on potential liver transplant candidates, explains that because most doctors are relatively unfamiliar with liver disease, approximately one-quarter of the transplant team's patients have been initially referred with the wrong diagnosis. Thus, they begin by attempting to identify the real nature of their disease, along with all of the related physical and emotional complications.

Rebecca Treat's evaluation at Presbyterian-University Hospital began with a series of blood tests to determine blood type (organs are usually not transplanted across the ABO blood type grouping), to evaluate the function of her kidneys and other vital organs, especially the liver, and to confirm the initial diagnosis of Non-A, Non-B hepatitis. A CT scan, a type of X-ray that utilizes a computer to produce cross-sectional views of the anatomical area being investigated, is next in the evaluation process. Also called a "liver volume test," this will determine liver size, and identify abnormalities that might interfere with the success of the transplant.

The transplant team will also examine the liver through ultrasound, an imaging procedure that arranges sound waves to create a picture of the liver and its surrounding organs. They will learn how effectively their patient's liver is working as a refinery by injecting a special dye (Indocyanine Green Test), and measuring how it was processed and cleared. They will conduct an endoscopy, in which a lighted tube is passed through the patient's esophagus and stomach to see if varicose veins, which might cause fatal hemorrhage during surgery, are present. They will do an electroencephalogram (EEG) to record changes in brain waves that might have occurred because of liver disease. An ophthalmologist is called in to evaluate the effect of liver disease on the eyes (color changes will often occur). The patient will also receive a series of pulmonary function tests to measure lung capacity and ability to tolerate a lengthy operation under anesthesia.

At some point the patient will also receive a neuropsychiatric evaluation, a series of tests to determine the impact of liver disease on the patient's perceptions, judgments, reflexes, and memory. Heart and heart-lung transplant patients might undergo a similar battery of tests, but more often than not the liver transplant evaluation is considerably more technical because of doubt concerning the referring physician's initial diagnosis.

"Everyone who comes here for evaluation," says Sandee Staschak, "has trepidations and anxieties; they are afraid of what might happen to them if they are not accepted for transplant, as much as they are afraid of what will happen if they *are* accepted. Sometimes it is a very secure feeling for them to be here and to discover that they are the tenth patient on the unit suffering from a particularly rare liver disease because they were kind of a novelty at the hospital where they were originally diagnosed. Other people become very put-out because they are not getting the kind of personalized attention they are used to. That doesn't usually happen here. We do not have time to sit and talk to people for too very long. It's incredibly busy—and you never know what is going to happen next—or when it is going to happen." Working at the world's major organ transplant center, says Staschak, is like living life inside "a twenty-four-hour time bomb."

Chapter 10

FACE TO FACE

The woman has brought her nine-year-old child to Pittsburgh from Ohio, despite strong objections from her husband.

"We've known that Lisa has been dying [from PPH] for a long time. My husband is resigned to it—in fact that's why he refused to come with me—but I wanted to find out about heart-lung transplantation. If there's hope . . ."

Robert Hardesty leans forward in his chair. "It's never been done on someone so young, and I can't offer much hope that it will be attempted in the near future. Organs are the big problem. How often will we get a heart and lung Lisa's size and blood type to use?"

"But it's possible," says the woman.

"Possible," Hardesty admits, "but let me tell you. There are things worse than death. I am referring to putting her through the operation. It could be a devastating procedure."

The woman is near tears. Her shoulders are trembling. As she talks, she wraps a lace handkerchief tightly around her fingers, then wipes her palms repeatedly against her knees. "If we do transplant her, what do we have to look forward to?"

Hardesty's face shows no emotion. His voice is soft and respectful. "There's little information as to how much time we can buy her. You have to understand, no one who has had a heart-lung transplant here or anywhere else has remained alive more than four years. There are many questions we can't answer: Will a transplant extend her life for a significant amount of time? Will it improve the quality of her life over and above the life she leads now? Will the heart and the lungs grow along with the rest of her body, or will she have to have another transplant down the road?"

("There are good indications that the heart and lungs will grow along with the child," Bruce Reitz reported in 1986. "The animals, like calves, that are transplanted at a 100 pounds will grow to a 1,000 pounds. Basically, the child's heart has as many cells as does an adult's heart. It grows simply by enlarging individual cells rather than adding new cells.")

"What if I wanted you to do it anyway?"

"We would consider it," said Hardesty, "but what I am talking about is whether you should put her through it in view of the limited potential gain. The question is: Are we extending her life by transplanting her—or prolonging her death?"

While Robert Hardesty is attempting to dissuade the mother from committing her child to the hazards of transplant surgery and the difficult immunosuppressive course that will follow, he is also conducting a second level evaluation—one in which the candidate's age makes a great deal of difference. In contrast to pediatric patients for liver transplantation (Starzl's program boasts a one-year 80 percent survival rate), children as a rule cannot endure the trauma of cardiac transplantation. At the time Hardesty interviewed the nervous mother, only a very few infants and perhaps a couple of dozen children worldwide had received heart transplants. Three years later, those totals would be quadrupled—still not a very substantial number, especially when only half that number had survived a year post-transplant. In 1984, no one under nineteen years had received a heart-lung transplant. But by 1987, Hardesty and Griffith would have transplanted children fourteen, seven, and three—the youngest ever to receive a heart-lung transplant in the United States.

While some patients can be too young for transplantation, it seems that under certain circumstances they can also be too old. In England, there was a tacit, unwritten understanding amongst physicians that individuals over the age of fifty-five suffering from end-stage renal disease not be referred for dialysis or transplant, a practice that, a researcher discovered in 1984, led to 1,500 to 3,000 unnecessary deaths annually. In response, the National Health Service significantly expanded its budget for dialysis and transplant services. In the United States, not only is age discrimination illegal, but as George Annas, a bioethicist at Boston University, has said: "It is not medically logical to assume that an individual who is forty-nine years old is necessarily a better medical candidate for a transplant than one who is fifty years old."

Dr. Eric Rose of Columbia-Presbyterian Hospital in New York tells of one heart transplant candidate who gave his age as "fifty-eight" after being told during his evaluation that the general upper age guideline of the program was fifty-eight. A few months later, after he had been successfully transplanted, he was told that the age limit had been increased four years. "OK then," the patient replied. "So now I'm sixty-two."

As far as Hardesty could see, men and women in their late fifties and early sixties could look forward to many years of reasonably active lives through heart transplantation—a technique of proven therapeutic value. But he had serious and significant doubts about putting children through such a delicate and dangerous procedure as a heart or heart-lung transplant, not only because of the obvious pain and suffering to the child, but more so because of the potential damage done to the family unit. By offering the family such a vague wisp of hope, he and Griffith were not giving the mother and father the time necessary to prepare for the almost inevitable death of their offspring.

There are, however, other surgeons who disagree with Hardesty's position, including Dr. Leonard Bailey of Loma Linda, who has transplanted hearts into babies from four days old to three months, five of whom remained alive anywhere from three to eighteen months after surgery. "We know from experience that the younger they are, the better. Newborns are far more tolerant of their grafts than adults or even older babies."

"Look," Hardesty said, after a while to the woman facing him across the room, "if this were a heart, it would be a totally different story, or if she was a little bit older. But there's no way I can explain to you what someone, especially a child, would have to go through for a heart-lung transplant."

The mother looked at him and nodded, wiping tears with her lace handkerchief from her eyes.

"The best thing I can tell you is that if I were in your position, if it was my nine-year-old daughter, I wouldn't do it."

"I understand what you are saying, but many people, other parents especially, think that we, my husband and I, are terrible for not trying to do anything to help Lisa."

"You're doing the best you can."

"But they don't understand. I feel guilty."

Hardesty shakes his head: "She isn't my daughter. I don't see her suffering day in and day out, and I don't relate so much to her dying in the same way that you do." He peered out the door toward the nurse's station, where the little girl was waiting.

"I don't have a nine-year-old daughter sitting in a wheelchair, breathing in oxygen, clutching a babydoll in her lap that she calls a patient. I'm not in your position. So," he says, softly, with a sigh, "if you want to consider transplanting her, we'll consider her for the list."

"I can walk a little bit, but any distance I go, I get out of breath," says nineteen-year-old Cindy Sprague of Mexico, New York. She is slender, pale, and blonde, sitting in a wheelchair with plastic nasal cannulae plugged into an oxygen bottle in her lap.

"How often do you use the oxygen?" asks Hardesty.

"Continuously."

Cindy's mother explains that Cindy went to Austria the summer after high school to study German, but when she got sick, she was airlifted home.

"The good news," says Hardesty, "is that we've had a 75 percent survival rate with patients with PPH."

"The bad news is how much it costs," the father says.

"It is expensive," Hardesty acknowledges, "anywhere from $90,000 to $140,000, depending upon how long she stays in the intensive care unit." A quarter million dollars for a heart-lung transplant would not be considered unusual, however; $500,000 is rare, but it happens. Most of the charges are for hospital services, tests, and medications; the transplant team's fees rarely exceed $12,000. Costs of liver transplantation are comparable.

"The bad news," Hardesty continues, "is the reality of the waiting period. It's not that our list is very long, but your blood type, A, your size and weight (around 100 pounds) are very common on our list, so there are a lot of people ahead of you."

"Cindy postponed her marriage until next August so she could get through her problems." Mrs. Sprague motions at a tiny engagement ring on the girl's slender hand. "As far as schooling, we figure she can make up college later."

Hardesty pauses, nods, smiles slightly. "Five years ago, we wouldn't have been able to do anything. Now, if we can get you transplanted, you have a 75 percent chance of someday lifting yourself out of the wheelchair and pursuing a relatively normal life."

"Yes," Cindy's mother says, softly. "That's *if* we can get her transplanted."

Hardesty shakes hands with Mr. and Mrs. Sprague, smiles at Cindy, says goodbye, and leaves them alone in the room.

"You mean *if* we can get the money," Mr. Sprague says to his wife, sighing, shaking his head slowly back and forth.

Mr. Sprague knows that in Pittsburgh, or at any other major transplant center across the United States, "evaluation" means, more than anything else, money. No matter how near to death Frank Rowe, Winkle Fulk, Cindy Sprague, or any of the hundreds of people who come to Pittsburgh from all over the world each year, they will not be transplanted unless they can pay for it. In Pittsburgh and other transplant centers, a prospective patient must prove adequate insurance coverage, or, failing that, deposit anywhere from $100,000 to $200,000, cash, in advance.

Basically, according to Edward Berkowitz, manager of credit and collections at Presby, there are five possible methods of payment for a transplant patient. The first option is the federal government. Berkowitz explains that in 1972 Congress authorized payment under Medicare for patients taking dialysis or receiving kidney transplants, a decision many legislators feel was disastrous because it turned out to be so expensive. At the time, Congress estimated an expenditure of $140 million per year. Today that program exceeds $2 billion annually. Medicare has continued to cover kidney transplants, and in 1987 has introduced an experimental and very limited trial program of compensation for heart transplantation, which includes patients over sixty-five and patients who have been on disability for more than two years—in total less than 5 percent of all extrarenal transplant patients. But possibilities of expanded transplant coverage under Medicare are unlikely in the foreseeable future.

Coverage by "the Blues" (Blue Cross and Blue Shield) is quite possible, but each Blue Cross association, and there are hundreds of them across the United States, has its own policy regarding both *whether* it covers transplantation, and if so, *which* transplant procedure might be included. In the Pittsburgh area, for example, Blue Cross will cover all transplants, whereas across the border, fifty miles to the west in Ohio, some Blue Cross associations, but not all of them, will cover heart and liver transplantation, but only when done in Ohio. Presently in Ohio, a person dying from heart or liver disease must look for therapy in his or her own back yard—or do without it.

Commercial insurance, the third way in which a transplant might be paid, most often has to do with the generosity of the organization for which the patient works, for very often, transplant coverage is not automatic in health care policies; it is an option that must be purchased separately. According to a survey of sixty-five companies, conducted by the Health Insurance Association of America (HIAA), most companies are beginning to routinely pay for transplants under group health insurance contracts. "All sixty-five companies will pay for cornea and bone marrow transplants, while sixty-three reported their willingness to reimburse for kidney and skin transplants. Bone transplants are reimbursed by sixty companies, heart transplants by fifty-five, liver transplants by fifty-two companies, and heart-lung transplants by forty-five. Pancreas transplants proved the least eligible for payment—thirty-seven companies said that they are willing to pay for this operation, twenty-one of them as standard practice and the remaining sixteen on a case-by-case basis."

The fourth and perhaps the most erratic and difficult area of coverage is through state medical assistance. But many state welfare agencies are very hesitant to cover transplantation, says Berkowitz, especially those in the deep south, such as Alabama, Georgia, Florida, Arkansas, and Louisiana, which are also the states in which the "Blues" are most conservative. It is not at all an understatement to maintain that whether some people live or die often depends upon where they happen to claim residence.

In 1983, Judy Tazelaar, a forty-year-old Detroit mother of four suffering from cirrhosis was admitted to Presbyterian five times for treatment, and five times she was subsequently discharged because the only therapy remaining for her condition was a liver transplant, and she lacked the necessary coverage or cash deposit.

Tazelaar eventually appealed directly to White House Transplant Liaison Michael Batten, who convinced the Governor of Michigan to authorize Michigan Medicaid coverage. But a few months after being successfully transplanted, Michigan Medicare declined to pay. Presbyterian-University was thus forced to absorb the charges, a situation that has led to a hardening of position as far as admitting transplant patients with questionable finances. (The hospital lost more than $1 million on its transplant program in 1983 due to transplant research and bad patient debt.) Children's Hospital has also recently instituted a policy of initiating court action against parents who refuse to pay bills.

A few hospitals, which includes Children's in Pittsburgh and Columbia-Presbyterian in New York, have used their endowment to help absorb and defray the overwhelming expense to less-fortunate families. Eric Rose has said that it is "intrinsically unfair" to deny transplant therapy to anyone who pays taxes, simply because taxpayers' money has been essentially responsible for research that has developed heart transplant techniques, while bioethicist George Annas of Boston University has pointed out the inequities of such a system, which favors the white middle class. "It is another example of how we as a society are doing more and more things for fewer and fewer people at higher and higher cost."

The fifth financial option for transplantation is both the most obvious and the most impractical: direct payment, beginning with the submission of a cash deposit before being admitted to the hospital. Based on the average transplant charges for 1985–86, this means $40,000 for kidneys, $85,000 for hearts, $130,000 for livers, and $135,000 for heart-lungs. Berkowitz estimated that under 5 percent of patients paid for transplants in this manner. "Primarily these are foreign patients or those who have had massive fund raising events."

Reverend Leslie Reimer strongly disagrees with a "money first" policy, but doesn't see any way around it at this time. "I recently had a conversation with a Presby administrator, who said, 'If we didn't worry about money, then nobody would have a chance at transplantation, for nobody would be here for transplant if somebody didn't pay the bills.' That is an interesting piece of rationalization, but I'm not sure I buy it. I don't know who is going to pay, but I do know that it is not good to let money determine who lives and who dies, and that is exactly where we are."

The past few years, public appeals for large sums of money to subsidize transplant surgery in life or death situations have been incredibly successful, but Reimer worries about what might happen when the uniqueness of transplantation wears thin. "Transplantation is still new enough that most people who do local fund raising are first or one of the very first to attempt it in their area. But how many times will it be possible to convince people to give money when this first wave is over? Then what do we do? Where do we go from there?"

Because of its socialistic National Health Service, which automatically assumes responsibility for all health-related therapy and medication, the United Kingdom has a somewhat different situation for funding new surgical procedures. When the cardiac transplant program was initiated at Papworth Hospital in 1979 by Dr. Terence English, neither the government

nor the patients objected. English was told that if transplantation was viable and he felt up to the challenge of the surgery
and the management of immunosuppression, he could have
a go at it—provided he could fund it on his own. English
relied on the generosity of a local millionaire, who graciously
supported the first three transplants, procedures that eventually demonstrated to the government that transplantation was
worth subsidizing.

A few minutes after Hardesty departed, Griffith came in to
visit with the Spragues. It is at moments like these when
one can see the primary difference between the two young
surgeons. Hardesty is nearly always controlled. He deals with
each situation evenly and objectively while Griffith cannot
so easily hide his compassion for the patient or his disappointment with himself at not being able to provide immediate
help. Even his voice telegraphs his distress.

"How long have you been sick, dear?"

Cindy doesn't answer.

"A year," her mother says.

"Have you experienced any bleeding?"

Cindy still doesn't answer.

"Was that really scary for ya? The bleeding?" He reaches
out and feels her abdomen gently.

"Have you had any swelling? Does your waist swell?" He
pauses, looks at her, smiles. "I guess that's a dangerous question to ask a young lady."

Again, Cindy doesn't answer, but neither does she avoid
his gaze. Tears begin to slide down her pale cheeks, but she
is crying silently.

"What did Dr. Hardesty tell you? What did you hear? You've
got to talk about this. It's OK to cry," he reaches out and
touches her cheeks, "but you've got to talk about it anyway.
Remember," he says, "we're in this together."

Cindy opens her mouth, but the words just don't seem to
be coming. Griffith waits, gives her time to compose herself.
She sniffs, continues to stare.

There are no chairs or windows in this room, and both
parents are standing and leaning against the cream-colored

vinyl-covered wall, stiffly and uncomfortably, their faces frozen in a strained and congenial kind of smile. A low buzz of activity can be heard outside in the corridor. Cool air whistling through the ceiling duct blows down on them.

Cindy shifts in her wheelchair, lifts and then replaces the oxygen bottle in her lap. She will have to get it refilled for her trip home that afternoon. Her voice is almost inaudible, and Griffith cocks an ear and leans forward to listen. "He told me I have a 75 percent chance," she says, finally.

"How long did he say you can live after the operation?"

"He doesn't know."

Griffith shakes his head. He speaks even more softly. "It's not easy. It's rough. Tough medicine. I wish you were a little bit older, so that you've been out and around more and can make a stronger decision." He shrugs. "Is that an engagement ring on your hand?"

"Yes, but we've decided to wait."

"That was wise," says Griffith, nodding. "It just means that we will have to get you a donor quickly."

Now he is ready to leave. He picks up a file that he had carried into the room, tucks it under his arm, and stuffs his stethoscope into the pocket of his white lab coat. He shakes hands with the Spragues and opens the door, then, almost as an afterthought, he turns back to Cindy who, for the first time, smiles back at him.

"Live every day," Griffith tells her. "Don't live for the waiting list."

Cindy lived several months after visiting Hardesty and Griffith that summer afternoon—not long enough, however. She died at home in Mexico, New York.

Chapter 11

BEYOND THE "GOD SQUAD"

In a panel discussion coordinated by Presbyterian-University Hospital personnel, focusing upon ethical issues in transplantation, one participant urged surgeons to more thoroughly examine "the psychological makeup of the recipient" during the evaluation process, prior to transplant.

"It is important to get someone really hungry for that organ," he said, "someone who will stay hungry after they have received that organ. I always use the example of my uncle who had a double bypass operation a couple of years ago. Immediately upon release from the hospital, he went to smoking two packs of cigarettes a day. That was a tremendous waste of talent on the part of the surgeon, of medical effort on the part of the staff, and a tremendous waste of money—and for what? My point is that organ recipients have got to want to take care of that organ. You've got to be really hungry—because you want this organ. You have got to be psychologically ready. It's a gift," he concluded, "and in the same way that you must cherish a gift, you must cherish the transplant."

After the man had finished his part of the discussion, the audience, a group of upper-middle-class men and women involved in volunteer work, applauded—not only because of the statements he had made, but perhaps more so because of who and what he was. This man, a forty-two-year-old Catholic priest, had, over the past ten years, received three kidney transplants. He later reflected that his point of view regarding transplant candidate screening probably represented the feelings of a vast majority of his fellow recipients. Once again the audience indicated its approval with scattered applause.

Although the priest's opinions were interesting and important, what was truly fascinating was the startling contrast between what was possible in the present and what had been in the past. A quarter of a century ago, the concept of kidney transplantation was a brave new experiment launched by a small and dedicated cadre of scientists, while prospects for extrarenal transplantation were the distant hope of a few scattered dreamers. Today, kidney transplantation has become routine surgery, while one-year survival rates in extrarenal transplantation range from 65 percent for liver and up to 85 percent for cardiac transplant recipients. And yet, many of the ethical problems debated in Pittsburgh amongst social workers, religious leaders, surgeons, and recipients on that afternoon were identical to the problems confronted by the pre-transplant medical community twenty-five years ago. Surgeons and scientists have made remarkable strides in transplantation since then, while the ethicists, who in many ways have had the much more difficult job, continue to struggle for answers.

It began in the basement of an out-of-the-way annex in Swedish Hospital in Seattle, Washington, in 1961, where the world's first Artificial Kidney Center was located—a few machines that, at any given time, could offer an indefinite extension of life to approximately six of the many needy people dying of incurable kidney disease. But who would be selected? The hospital's medical board created an Admissions and Policies Committee of seven people—a clergyman, a housewife, a banker, an attorney, a labor leader, a surgeon, and a governmental official—a group that came to be known as the "Life and Death Committee" or later, "The God Squad." The labels accurately reflected the Committee's basic role: to play God, to decide who would live with dialysis and who would die by assessing the relative worth (or worthiness) of each and every individual who had applied.

Although there were no kidney specialists as voting members of the Committee, the medical board had simplified matters to a certain extent at the outset by establishing age limitations based upon medical criteria, eliminating children as candidates, as well as adults over age forty-five. Considering lack of knowledge about dialysis as therapy, it was felt at the time that older patients were too susceptible to potential medical complications caused by dialysis, while children were too naive to be connected to such a frightening apparatus, and to be forced to conduct their lives under such stringent restrictions.

During its first couple of meetings, the God Squad established further limitations, according to veteran journalist Shana Alexander, who wrote an in-depth profile of the group ("They Decide Who Lives, Who Dies") for *Life* Magazine in November 1962: ". . . they agreed to consider only those applicants who were residents of the state of Washington . . ." They justified this stand on the grounds that since the basic development of the Kidney Center and some of the technological innovations "has been done at the University of Washington Medical School and its new University Hospital—both state-supported institutions—the people whose taxes had paid for the research should be its first beneficiaries."

Age restrictions can be partially justified on medical grounds, but in today's modern world, especially considering the tremendous scope of organ transplantation, preference to the "hometown kid" would be an unacceptable concept. Can local candidates be given priority in Pittsburgh, for example, if the organs being transplanted into them come from Illinois or Alabama? If a transplant can save a life, what does it matter where the patient resides, unless the patient's location diminishes the prospects for successful surgery? Currently, the United Network of Organ Sharing (UNOS), the organization designated by the Department of Health and Human Services to establish a national organ distribution system, is examining a proposal by Tennessee Senator Albert Gore, to give local candidates priority with local donors only, and in nonemergency situations.

The concept of giving preference to candidates because of where they live has been rendered even more complicated by the emergence of the hotly debated foreign national issue brought to the forefront of the national medical news by the allegations and revelations of the *Pittsburgh Press.* Considering the dearth of donor organs and the ever-expanding list of prospective recipients from all across the nation, should valuable resources be expended upon patients coming from other countries for transplantation?

Robert Gordon, director of Starzl's kidney transplant program, recognized the problem, but he also did not think that he could effectively function under a system that denied foreign patient access. In the summer of 1985, within a few months after the *Press* articles were published, Gordon developed a quota system that would allow foreign nationals to receive an equivalent of 5 percent of the number of kidney transplants performed at the hospital during the previous year. Under this plan, adopted by Presbyterian, after foreign nationals became accepted as patients and established on the waiting list, they would be treated as equal to Americans.

A proposal for a similar system of nonresident alien allocation was made public in April 1986 by the federal Task Force on Organ Transplantation, which recommended that aliens receive no more than 10 percent of the kidney transplants at any hospital, and that Americans receive priority for all extrarenal organs. The ongoing controversy triggered by this issue is symbolized by the statement of exception, signed by a minority of the Task Force members, who believed that the 10 percent quota for kidney recipients was unfair to Americans seeking transplants. The statement opposed any priority treatment of foreign citizens.

Bioethicist Arthur Caplan might argue with the direction of the Task Force in these issues, but he supports government intervention in the initial decision-making process. "The patient's race, nationality, or the extent of his patriotism should be none of the doctor's business. That is a society's decision, a governmental decision; it's not a medical decision." It is also unfair and inappropriate to rest the responsibility for these decisions on the shoulders of surgeons and then to criticize them for doing it wrong. In fact, Caplan has labeled the foreign national issue "a red herring," and contends that, "It is not foreigners, but wealthy foreigners that people object to getting priority and special treatment."

Subsequently, Pittsburgh's surgeons devised a computerized "multifactorial" system of selection for renal candidates which assigns candidates "credit units" based upon the essential aspects generally considered during the recipient selection process: waiting time, medical urgency, and additional (scientifically oriented) criteria. While children do have priority over adults, the questions of lifestyle (smoking, drinking, etc.) are not considered in the selection.

"Introduction of an objective method for renal recipient selection has had a positive effect on our program," Starzl and his team subsequently explained in a 1987 article in the *Journal of the American Medical Association* (JAMA). "Ad hoc case selection at odd hours, guided by the often faulty memory of a transplant coordinator or by incomplete tabular information has been eliminated. During the course of the trial year [1986], waiting lists [in certain blood types] have been completely eliminated, and the duration of waiting [for other blood types] has been greatly shortened. A decision to proceed with transplantations still rests with the responsible surgeon, with the only provision being that an explanation must be sent to the Director of the Organ Procurement Foundation and to a community oversight committee when there is a deviation from the standardized process."

This "Oversight Committee," made up of high-ranking corporate executives, influential political leaders independent of the medical community, has been established in Pittsburgh to open the recipient selection process to public examination (as Caplan, Denny, and others have urged), and to respond to candidate complaint or criticism. This is a retrospective group; the God Squad, in contrast, had been a "prospective" group. At present, this Committee reviews the applications of all nonresident aliens accepted by the transplant team to assure that the system is in compliance with established policy. In 1988, Thomas Starzl introduced a similar but more sophisticated mulifactorial system for selection of liver recipients.

Despite the fact that the controversy over transplant allocation ethics revolved around the system in Pittsburgh, it is important to point out that Pittsburgh's response to the criticism has become the nation's standard. The distribution system introduced by the UNOS federal network in October 1987 is based upon the Starzl-Gordon "multifactorial" creation, while the UNOS policy concerning foreign nationals is, if anything, less severe than Gordon's original suggestions.

In general, UNOS has decided that nonresident alien transplants should account for no more than 10 percent of the hospital's transplant patients *in each category*, according to Gordon, a member of the UNOS committee that will monitor these guidelines. The situation is loosely structured so that some large hospitals, such as Presbyterian-University, with a history of transplanting organs into foreigners and an expanding surgical training program, may be allowed to exceed the 10 percent, while smaller centers could be penalized for transplanting at a 10 percent foreign national rate if they cannot show precedent for such action.

By far the most difficult of the questions confronting the God Squad in 1961–62—closely mirrored by the questions being discussed by the priest and his fellow panel members in Pittsburgh that afternoon—were the psychosocial issues. As a dramatic demonstration of the subjective and value-laden manner in which the God Squad functioned, Shana Alexander interviewed each Committee member and pieced together a facsimile transcript of an actual discussion, excerpted below. At this point in the conversation, the lawyer, who is the Committee chairman, has announced that the Kidney Center has two more vacancies and that the Committee must choose from a list of five finalists.

> BANKER: Just to get the ball rolling, why don't we start with Number One—the housewife from Walla Walla.
> SURGEON: This patient could not commute for treatment, so she would have to find a way to move her family to Seattle.
> BANKER: Exactly my point. It says here that her husband has no funds to make a move.
> LAWYER: Then you are proposing we eliminate this candidate on the grounds that she could not possibly accept treatment, if it were offered?

MINISTER: How can we compare a family situation of two children, such as this woman in Walla Walla with a family of six children, such as patient Number Four—the aircraft worker?

STATE OFFICIAL: But are we sure that the aircraft worker can be rehabilitated? I note that he is already too sick to work, whereas Number Two and Number Five, the chemist and the accountant, are both still able to keep going . . .

HOUSEWIFE: If we are still looking for the men with the highest potential of service to society, then I think that we must consider that the chemist and the accountant have the finest educational backgrounds of all five candidates.

SURGEON: How do the rest of you feel about Number Three— the small businessman with three children? I am impressed that his doctor took special pains to mention that this man is active in church work. This is an indication to me of character and moral strength.

HOUSEWIFE: Which certainly would help him conform to the demands of the treatment . . .

LAWYER: It would also help him to endure a lingering death.

In the end, the aircraft worker (because of the size of his family?) and the small businessman (because of his dedication to the church?) were selected by the God Squad. It is difficult to know how much these selections were tainted by personal prejudice, but clearly, despite the well-intentioned nature of the Committee members, the God Squad as a concept was an imperfect solution to a very muddy ethical dilemma, as demonstrated by the retrospective reflection of one Committee member, quoted by Fox and Swazey in their book, *The Courage to Fail*, in 1974:

" 'I remember voting against a young woman who was a known prostitute. I found I couldn't vote for her, rather than another candidate, a young wife and mother. I also voted against a young man who, until he learned he had renal failure, had been a ne'er do well, a real playboy. He promised me he would reform his character, go back to school, and so on, if only he were selected for treatment. But I felt I'd lived long enough to know that a person like that won't really do what he was promising at the time.' "

Sooner or later during evaluation, Frank Rowe, Winkle Fulk, Rebecca Treat, and all other candidates coming to Pittsburgh will consult with a transplant social worker, whose mission is to explain more about the experience through which they will soon be traveling, and to determine from a psychosocial point of view, whether the patient is acceptable for transplantation. Although she feels that the selection process is usually above reproach, liver transplant social worker Donna Rinaldo, who has been working with transplant patients since the inception of the program, has, on occasion, registered her doubts. "Looking back on it we've had some patients who really shouldn't have been transplanted, but," she adds, "that is so terribly difficult to determine beforehand.

"I have one patient I am thinking of particularly who had a drug and alcohol problem," says Rinaldo. "We talked a lot about that before the transplant. She wanted to commit suicide in the hospital, she was so uncomfortable with her illness. But we figured, 'Once we transplant her and make her life more tolerable, she won't need the drugs and alcohol so much.'

"On paper, there is a policy as far as abstinence—a patient has to be drug or alcohol free for at least six months. But most of our patients are drug and alcohol free for that time simply because they're too sick [to drink], they've been hospitalized, etc. But after they begin to feel healthy again, the problems which caused their dependency are still there. They revert to their previous habits."

In this particular case, the woman had been chemical free for a long enough time. "The husband presented himself as being extremely devoted and really caring about this lady's future and their life (they had a small child) together," said Rinaldo.

"She had the transplant, and another surgery beyond that for complications; in fact, she had two liver transplants, and she was in the hospital for about six months. But when she was discharged, her parting statement was 'I'm going to the first bar on my way home and get drunk.'

"We thought she was joking, but her life continued to fall apart. She went home, couldn't take care of the little girl, was not emotionally strong enough to handle some of the changes that had gone on in her life. She had been a model before, so the side effects from cyclosporine and prednisone really took a toll on her, and she couldn't handle any of these things. She and her husband sought psychiatric counseling. There were many problems. She started to drink at home. The husband started to drink. They fought; he would throw beer cans at her . . . that kind of thing. She came into the Emergency Room once after being hit by a couple of beer cans, and he was arrested and thrown in jail. Her life is meaningless right now. She's had another child in the meantime, but she can't take care of either one of her kids. She doesn't want to go to work, and there are many financial problems.

"You know, you sit there and think, 'Well, who am I to make a value judgment and say that this person shouldn't be transplanted? But then again, at the same time, you wonder, what is the quality of life after the transplant? What was the purpose of it all?"

Arthur Caplan observes that "quality of life" is sometimes not an easy state to define or to predict. During the evaluation process, members of the transplant team—surgeons, nurses, social workers, etc.—must carefully weigh a number of factors in relation to the potential recovery of a particular candidate.

"I think that part of quality of life is being able to have cognitive mental awareness, so for me, people who are so severely retarded, having no intellectual function, or people in a coma, who are in permanent vegetative state, should not receive aggressive medical care." In other words, says Caplan, no transplant.

"A second component is, can you make it possible [with a transplant] for the person to function at a level somewhat comparable to what they had before they were afflicted with the illness? I've been a critic of the [permanent] artificial heart because it seems to me that by tying somebody down to a bed with a 350-pound console, your quality of life is so limited in terms of what you can do, compared to what you had been able to do, that it is not justifiable.

"A third quality of life thing is pain. If you are in constant, chronic, terrible pain, it is not a very good way to live. For example, a cancer patient. Would I transplant them? No—not if it meant keeping them alive for more constant chronic pain."

Finally, says Caplan, quality of life means "an ability to form personal relationships and contacts. If you are so encumbered by the technology of a transplant that you have to be bed-bound and under constant professional care, your quality of life is limited because you can't make friends. Let's say you have to have a tube down your throat all the time—you can't talk, you can't engage with others. We are special creatures and that dimension is important to what we would call 'the good life.' "

Caplan sides with physicians, who are practically alone in their belief that psychosocial issues, such as drug addiction, alcoholism, should not enter into the selection of transplant candidates. "Alcoholism may be relevant if the guy is still drinking and he has no chance of preserving a transplanted liver. But if he says he is cured and to the best of our knowledge he looks cured, he should be as able to get a transplant as anybody else. I don't think that physicians should get into the business of making moral character judgments about why people get sick—they should respond to need for treatment—not the cause of the need."

Gastroenterologist David Van Thiel, who stresses that only one liver in ten is susceptible to alcohol-induced cirrhosis, says that initially he was opposed to the idea of transplanting alcoholics, but since becoming deeply involved with Thomas Starzl and the liver transplant team he has changed his mind, although his reasoning differs from Caplan's. "If there is meaningful life to be expected with or without their alcoholism in the future, it is worth doing." He offers as an example the possibility of a renowned novelist, who drinks himself to the edge of death. "I think we would transplant him if we could. He could write a couple more books . . . hell, that's worthwhile. Lots of very worthwhile human beings have alcoholism as a problem, but as long as they have meaningful life with their alcoholism, then it is worth doing. We can't tell people who drink or smoke or overeat to die in the streets, particularly if they have a potential for meaningful life," he adds.

Mary Burge, Stanford's cardiac transplant social worker, explains that before accepting a suspected addicted personality into their transplant program "we look at what role we think alcohol or drugs play in that person's life. If it's a social drinker, say a construction worker who usually stops off with the guys and has a couple of beers, or more than a couple of beers, and it's part of his lifestyle, that's one thing." The situation would be different, however, if it "would be somebody who regularly medicates himself with alcohol as a substitute for other kinds of coping."

How to tell one personality from another? "One way is to see how open they are in describing their drinking habits. A continuing alcoholic will, of course, cover up and say whatever he thinks you want to hear, but somebody else . . ." She interrupts herself to describe a recent case, "a man in his early thirties, who said during the evaluation interview that when he was seventeen or eighteen, he had drunk a case of beer a day.

"I said, 'You mean a six pack?'

"He said, 'No, I said a case.'

"I said, 'Was that a period in your life when you were trying to find yourself?'

"He said, 'Hell no, I was trying to lose myself.'

"I said, 'Do you still do that?'

"And he said, 'I don't feel the need for it anymore.'

"His honesty seemed to me a good sign of somebody telling the truth about what his habits are now."

Although transplanting alcoholics remains a controversial area of discussion (at this time, no valid scientific data exist which track the use of alcohol and drugs after transplants), the question of transplanting AIDS victims—or even those patients simply exposed to the AIDS virus—is so controversial that most surgeons will refuse to discuss the matter at any length. At a seminar in Pittsburgh in March 1987, however, Thomas Starzl, who seems to gravitate to and thrive upon volatile minority points of view, once again became a prominent name in the national news by maintaining that patients exposed to AIDS, who have not yet developed the severe form of the disease, ought to be accorded the opportunity for transplantation. "To me, it's as much a philosophical issue than anything else. The first real question is, should AIDS be treated? Having made that decision (if affirmative), the second question is, should we treat the patient with the best modality available?"

Not only is it incumbent upon the surgeon to transplant potential AIDS victims, Starzl continued, but it is safer than not transplanting and permitting them to remain on dialysis where, because both patients and employees must handle blood and other fluids, an excellent opportunity for the spreading of the highly contagious virus exists. "Isn't it almost an exercise in medical sophistry to maintain these AIDS patients in a system where the danger of spreading [the virus] is greater?"

Mary Burge of Stanford is "perplexed" by the AIDS problem, but she agrees with Donna Rinaldo that most therapies, including transplantation, will not permanently change a person, although they might influence their habits temporarily. "Early experience in the transplant program was that people who were alcoholics before their transplant, even if they stopped during the time they were in the hospital, usually went back to that when things in life got rough. So we are likely to hold out and not accept a candidate who has a major history, a real dependence, upon alcohol. We are not doing some kind of 'witch hunting,' we just want to be sure that these people will be compliant and will be able to cope. Compliancy is the main thing we are looking for; we are not trying to decide who should live and who should die, but who has the best chance of living and surviving and doing well."

Although it is not always possible to predict with any accuracy that a diminished quality of life due to social problems will occur after transplant, sometimes, Donna Rinaldo says, there are "red flags."

First, there are patients who may feel they don't need to take their medications as prescribed. "I have a man who is a 'born again' Christian, and he feels God is going to keep him healthy, and if He doesn't, then there's a reason for that. He told all of us, even before his surgery—during his evaluation—that when he was discharged, he wasn't going to take his medications. The doctors knew that," says Rinaldo, "but they transplanted him anyway. He's out; he's discharged, but I'm not sure how carefully he is following his routine." One of Presbyterian's early heart transplant recipients also ignored the notion of regular medication, and after three years of relatively good health, his heart went into sudden and severe rejection. Near death, he was subsequently retransplanted, which meant, in essence, that because of his noncompliance, someone else was denied the rare donor organ—the second organ—that might have been unnecessarily transplanted into him.

Another important red flag has to do with financial problems—not in paying for the transplant, which might be covered by insurance, but paying for medication (as high as $10,000 for cyclosporine and prednisone, annually) and self-support after transplant. "There aren't too many options for people if they don't have finances; they are going to have trouble, unless they do independent fund raising, or they happen to be very indigent and qualify for medical assistance," says Rinaldo.

Are there other indications to take into consideration? "An ability to deal with stress. An ability to be out of control. There's just no way people can be in control in this kind of situation. And if that's a difficult thing for somebody to deal with, then they're going to have a horrible time. I had a guy from New York, a prestigious investment banker, and he had a hard time because he was used to being the one to call the shots, and you simply don't call the shots on this liver service. Even the surgeons don't know what is going to happen from one minute to the next."

Most extrarenal transplant surgeons and social workers will confirm Rinaldo's observations, including surgeon Eric Rose of New York's Columbia-Presbyterian. "To some extent we have had some of our biggest problems with patient compliance in the high-powered executive types that have been transplanted. They think, 'I've controlled my life since before this all started, and now that I am feeling fine, I am going to control my life again.' We have had two like that who have died because of noncompliancy. One was an AT&T executive who called me one Sunday morning and said, 'I've had fever, and I've been short of breath for a week,' obvious signs of rejection. He knew that, but he wasn't willing to give in to it. I had another high-powered type who sat home showing all the signs of rejection that I and my staff talked with him about. But he did not call me for two weeks. They were both dead within forty-eight hours."

After all medical, economic, and psychosocial tests are conducted over the course of evaluation, each liver patient's history, tests results, and prognosis are presented to the transplant team—coordinators, social workers, clergy included—at a group meeting each Tuesday. "We discuss the patient," says David Van Thiel, "what's wrong with him, how seriously ill we think he or she might be, whether they've reached the end of the line in terms of liver function. We try to determine when that point of no return might occur—when their disease becomes critical enough for immediate transplant." A similar discussion centering upon heart transplant candidates takes place on a more informal level between Hardesty, and Griffith.

At the Tuesday liver conference in late January 1985, the transplant team estimated that Rebecca Treat could probably live a limited but normal life for as long as a year before a transplant became a high priority. At that point—or if she took a turn for the worse sooner—she would be called back to Pittsburgh.

P A R T IV

THE WAIT

C h a p t e r   12

HOPE AND DESPAIR

Returning to Kansas City after the evaluation, Dave Fulk counseled his wife to maintain perspective, not to expect too much from the transplant team, too soon. "When we were in Pittsburgh in August, they said that we would have to wait for an organ, and that they would be calling us anywhere from tomorrow to eighteen months." He averaged it out. "I figured we'd be going to Pittsburgh in February." Recognizing the wisdom in her husband's advice, Winkle resigned herself to a long and frustrating winter. But then one afternoon in November, the phone rang. Winkle, alone at home in her bed, answered.

"Mrs. Fulk?"

"Yes."

"This is Joanne, Dr. Griffith's secretary. So how are you doing?"

"I'm OK," Winkle said.

"We understand that you have a means of coming out to Pittsburgh," Joanne said.

"Yes, we have arranged for a private airplane."

"Fine. I would like you to call me back in fifteen minutes with the tail numbers and the colors of the plane." The woman paused, and then said, matter of factly, "We have a possible donor for you."

Joanne began providing additional information, about the Allegheny County Airport where they would be landing, about clothing to bring, instructions about not eating, ambulance service from the airport to the hospital, but Winkle couldn't seem to move or even think fast enough. "Wait a minute," she said, "I think I better write this down." She went over to the desk for a pen and paper. But the significance of the phone call had not penetrated, not yet. She hesitated. She was beginning to feel funny, lightheaded. Then all of a sudden it hit her.

"They had a person for me. I was going to be transplanted. This was November 15, 1984. It was 1:20 in the afternoon, and I was shaking. I was just shaking like a leaf. My mother was there. And she saw the look on my face, and she went totally white. I'll always remember that."

Winkle sat down at the desk, listened to Joanne carefully, wrote down all of the instructions and information, then hung up and dialed Dave at work. She couldn't wait to tell him. And she needed to hear his voice, which had always calmed and settled her. But at first the telephone call did not go through. Maybe she hadn't dialed properly, or the lines were tied up, she didn't know. But this was not the time for anything to go wrong. She could feel the panic beginning to well up inside of her as she listened to the emptiness at the other end of the line. She took a deep breath and dialed again. This time, mercifully, it rang, and Dave answered.

She told him that Pittsburgh had called, and that they had a donor. He was to phone the air charter company that had promised to have a jet ready within an hour, at any hour. Then she hung up and began to pack. "Everything for Dave," said Winkle. "I don't think I missed a thing for him. Then there was me. What did I need? A nightgown. I was going to be in the hospital, but I can't remember what else I threw in for myself." All she can recall is the fear and the excitement, the mixed emotions.

"I couldn't stop shaking. And I was excited. And I was happy. But I was crying. And I kept saying, 'Do I really want this?' I had talked about this for so long, with Dave, my mother and the kids, and the moment of truth was finally here, but did I really want it?" Even then, she realized that there could be no hesitation because, in fact, there was no other alternative. This *had* to be what she wanted. There was nothing else.

She looked over at her mother once again. White all over. She would settle down after Winkle and Dave left for Pittsburgh. She would cry, then pray; she would make dinner for the kids, clean up the house. But now, there was nothing Winkle could do to help. There was little to say.

"I got packed and Dave came in—he was home in five minutes—and he sat down, and the first thing I noticed was that he was also shaking. It was the first time in my entire life that I have ever seen him nervous. And that bothered me. That shook me up. To think that he was upset. He's always been my Rock of Gibraltar."

"I was just sort of shocked that they called so early," he says. "It was like calling to tell me, you gotta go to Caracas, Venezuela."

Winkle had regained her composure by the time they reached the airport, although the excitement, the elation, the relief after waiting those months churned inside of her. "All these people were busy working there, and I just wanted to tell them, 'Hey, I'm going to have a heart-lung transplant.' I wanted to tell everybody, but I didn't. I don't even think the pilot and the copilot knew who I was or why I was going to Pittsburgh."

An hour and a half after the initial phone call from Dr. Griffith's office, the chartered jet lifted them off the ground. Dave and Winkle talked off and on through the flight. It will be nice to have the transplant done now, just before Thanksgiving, they decided. What a nice Christmas present—a heart and two lungs. If all went well, they would be home by the new year.

On the plane to Pittsburgh, Dave Fulk decided to keep a journal, charting their transplant experiences. This is part of what he wrote back then:

When we arrived at Pittsburgh it was raining—we were immediately met by ambulance and taken to the PUH [Presbyterian-University Hospital]—about a 10 minute trip. Upon arrival, we received priority treatment in the ER. X rays were taken and

Winkle was taken up to the 7th floor for a quick physical,—blood samples were taken and she was shaven from the feet to her chin. We were told that Dr. Hardesty (one of the surgeons) had gone to Miami, Fla., to harvest the organs. The donor (potential) was a man in his early 20's who was a cab driver and had been shot in the head—he was clinically dead but was being kept alive on life support systems.

At approximately 9 P.M., we were told that the surgery was to be scheduled at about midnight.

"When I got there, I phoned my mother to tell her to call everyone on my list and to tell them I was having an operation," said Winkle. "Because now I was ready. There was no longer any doubt in my mind. 'Now I'm ready,' I told her. 'This is what I want.' "

A heavyset black woman came into Winkle's room to wash her. "She was so nice, so friendly, just joking around. She's the one person I can really remember and enjoy because it took away almost any fear that I might have had left."

Not long after, a young man came in to complete a medical history they had started in the emergency room while being admitted. She answered his questions carefully. There weren't that many, he assured her. Before they could finish, another man came into the room, a resident, in blue scrubs and white lab coat. "I need to talk to her," he said.

"I'm almost finished with this history," the young man answered. "Wait a minute."

"No," said the resident, "I need to talk to her now."

He was silent until the young man left the room. "I have some very bad news for you."

"What went through my mind," said Winkle, "was that Dr. Griffith had been in an automobile accident, or that he had suddenly taken sick and couldn't do the operation. I never gave the donor any thought."

But the donor was the problem. Standing and looking down at her in the bed, the resident told Dave and Winkle Fulk that Dr. Hardesty had determined, upon examining the donor at the hospital in Florida, that the lungs were simply not good enough to be used in a heart-lung transplant. Which was entirely true. What the resident did not tell the Fulks—and perhaps did not know himself—was that even if the lungs had been acceptable, they could not have been implanted into Winkle. Somehow, the procurement coordinator in Florida had miscalculated the donor's weight when he had first contacted Pittsburgh. Winkle weighed 127 pounds. The prospective donor was near 200. In either case, a heart-lung transplant was impossible.

"So the resident told us we could leave," said Winkle. "And there I was at 9:30 on a Thursday night in a strange city, Pittsburgh, with no place to go."

> Needless to say, we were very disappointed. Apparently, this has happened before, but this is generally the exception rather than the rule. Winkle spent a long sleepless night since her roommate was in very bad health and kept everyone awake with her constant moaning. I slept on a couch in a small lounge area near Winkle's room.

False alarms, such as the one experienced by Dave and Winkle Fulk, are unfortunate, but not uncommon during the waiting period which, says Virginia O'Brien, "many patients declare is the most difficult period of all."

While Bob Hardesty was jetting to Miami for Winkle Fulk's heart-lung bloc, Shun Iwatsuki of the liver transplant team was en route to Tallahassee, Florida, to retrieve the liver of a boy who had drowned in a boating accident. But later, halfway through the *hepatectomy*, the process of surgically removing the liver from the donor, Iwatsuki hesitated. "This doesn't look right," he said.

Iwatsuki asked the anesthesiologist a couple of pointed questions, then looked up at the Pittsburgh Transplant Foundation coordinator who had accompanied him, Bob Duckworth. "The liver is spoiled," Iwatsuki stated. For some reason, the ventilator and IV fluids had not been maintained during the transfer of the donor from ICU to the operating arena, he concluded. "There's no reason to go any further."

Both procurement teams returned the following morning empty-handed, but Duckworth was accepting. "Foul-ups, of one sort or another, are part of the job, although relatively rare. Something like this happens, usually, about 10 percent of the time."

A few days later, and during the same week that the Fulks had rushed to Pittsburgh, a similar drama involving two women, both Winkle's age, and both, coincidentally, from Florida, was unfolding.

In August, Mary Katherine (Kay) Smith, and her husband Frank, a Chief Petty Officer in the U.S. Navy (retired), had boarded up their house in Blountstown, in central Florida, and moved to Pittsburgh to await Kay's liver transplant. Although Hardesty and Griffith prefer that patients remain at home until an organ becomes available, Starzl often requests that patients whose liver diseases are particularly unstable, such as Kay's Primary Biliary Cirrhosis (PBC), relocate in Pittsburgh, so the transplant team can regularly monitor their condition.

Kay suffers from a complication of liver disease called "varices" which, in elementary terms, are varicose veins (distended) inside the body. As her liver becomes increasingly damaged, thus limiting the supply of blood that can be filtered through it, the blood begins to back up. Because her veins are varicosed, they will begin to leak, and after a while, without warning, she will hemorrhage, or bleed internally. Often, she will be hemorrhaging—bleeding—and not know it, until she becomes weak, and suddenly, near death. She must then receive instant and massive transfusions.

It is an unending circle for Kay Smith. The hemorrhage releases the pressure in her veins, and with the transfusion, the liver then begins to function normally, albeit inefficiently. But sooner or later, the pressure will begin to build up in her veins until the internal bleeding begins once again. Twice over the past nine months, she had almost died because of massive blood loss.

"The problem is that as soon as I get a transfusion, I begin looking real good. My energy is restored. My jaundice goes away. The doctors think I'm better, I'm not so sick. They don't believe my need for a liver is as critical as other patients. When a donor becomes available, maybe I'm passed over. The other part of the problem is that I don't know I'm losing blood until I suddenly keel over. First I'm healthy, and then in the next minute, I'm about ready to die. Someday, maybe, they won't be able to help me in time."

Kay Smith's wait was further exacerbated by her rare blood type "B," shared by only 5 percent of the population. ("AB" is also rare, while the other two blood types, "A" and "O," are very common). Liver transplant surgeons will cross donor-recipient blood types in life and death situations, but since each blood type contains antibodies against opposing blood types, organ tissue becomes sensitized to the blood with which it feeds. Adjusting to other blood types, especially in a body that has been heavily immunosuppressed, can cause a myriad of complications. As long as Kay Smith remained relatively stable, Starzl had determined, the transplant team would hold out for the B. Blood types are not crossed in cardiac transplantation.

The Smiths were living at Family House, a thirty-nine-room outpatient facility used primarily for cancer patients or patients recovering from or waiting for transplant. Located at the foot of Cardiac Hill, Family House opened in late 1983 after a $1.2 million renovation, remodeling and connecting two existing old and vacant Victorian houses—and just in time. Thomas Starzl's arrival in Pittsburgh from Denver, and the sudden success of both the liver and heart transplant program, had exerted an unwieldy burden on the health center, and on the families who, necessarily, accompanied the patients.

Before Family House, most families unable to pay for motel rooms each night, had lived like backpackers, sleeping in patients' rooms, sneaking into empty rooms nearby, curled up in chairs in lounges and waiting rooms or sprawled along the walls in hospital corridors. Local churches had sometimes helped out. Joan Humphrey, a member of the congregation of the First Presbyterian Church in Mt. Lebanon, a suburb of Pittsburgh, formed the organization, "Those Who Wait," a kind of clearing house for Pittsburghers willing to open up homes to transplant families. Also, since 1979, there had been a Ronald McDonald House, initially financed by the Kroc family of McDonald hamburger fame, subsequently operated by the University Health Center. Although Ronald McDonald accepted transplant children and their families, it had been operating at capacity even before Starzl arrived.

Financing for Family House had come primarily from traditional Pittsburgh benefactors: the Richard King Mellon Trust; Frank Fuhrer, a successful local businessman, former owner of the Pittsburgh Triangles, a tennis team; the Pittsburgh Pirates baseball team. The local chapter of the American Cancer Society had also contributed a substantial sum, and its Women's Auxiliary took an active and integral role, pledging to do whatever necessary to preserve the characteristics of the two old houses from which Family House was formed: the stained glass, beamed ceilings, oak bannisters. "This was not going to be a dormitory," said one of the founders, Mary Lou McLaughlin, today director of Family House. "What we wanted for these people was a real home."

Mary Lou McLaughlin explains that at first the women committed themselves to furnishing and decorating the entire facility, estimating that it would cost $50,000. Within the next six months, they sponsored a charity ball, which generated $35,000 profit, and a wine auction, which earned another $15,000. This didn't prove to be nearly enough for the comfortable home-away-from-home they had conceived. To make up the difference, they approached local merchants, labor unions, gardeners, anyone who could donate goods and/or services, and the results of their efforts were very positive. "There wasn't anything that we asked for that we didn't get," says McLaughlin. "In fact, sometimes we got too much. We put out a call for bathroom fixtures and before we knew it, we had ninety-nine extra commodes we had to return."

The Auxiliary also decided to put a price on each and every room in the house—what it would cost to make it perfect, from paint, to carpet, to furnishings—and "sell" them to contributors. The library, for example, would cost $4,500. There would be a plaque on each door, dedicating the room on behalf of the donor. Every single room has a story, says McLaughlin, beginning with the room above the library, 212, in which Kay and Frank Smith were staying.

"The father of a friend was an executive vice president of Corning Glass, and I originally approached her with the idea of getting her father to donate dishes for the Family House kitchen. He agreed to give us ninety-nine complete place settings, but in the meantime we had received three other complete sets of ninety-nine, so everything was left up in the air for a while, as to what, if anything, he would contribute, until the following summer when he came to Pittsburgh for a wedding. I knew that he was going to be in town, and I called him and asked him if he'd like to see the facility, which was, at the time, still being remodeled."

She picked the man up in her car, and as they neared their destination, he noted in passing that he was a former Pittsburgher, that he had grown up in this very neighborhood. And, as they turned down McKee Place, where Family House was located, he said, according to McLaughlin, " 'You know, I was raised right on this street.' And then we pulled up in front of Family House, and he pointed to one of the Victorians, the one on which we had worked hardest to preserve, and he said, 'In fact, this is my house.' And then we came in, and I showed him around and we walked into 212, and he said, 'And this was my room.'

"Later that evening, he called me at home and said, 'I'd like to have my room back now. I'd like to dedicate it to my son, who died a few years ago from cancer. I lived for three months in a hotel in Boston while he was being treated, and if there would have been a Family House there, that's where we would have stayed.' "

Facilities based upon the Family House idea are beginning to spring up at a number of transplant centers across the United States, and even at Papworth in England, where a tiny Victorian house in Papworth Village on the outskirts of Cambridge—25 Irma Street—has just begun to accept waiting and recovering transplant families. Research by Noreen Caine, an administrator in the Papworth transplant program, has demonstrated that a patient will recover just as quickly in such outpatient facilities as in hospital, while costs are significantly (as much as 50 percent) lowered.

The kitchen of Family House, along with the adjoining

TV room in the basement, was funded ($30,000) by Presby's transplant surgeons. Here, residents of Family House can cook their own meals—there are two stoves, two large refrigerators, and two dishwashers, a modicum of cupboard space—and a long bar/counter with high stools. This is also where people will gather to sip coffee, smoke, snack, and talk. There is hardly a moment when there isn't a fresh pot of coffee and at least one transplant-oriented conversation going on, no matter what time, day or night.

It was here, in the Family House kitchen, on Tuesday of Thanksgiving week, that Kay Smith received her first phone call from the liver transplant team. There was a "possible donor," Kay was told. Nothing certain, but all indications were promising, *and,* at long last, it was a B. "Don't go anywhere without your beeper," she was cautioned.

Kay was more relieved than excited. All along she had realized that waiting three, four, even six months was a possibility . . . and after all, waiting wasn't exactly a new experience for her. Hadn't she waited and prayed for Frank when he had served his tour of duty on the aircraft carrier *Saratoga* off the coast of Vietnam? "Of course, this was different," she observed, "not so much because my life is at stake, but because, when Frank was away, there was always a day I could look forward to when he would return." She could put her finger on the month and the date on the calendar, hanging on their kitchen door. But since coming to Pittsburgh, "I had nothing concrete to look forward to, nothing to aim at—only a vague hope that the transplant dream will come true, at least up until now."

Later, back in room 212, Frank said, "Are you really ready for this? Do you really want to go through with it?"

"I am. I have been. How about you?"

"I've been ready," said Frank, and he joked: "If this don't work, I'm going down to the zoo," a reference to the recent Baby Fae transplant, in which the heart of a baboon was placed into an infant child.

"If I find out that's the only way I will be able to live," said Kay, "then I won't turn it down."

Nearly 2,000 miles away, at the Mayo Clinic in Rochester, Minnesota, Mrs. Eva King, of Tampa, Florida, a reservationist for Eastern Airlines, was being told that liver surgery to remove a recently discovered malignancy could not be attempted. The surgeons concluded that the mortality rate of the surgery required to try to deal with the cancer was 80 percent, and consequently, they decided, after a great amount of thought, not to attempt the operation.

"So what recourse do I have now? What are you recommending that I do?"

"They told me," said Eva, 'You go back to Tampa, take some chemotherapy.' "

"Will that cure it?"

"No, chemotherapy will not cure it, but we hope that it will put it in remission and give you a little bit longer to live."

According to Eva's husband, Don King, the idea of a liver transplant was discouraged. It would not work, they told him, and it would cause unnecessary suffering, even to try. In desperation, Don phoned a family friend, a physician, who arranged an emergency evaluation with Thomas Starzl in Pittsburgh—and not a moment too soon. "On the plane to Pittsburgh, Eva was extremely disoriented. She did things that were really out of character for her, especially considering that she was an employee of the airlines. She gave some man on the plane 'hell' for trying to sit down beside her. She said, 'I don't care if he's got this seat or not, he's not sitting down with me. Find another one.' "

Don and Eva King stayed in a nearby motel Monday night, checked into Presbyterian-University Hospital on Tuesday, and sometime during that day, Eva lapsed into a coma because of the ammonia that had been trapped in her system. Eva's liver was clearly failing. Her condition worsened as the hours passed.

Late Wednesday afternoon, Eva King was rolled into the operating room for exploratory surgery. About three hours later, Bud Shaw of the liver transplant team, in his blue surgical gown and blood-stained scrubs, walked into the ICU waiting room and explained to Don King that a liver resection (cutting out the tumor) was not the answer to Eva King's cancer. Her liver was too far gone, and she was deathly ill. Only a transplant would save her life.

On any other day, the possibility of an immediate emergency transplant under such circumstances—the patient was already "opened-up"—would be unlikely ("We don't keep livers in stock, like ketchup or soup," Starzl once told a naive reporter), especially considering Eva's rare blood type, but luckily—miraculously—a B liver, Eva's size and weight was available, Shaw told Don King. It had been slated for someone else, but Eva, because of her deteriorating condition, clearly had the priority.

A month later, from her hospital bed, Eva King confessed that at first, when she had found out how she had gotten the liver that had saved her life, "I was a little reluctant to even speak to Kay, because I felt so bad. The first time I saw her, I could see that her skin and eyes were yellow, and she was not feeling well at all. My daughters told me that Kay and her husband sort of gave them a hard time at Family House about me getting the liver that should have been hers, because she had been here for so long, waiting. But when they found out that I just had a matter of hours to live, they accepted it. I felt very bad that she didn't get her chance to have her liver, but I guess that's life."

Kay Smith, blonde, slender, pretty, with a dazzling smile, and a very gentle and polite traditional southern manner, was the "mother figure" at Family House during that time, even though she was becoming increasingly weakened from her condition. Previously, she always seemed to want to try to comfort people, help new arrivals to get situated and talk out their problems. She had been especially helpful to a tall, fragile seventeen-year-old from Dallas, Texas, Mary Cheatham, who had come to Pittsburgh with her mother, Joanne, and her father, Russell, to undergo an historic heart-liver transplant, Pittsburgh's (and the world's) third attempt at this difficult double transplant. Mary, who had been featured in a *Time* Magazine article focusing upon heroic, high-tech, high-cost surgery, suffered from homozygous familial hypercholesterolemia, a rare genetic illness, in which the liver cannot process fatty cholesterol, which then accumulates in the blood vessels and causes acute heart disease, leading to the eventual destruction of both organs. From the very first day of their arrival, Kay had become kind of an adopted godmother to Mary, helping Joanne console and lift the spirits of her frightened daughter, who, because of her combined heart and liver ailment, had never lived a normal day in her life, never even gone out on a date.

But the false alarm had clearly jolted Kay Smith's confidence and weakened her spirit. "I understand the situation," she said. "Eva was going to die, and I don't wish death on anybody. But I'm getting desperate. I want my liver. I know I'm being selfish, but I can't help wondering: When does it get to be my turn?"

Triage is a term invoked by surgeons in combat or emergency situations in which casualties are categorized to determine efficient use of personnel, supplies, and equipment. Treatment of those patients who will live (temporarily) without therapy of any kind is delayed, while treatment of those patients expected to die, despite therapy, will not be attempted. Maximum resources are consequently directed toward the third category: those patients who will probably survive, if given immediate and concentrated care. Because of the scarcity of donor organs, triage is an obvious necessity of transplant life. Although Kay Smith had been waiting considerably longer, and she would suffer a great deal physically and emotionally without a transplant, she was not at the point of death, as was Eva King. Without the emergency transplant surgery, it is quite possible Eva King would not have lived out the night.

Social worker Donna Rinaldo explains that the system of selection is complicated not only by the scarcity of donor organs, but also, ironically, because of the talent of the liver team—the surgeons and the gastroenterologists—and their experience treating people suffering with end-stage liver disease.

"We have patients who have been on our waiting list for two, three years, who were very sick when they came here, ready to die, but were treated and brought to a more stable position. "Therefore, they don't need a transplant as badly as they did when they first came here. They still need the transplant, don't get me wrong, but it isn't necessarily crucial at that moment. Then we have somebody who might come in today in pretty bad shape, like Eva King, get halfway through the evaluation—and crash. People with liver disease do that. They seesaw. They go up and down real rapidly. There's no way to predict who's going to be able to hold out and who isn't. It's a day-to-day change. I don't know what you do about that.

"Someone who is more stable tends to get pushed aside, even though they could probably get through the surgery and do very well and ideally should be done when they're stable. They often aren't done because of the great needs that we have here. There are just so many doctors, so many hours, so many livers . . ." The ever-increasing number of patients, arriving day and night, sometimes without warning, creates a situation that makes any semblance of planning or organization nearly impossible. "Often it feels like we're a liver factory," Rinaldo says.

Gastroenterologist David Van Thiel is primarily responsible for this "Catch-22": He monitors the sickest of the liver patients, juggling their treatment, extending their lives while also extending their suffering. "It's true, I do this, but if Tom Starzl was not in Pittsburgh, if transplantation was not available to my patients, I don't think I would. There would be no reason to do that to people if we weren't going to transplant them. But if I can keep them alive, just until a donor is discovered, and they can get a transplant, then these people can possibly live and be happy. You have to ask yourself, 'What's the goal?' If the goal is a brand new life, then it is worth a little suffering."

It is much more than a little suffering, however. "It's a very bad time," according to Maureen Avery of Seattle, Washington, whose husband, Terry, suffering from end-stage liver disease, waited four months in Pittsburgh before being transplanted. "Terry couldn't take a shower by himself. He had to sit in the bottom of the shower. He couldn't stand by himself. He was afraid to be alone. He needed that security of knowing there was a normal person around him, someone who could speak up for him if something needed to be done, because he couldn't verbalize what was happening. He couldn't call a nurse to come in and get something for him, or if he called one, by the time they answered, he'd forgotten what he wanted. It scared me to see him in this situation. He would just lay in the hospital bed, in a dream world part of the time. He didn't care what was going on. He didn't have the strength to care. Unless you have someone here to protect you and to look after your best interests, you're lost; forget it.

"You don't live here—whether you are at Family House or anywhere else—you exist here," Maureen Avery continues. "You've left your family, you've left your life at home, and you just sit and wait. You try to make the best of it, though there are times when you just can't do it. You erupt at somebody or go into the shower and scream your lungs out. You have to get your mind off it, you get so sick of hearing 'liver' and 'biopsy' and 'diseases' and 'whatever' and 'beeper,' that darn beeper that never goes off. You get so sick of that, and you can't leave the house without turning that dumb thing on. That really was the worst. Once we got past the evaluation, 'OK, they're going to accept you,' then it was the sitting around and marking time that is so terrible. I wouldn't wish it on my worst enemy."

Months after his successful transplant surgery, Albert Lilly of Scranton, Pennsylvania, whose liver transplant odyssey was documented in a 1985 CBS Reports focusing on transplantation, "The Gift of Life," remains haunted by the agony of the waiting period. "I was told initially at my evaluation that I would have to wait several months for a liver, but then I would come out here every four to six weeks, walk into Starzl's office. He would say, 'You're a blood type A. How you feeling?' I would tell him. Then he would say, 'Don't worry about coming back here again in six weeks. Before that time, we'll have you transplanted.' That went on all the way up until August [nine months after becoming a candidate]. It was the most frustrating thing in the world."

Lilly says that he was often made to feel guilty about wanting a liver so badly. "Every time we would come out here and talk to Starzl about pushing to get an organ, the story would always be, 'Well, you are on the list, but there are more critical people here.' As soon as he says that to you, the first thing you say to yourself is, 'Gee whiz, I don't want somebody else to die so that I can have a liver. I was never feeling that bad.' "

According to Greta Coleman, heart transplant social worker at Presby, patients do not usually allow themselves to regard the organ that will be transplanted into their body as if it were something they are taking from someone who would die without it—or from someone who is living, but who has to die in order for them to live. "They hardly ever deal initially with the fact that someone has to die. They know it, of course, but they don't want to have to think about it. This comes later, after the heart is in their body. But first and foremost, what they want to do is live—and at just about any cost."

Joan Miller, an RN and heart transplant coordinator, who has worked under Shumway at Stanford for nearly fifteen years, observes that the subject of someone having to die in order for the patient to live has been dwelled upon primarily by people unaffected by the transplant, "reporters mostly" but not the recipients, who "have other more important things to think about. For them, it was just terrific to be able to breath again, to lay flat in bed and to feel well all the way out to their fingertips. That's what they wanted to tell somebody. They really hadn't gotten around to thinking about whether or not the heart was theirs—or whose it was before it became theirs."

Patients waiting for heart transplants over a two-year period interviewed by Presby social worker Mary Gibbons, also avoided the "death for life" issue and showed most concern with questions concerning what Gibbons refers to as "the mythologies of transplantation, such as 'You think I'm going to get a woman's heart?' And 'How were they [the donor] sexually?' or 'Will it affect my personality?' " The patients required regular assurance that they would be the "same person" after transplant, except that they would have extended life expectancy.

There is only one well-documented case in which a transplanted organ—a liver—caused the recipient, a thirty-eight-year-old alcoholic male (the transplant took place in 1978, prior to strict evaluation procedures), continuing psychological problems based upon what he described as being "pieced together" with his "new wife [the donor was a female], an alien piece of meat." Referring to his malady as a "Frankenstein Syndrome," the man began wearing earrings that contained engravings of the Virgin Mary. Two years after his surgery, he said that although he and his liver "have grown attached to each other," he did "not feel like an integrated person." He soon began to drink heavily once again, returning to his old alcoholic "binge" patterns, and damaging his liver once again. Not long after, he died.

Gibbons's research reinforces Brian Broznick's observation that hearts have certain spiritual and symbolic meanings that affect patients differently than pancreas, liver, or kidney transplants. Said Gibbons: "One child of a rather fundamentalist Christian family said to her mother, who is a nurse, 'Mom, they teach us that Jesus is in your heart and if they take out your heart, then will the devil get in?' "

By far the most difficult part of the waiting process for the patient, says Greta Coleman, is contending with the fear "that they will die before a donor is found. First, they make up their mind that this, transplantation, is their second chance . . . 'Yes, I'm going to go through with this; I want to live;' they are past the 'Why did this happen to me?' period, past the euphoria of being accepted as a candidate, past the stage of acceptance of their illness. But then comes this fear that they are going to die before a donor is found. 'I've been here for so long,' they often ask, 'did the doctors forget about me?' "

The week before Christmas, Kay Smith learned through the Family House grapevine that two B liver patients had recently been transplanted. The story turned out to be true, but both patients were men, much larger and heavier than she, but for a while, Kay became convinced that Starzl was not being completely straightforward with her, that he was transplanting other people behind her back. "All Starzl and

I have between us is honesty. Now that's gone. What do we have left?"

As her condition continued to deteriorate, she began to consider leaving, although months ago she had concluded beyond a doubt that transplantation at Pittsburgh by Starzl's team was her only real chance. But she was losing her grip.

"If you would only wait a little while longer," a friend at Family House cautioned her as they sat in the kitchen sipping coffee.

"They're great doctors," said Kay. "But I'm a unique case. I'm hung up in the B system. There hasn't been a B that's come along that's fit me for months—except for one. I don't blame them for doing Eva; she needed it. But if anybody else comes in, in a coma, they're also going to do them instead of me. I'm stuck."

"If you would only explain your position to them . . . if you would insist that they listen . . ."

"Then they'll run out and get me a bad one [liver]."

"They won't do that."

"You've got to understand," Kay began to cry. "I had such high hopes, such strong beliefs. And now, this is a failure of my faith. I'm not saying that God promised me, but I believed so much in a second chance . . ."

"But it isn't over yet, Kay."

"Don't you remember me when I came here?" she asks. "I'm a different person now. Even my family [two daughters and a son] can see when they visit I'm a different person than the one who left home."

This is the rhythm of life at Family House or at Presby and Children's: Someone will be very sad, afraid of dying before a donor is found for them. Another will be happy with the announcement that a suitable organ has been located. Others will be confused and punch-drunk because suddenly, after nine months or six months or two years post-transplant, they have had to return to do it all over again. There is also a group of people like Rebecca Treat, who have come for evaluation with great expectations, and then the unusual case like Winkle Fulk, who was summoned to Pittsburgh with the promise of salvation, only to be met with a thundering disappointment.

While transplant patients and their families most often draw strength and practical help from one another, there are drawbacks to being in such close proximity at Family House. According to Thresa Fortner, whose seventeen-year-old son, Mark, is waiting in Pittsburgh for a retransplant less than a year after his first liver graft lapsed into slow and irreversible rejection, it doesn't take long until you are terribly confused and don't know what to think about all the other patients and their particular problems, and how those problems impact on your own situation. "You don't even know how you are supposed to feel about these people, especially if they have the same blood type and body size as your son's." There are always at least two answers to every question:

Do you want your son to get sicker than he is? "No," because then he will be closer to death. And "yes," because the sicker he gets, the more Starzl and the transplant team will concentrate on his particular case. Would you like to see a big automobile accident in front of the hospital, with many fatalities? "No," I don't want to see anyone die. But "yes," if someone dies then maybe my son will live.

Frank Rowe, the heart-lung transplant candidate so insistent with Bartley Griffith during his evaluation, and so enthusiastic about his dream of salvation through transplantation, had also changed significantly over the course of his waiting period, which was to eventually extend through 1985 and 1986 and into 1987. One pessimistic nurse who had talked with him briefly at his evaluation had observed: "He's hopped-up right now with transplant fever. In a few months, he'll 'crash' like all the rest."

Most candidates do crash with the agony of the arduous wait, but not Rowe—or at least not for a very long time. On the contrary, he became very influential and committed to an organization to which he might never qualify for membership: TRIO (Transplant Recipients International Organization), and through the next year of his waiting, he dedicated himself to writing brochures and proposals for foundation funding for TRIO, making speeches at high schools and colleges about transplantation, initiating organ donor awareness drives with the Rotary Club and other civic and religious groups, and presenting papers at conventions, focusing upon the transplant patient's perspective. Organ transplantation became a religion and a "cause celebre" for Frank Rowe. More than any other patient waiting in Pittsburgh for transplantation, Rowe kept himself productive on behalf of transplantation as long as possible, until the effects of his disease, PPH, began to slow him down. A wheelchair became a permanent fixture in his and his wife Joyce's rented house. And as Frank's energy slowly diminished, he found himself slipping gradually into a severe state of depression.

Joyce watched helplessly, as the waiting took its toll on the man she knew to have been so spirited and so committed to transplantation and to life: "The Christmas holiday, our *second* Christmas waiting in Pittsburgh, was awful," said Joyce, "because Frank became convinced it would be his *last* Christmas. He thought he would die before they found a heart-lung for him.

"Frank's family, his parents and his kids [from a previous marriage] came to Pittsburgh the 28th of December. The tension of having all those people around seemed to bother Frank more than it usually does. Frank's not a real gung-ho person where any of the kids—mine or his—are concerned, but he talked to his own kids very little this time, which is unusual. He usually spends more time with them, playing games and doing things with them. That whole week that his parents were there, it was like he was a robot. He remained frozen in front of the TV set most of the time.

"And New Year's Eve was bad. New Year's Eve was real bad. He sat up and drank a whole bottle of champagne by himself, downstairs. He had on one of the New Year's Eve programs, and he just was in such a funk, I mean, he was depressed, talking about, 'What's the use of going on?' I was really worried. He just lost all will. I don't know if it was the significance of the 'end of the year and the new year doesn't look any brighter for me' . . . I don't know what it was . . . but he wouldn't come to bed that night. He just sat in that chair and kept saying, 'Get away from me.'

"The weekend after New Year's was probably the worst. He told me he didn't want to be married anymore, he didn't want the commitment of marriage, he didn't love me anymore, he wanted me to get out. And he carried it further than that— it was not just one of these twenty-four hour deals—it went on for days, and it worried me to the point that I was afraid that Frank was slipping too deep, and I didn't know how—if ever—we were going to get him out of it."

Neither will Frank ever dissolve the image of the pain and emptiness of those holidays because it was a time "when I felt the panic come on 'hot and heavy.' You get knotted up in your gut, as if you have been terrorized by something—I mean, you feel absolute fear. And inexpressible exhaustion. That's how you feel.

"And that night, I felt so tired—I had no more fight left in me. If death was inevitable, then why wait another year? Let's get it over with and let everyone else around me go on with life. Joyce kept coming down to the living room to try to persuade me to come upstairs, and I kept saying, 'Get the hell out of here, go on with life. Why keep associating yourself with a futile situation? Go and be productive and forget about me.' I was almost catatonic—that's how it feels, that's how I felt that night. I sat on that chair, with my feet up on the stool, and with the single exception of lifting my arm to drink the champagne out of the bottle, I did not move for three hours. I was wiped out. I was tired of being so fucking hopeful for myself and for everybody else."

Rowe is extraordinarily appreciative of the support and love he receives from his family and friends, but he feels that their overwhelming dedication during this agonizing waiting period is sometimes more of a hindrance than a help. "Joyce has confessed to me some days that she is trying too hard, overcompensating, which makes life even more difficult, for in my situation and in every other similar situation, the patient carries everybody else.

"When the family is down and sad, I feel guilty that they feel that way, knowing that it is probably due to a situation which I have generated, and the way I get through that guilt is to try to jack everybody up again. In so much as everybody patterns their day after how they perceive Frank feels, everybody will pattern their attitudes based upon what they see Frank doing. If Frank is up, if Frank is talking in terms of future, Frank is back on the track, and then we can all be more comfortable.

"But as the spring of my clock keeps winding down," says Rowe, pausing, lowering his voice down to a whisper, "it gets tougher to respond in this manner, and I guess that led to the worst of all weeks when I seriously began considering the possibility of suicide.

"That incident occurred at the dinner table. There was a big argument because my fuse was real short that day. I just blew up, and everybody hurriedly finished their dinner, except for Joyce. She and I were sitting there, and I got so mentally spent from the tension of that scene, that I was literally sitting there stuporous in my seat at the table. She cleared my plate, and my eyes were fixed on one of the little flower designs on the tablecloth, and I just sat there. Three-quarters of an hour, maybe—an hour, I don't know. I was muttering some things and she was trying to communicate to me, trying to make some sense out of what had just happened. And I said to her, 'Hey, I am too fucking tired to go on. I can't go through this anymore. The time has come to end it, and be done with it—I can't go on. I am going to kill myself.'"

Frank paused. He is quite articulate, an experienced and accomplished public speaker, comfortable in front of large crowds. It has always been easy for him to be candid about himself, if and when he considered it appropriate. "Understand, I wasn't just talking, saying something for effect. I meant it. I was pretty far gone. It wasn't until the next morning that I started to look back on it, my declaration, with a more sensible posture, and I realized that before it was too late, it was time to see a therapist."

Despite Frank's erratic behavior, his periodic hostility toward the family, Frank and Joyce continued to remain close—and committed to one another. "Certainly our relationship has changed," said Joyce. "Sometimes we're more of a parent-child relationship than a husband and wife type of thing. And as time passes, I find myself thinking more and more about how I want this to be over and our lives to be back to normal. I think I am spending less time dreaming about the future, now. We always used to talk about the house we were going to have after the transplant, the things we were going to do after the transplant, the travel. I am now not thinking about them as much, not talking about them. To me, it is getting through every day, just getting through what I have to do, day-to-day, making sure that Frank is comfortable, and trying to anticipate his moods and what he needs."

But Joyce realizes that Frank could not get along without her support. "Not now. I don't think he could. I think that if I left him he would lose all will. But, of course, I don't plan to leave him. As much as I hate him for what he has done to our family—the tension and aggravation—I still love him just as much, maybe even more than before this all started."

Chapter 13

NO MATTER HOW LONG THE NIGHT, THE DAY IS SURE TO FOLLOW*

A contrast between Pittsburgh and many other transplant centers, including Stanford, Papworth, and Addenbrooke's, is not one of effectiveness, but of philosophy. Pittsburgh's approach, especially from the point of view of the liver transplant team, was succinctly summarized by Dr. Shun Iwatsuki, who was heard to say, after interrupting a conference between one young surgeon and a patient during evening rounds: "Save lives first—explain later."

Iwatsuki's brief observation reflects stark reality: Pittsburgh is not only the largest and busiest transplant center in the world, but also the most pressurized. There are fewer attending surgeons, fewer ICU nurses and ICU beds, fewer social workers, fewer facilities and personnel, overall, per patient, than at any other major transplant center, anywhere. What is even more astounding is that Starzl, because of his superior experience, Hardesty and Griffith, because of their willingness to take chances, continue to accept patients into their programs that transplant centers throughout the world categorically reject—many of whom are eventually transplanted. "Sometimes I say to myself, 'This place is going to burst if we take one more patient,' " says Donna Rinaldo, "and then we take five more emergencies, and incredibly, we adjust." The liver

---

* A banner in a ICU waiting area at Children's Hospital.

transplant service will have approximately 100 patients in-hospital at any given time.

The "adjuster" for the liver transplant team, and perhaps the single most important presence other than Thomas Starzl himself, is senior liver transplant coordinator and RN Sandee Staschak, who has been the keeper of the transplant candidate list, and the conscience of the transplant team, ever since Starzl arrived in Pittsburgh in 1981. As the vital link between the patient and the surgeon, beginning with the patient's acceptance as a candidate and forever thereafter, Staschak and her associate coordinator, Vicki Fioravanti (pediatric), endure the waiting with their patients, 300 to 400 times each year.

Most prominent in Staschak's cramped office, the first in a row of offices in the transplant team headquarters at Falk Clinic, is a petite pair of pink ballet slippers hanging from the wall, draped directly above a poster framed in black and chrome from the Louisville Ballet: a pink pointed toe shoe standing elegantly on an upright egg.

Here also are baskets of fruit, bunches of balloons, arrangements of flowers that patients will often send her, a large jar of Tootsie Roll Pops for snacking, photographs of her husband Jeff Chicko, and her infant son, Zachary, a plaque made by one of her patients with "When you wish upon a scar" engraved in needlepoint, a computer, a comfortable visitor's chair with a panda so that her patients "don't feel lonely," and a sign that pretty much sums up the coordinator's attitude and unique perspective ("If you're calm, you simply don't understand the situation").

This room is the centerpoint and the pulse of the action for the liver transplant team. For twelve hours a day, five days (and seven nights; she is always on call at home) a week, Staschak rapidly fields phone calls from doctors, patients, and prospective candidates from throughout the world, people seeking a second chance—"their last chance," says Staschak. The liver transplant team's annual phone bill is estimated at nearly $100,000.

Thomas Starzl will also periodically buzz Staschak on the office intercom to tell her to pick up the phone and monitor one of his many telephone conversations. Later, she will be able to discuss the matter on his behalf during follow-up conversations or remind him what he might have agreed to do— or insisted that he could not do. "No one can think or speak for Starzl," she says. "No one dares. But he relies on me sometimes to remember for him and to point him in the right direction."

As she talks, lighting one Virginia Slim cigarette after another, the liver transplant attending surgeons, Starzl, Bud Shaw, Robert Gordon, Shun Iwatsuki, and Carlos Esquivel, continually interrupt, rushing in with a hurried question about a patient's status or to consult the ever-growing transplant candidate list. The list is computerized and updated with a hard copy printout weekly.

Slender, blonde, and very energetic, Staschak brings to the liver transplant team a great deal of spunk, for she is secure in her position and her relationship with the man she calls "His nibs." With the singular exception of Chief of Surgery, Dr. Henry T. Bahnson, she is perhaps the only person in the medical complex who has not been intimidated by Starzl. "Everybody is afraid of him, but I think he likes it when people talk back to him, because not many people do it."

Staschak is referring particularly to her return to the transplant team after a six-week maternity leave, to which Starzl had grudgingly agreed after an extended period of negotiation. "At first, I demanded six months. He countered by saying that he was only willing to give me two hours to have the baby before I returned for rounds. We worked it out from there."

When she returned from leave, Starzl was surprisingly distant and polite. "He was moping around to the point where I couldn't stand it anymore, especially since for the whole time I had been gone, he'd been calling me every day, telling me that the whole service was falling apart, asking when I would come back. Finally, I stomped into his office and started to scream and yell at him, called him every name in the book. The secretaries out in the hall were new, had been hired during my absence. So they didn't know me. You should have seen their faces. I don't know what they thought."

After about ten minutes of this haranguing, Starzl stood up and put his arm around her. He was smiling. " 'Now,' he told me, 'I feel better, because I know that you're really back.' " She has had a second child since that summer of 1985, and has often threatened to quit and become a full-time mother, but she remains a stalwart and loyal Starzl supporter.

Staschak can explain "the waiting game" from the transplant team's point of view better than anyone, for she is responsible for helping to create the system and making it work.

"Patients ready for transplant now, or who seem to be within a year of transplantation [such as Rebecca Treat], will go on the active list in chronological order, according to when they were evaluated. When there's a donor available, the procurement team will call one of the 'attendings,' usually Starzl or Shun." By "attendings," Staschak means full-time, tenure stream faculty members, as opposed to "fellows," surgeons who have already completed a residency and have come to Pittsburgh for advanced and specialized training, "residents," or "interns." The attendings "will contact me," Staschak continues, "or come in to see me, tell me what's available [the particulars of the liver], and then we look down the list and see who, according to blood type and size, can take that organ. We go through and discuss the possible patients, one-by-one."

There are certain patients who are higher priority than other patients, *"based strictly on medical urgency—who is the sickest—*but, realistically, nobody can be first or second or third on the list because of the many complications posed by the transplant situation. If, for example, we are offered a 10-pound B donor, and you are 100 pound O, then you are not the next person on the list because there's no way we can transplant a 10-pound B liver into a 100-pound patient and have it work. So, consequently, despite what patients might think, there is no first or second or third. Everybody is on the list, and the decision is made based upon the up-to-date facts at the time."

The degree of leeway in size, weight, and blood group depends on the disease and the urgency of the situation. "We will transplant across blood groups as long as the size is approximate, if it's an urgent, urgent case. The size range also depends upon how big the native liver is. We know that some diseases make the liver bigger, while other diseases make the liver smaller. Chronic active hepatitis [Rebecca Treat's diagnosis] shrinks the liver to incredibly small sizes. Primary Biliary Cirrhosis (PBC) [Kay Smith's problem] makes the liver big. So, say you had a woman that is 120 pounds, and she has PBC, she might be able to take a much bigger liver, maybe from a donor of 130 to 140 pounds. Rebecca Treat could take a smaller liver." Over the course of time, the other organs in the body accommodate to the changing size of a diseased liver.

"The height of the donor is also important. If you know that the donor is a male and he weighs 250 pounds and he's 5'6", then you know he is obese; if he's 6'2", then you know that he is taller and thinner. That guides us toward our decision. Right now, it just so happens that we have a few patients waiting in the hospital who are short and fat. But it is body fat [as opposed to muscle]. One lady is 5'4" and 280 pounds. She couldn't take a 200-pound liver, it would never fit because her actual requirement is probably a liver from someone who is 140 to 150 pounds. If she got a liver from a 280-pound donor, we'd need a shoehorn to get it in."

There is little flexibility in the case of donors for infants, according to Staschak's associate, Vicki Fioravanti, pediatric transplant coordinator. "You've got to be pretty much on the button, as far as size, and this makes the situation especially difficult, because we get very few infant donors, maybe four or five a year that are under fifteen pounds. You have to think about it. A kid that is nine, ten, eleven pounds is a newborn and newborns are not playing in the kitchen cabinets, not getting into mischief—they don't have accidents resulting in head injuries. And it is tougher for a doctor, nurse, or procurement person to approach the family of a newborn that is brain dead and say, 'The baby is dead and do you want to donate the organs?' That's extremely hard.

"For me, the hardest part of the job is when I get calls from parents, and they tell me how sick their children are. There's not much we can tell them. We tell them that we're looking and we're doing whatever we can, but it is tough.

There's nothing you can do to speed it up. You wish sometimes you can tell them it's going to be tomorrow, or it is going to be three days from now, but you can't. People call and ask, 'How long is it going to be to find a donor?' But I can't tell them that. I can't see into the future, as much as I would like to be able to do that."

Fioravanti says that during the waiting period "you frequently treat [psychologically] more the parents than the kids. There's a big difference between adult patients and parents of children who are patients. Parents want to know everything, while the adult patients will sit back and say, 'OK, this is what we have to do, and I'll try to be good about it.' The parents need more hand-holding. After all, that's their child lying there, and they can't easily deal with that fact." She remembers one child who would always "try to be real brave because Mom and Dad were having a hard time facing reality. We saw her first in clinic for evaluation, and she was very stoic, but when the social workers got her in a room separate from her parents, she broke down and cried. She was scared to death that she was going to die, but she couldn't let her parents see that because she knew they weren't emotionally stable enough to handle it."

Time and geographic proximity also impact significantly on the decision as to which candidate is selected, says Staschak. "First it depends upon how much time we get in notice from the donor hospital, and when we need to start the surgery. If we have someone on the list waiting in California and the donor is in New York and in unstable condition, that would force the procurement team to leave immediately for the retrieval, which means that it would be virtually impossible to organize the candidates to fly to Pittsburgh, get admitted to the hospital, and prepped for surgery." The liver would be in Pittsburgh, ready for transplantation, long before the patient could arrive from the West Coast. "So," says Staschak, "we have to bring in a local candidate, or someone staying and waiting in the area."

When the patient selected to be transplanted has liver cancer, a back-up patient is also brought in to Pittsburgh. Often when the patient is "opened-up," the surgeons discover that the cancer has spread to other parts of the body. If the back-up patient was not available, a valuable liver would thus have gone to waste. Kay Smith was actually Eva King's back-up candidate, if it had turned out that Eva's situation was not appropriate for surgery.

There are dozens of additional complicating factors. "Some of the surgeons are more proficient at doing harder cases than other surgeons, and if everybody, all 'the big guns' are flat on their back with exhaustion and can't do another case, then that may impact on who gets done. It may be a situation that, for example, may not be appropriate for one of the less experienced surgeons—unless Starzl is available to back him up." Sometimes OR or ICU space is at a premium. If there's nowhere to do the surgery or to treat the patient after surgery, then the liver will be turned down.

To alleviate the waiting period because of a scarcity of facilities, and to accommodate patients from distant parts of the country, a University of Pittsburgh satellite program was recently established at Baylor University Medical Center in Dallas, the nation's third largest hospital, directed by Dr. Goran Klintmalm, a Swedish surgeon who trained under Starzl in Denver and Pittsburgh.

When livers are available in the southern part of the country, or when a liver is available in Pittsburgh but OR or ICU space is not, Staschak will thus arrange for the transplant procedure to be done in Dallas. One of the first Pittsburgh-Dallas operations, for example, began when a procurement team from Pittsburgh headed by Starzl jetted to Halifax, Nova Scotia. The team removed a liver from a small male child and then jetted to Baylor in Dallas where the young patient who had been waiting was prepped for surgery and subsequently operated on by Klintmalm, assisted by Starzl. The entire procedure consumed twenty-eight hours from the time the procurement team departed Pittsburgh to the time the child was rolled into the recovery room. Said Starzl: "If we hadn't had our Texas satellite, the little girl would have died waiting."

Whether the transplant will take place in Dallas or Pittsburgh, the job of setting it up, arranging for operating space, contacting and helping to coordinate patient transportation—whatever it takes to bring the organ, the patient, and the surgical team together—falls exclusively to Staschak and Fioravanti. The process begins as soon as the donor has been confirmed and the procurement team has contacted Starzl, who will phone Sandee, *the keeper of the list,* at home if it is not during working hours, no matter what time of the day or night. Starzl has an uncanny radar system, says Staschak, which beams directly into her house. "He knows exactly what time I fall asleep because that's when he decides to phone me to discuss the candidates on the list."

Although intrusive, this is a significant measure of the confidence that Starzl has in Staschak, for there is no other coordinator at any other major transplant center with similarly awesome responsibilities. Most often, the transplants are coordinated by the procurement office, in conjunction with the surgeons. In Pittsburgh, for the liver transplant service, Staschak shoulders the entire load. The "load" includes the job of getting the patient into Pittsburgh, alive, and in advance of the liver. "So often the patients are in unstable condition and they need a 'Medevac,' an air ambulance with a nurse to keep them alive, or they are coming from some godforsaken place in the middle of nowhere, with only one flight to Pittsburgh with two connections and six hours of waiting. When we need them here for a transplant, we need them here now. So first we charter a plane, and then we find somebody to pay for it."

Neither Thomas Starzl *nor* Sandee Staschak will allow money or insurance company regulations to stand in the way of saving a patient's life. If the situation becomes untenable, the transplant team has been known to disregard Presby's or Children's policy and guarantee air charter payment themselves. "Look," Staschak will say to one of the attending surgeons, "we can't let this little girl die, waiting while someone from some insurance company somewhere in Oklahoma makes up his mind whether to pay $5,000 for her flight."

Staschak and the other transplant coordinators do not mind the harsh and stressful schedule [usually 10 A.M. to 10 P.M.], or even being disturbed in the middle of the night because the disturbance will often symbolize an end to a long period of waiting, not only for their patients, but for themselves, as well. "We are waiting, too," says Staschak, "whether our patients realize it or not, we are waiting with them."

Coordinator Joan Miller of Stanford explains that, over the years, the waiting became so difficult, so painful, that she eliminated it from her job. She only sees patients now after they have been transplanted. "In this business, you deal with a lot of death and dying and it takes its toll over time. I decided that I had to conserve my energy and my sorrow for those patients who died who had already gotten transplants. For the patients who died waiting, I was really sorry. And I was sorry especially that they never had a chance to try, but I had to stop meeting them and becoming involved with them or I knew I would eventually fall apart."

"Patients think that we tend to ignore them, but we don't ignore them," says Staschak. "The frantic level of activity here sometimes prevents us from being more attentive to their particular feelings at any given moment. I don't think they realize that. I don't think they realize that if we tried to deal with all of their aches and pains, all of their emotional problems, that we would be incapacitated by their agony and their grief.

"The burden of having their lives on our shoulders is so overwhelming that we simply refuse to think about it sometimes. But it is with us like an invisible hovering cloud. There are patients that you worry about all weekend; there are patients that you worry about all night long; there are patients that you are thinking about in the shower in the morning, how things must be done, what things must fall into place, in order for a life or lives to be saved."

There have been, however, patients and families in whom she has taken personal and obsessive interest. "There was one woman who touched me because she had no insurance coverage, so she fought the state and won, and I was touched by her tenaciousness; she was not going to let liver disease or the government get in the way of staying alive. Another person is a mother who lost both of her children during transplantation."

Staschak is referring to Judy Cochran of Birmingham, Alabama, whose two-year-old daughter, Kellie, will always be remembered by the transplant team, for she suffered simultaneously from incurable heart disease, cardiomyopathy (a disease of the heart muscle itself) and incurable liver disease. The natural beauty of most of the children on the transplant list is usually decimated by pain and disease by the time they arrive in Pittsburgh, but Kellie, with her deep blue eyes and brilliant irrepressible smile, somehow seemed to remain striking and beautiful despite the ravages of her illnesses, the mustard-colored jaundice and the bloated belly caused by the buildup of poisonous fluid. For more than a year she had weighed under fifteen pounds—and lately she had been losing weight steadily. The itching from the high bilirubin count was so awful, that Judy spent hours each day gently scratching the little girl's body with a hair brush, slowly, patiently, again and again, until Kellie's tender skin was nearly raw from abrasion. Judy observed that her hairbrush "was Kellie's all-time favorite toy," and caressing her daughter with it was the only time Judy knew for sure that Kellie would stop whimpering from the nagging and constant itching.

After being evaluated in Pittsburgh in July 1984, Kellie became a candidate for a heart-liver transplant, the same procedure that Mary Cheatham, Kay Smith's friend from Dallas, now at Family House, would undergo later that winter. At the time that Kellie and Judy Cochran had arrived in Pittsburgh, a heart-liver transplant had only been attempted once before. This had occurred on February 14, 1984, on six-year-old Stormie Jones of Cumby, Texas, who had been suffering from the same genetic disease—homozygous familial hypercholesterolemia—as was Mary Cheatham. Kellie's liver disease was different.

Less than a year before the surgery, Stormie had had a sudden heart attack, and doctors in Dallas, about sixty miles southwest of Cumby, had referred her to Pittsburgh. As in Kellie's case, it was Stormie's (and Mary's) heart that was most fragile, but Stormie's liver, nearly half eaten away at this point, would have probably continued to produce uncontrollable quantities of cholesterol that would soon plug the valves of a heart, if it had been transplanted singly, which was why a double transplant had been necessary.

The evening before Stormie's surgery, Thomas Starzl and Robert Hardesty had departed Pittsburgh on a chartered jet at 5:30 P.M., racing with Brian Broznick to Rochester, New York, where they began removing both the healthy heart and liver of a four-year-old who had been killed in a traffic accident. Meanwhile, Bud Shaw and Henry Bahnson were removing Stormie's diseased organs in Pittsburgh.

At 11:21 P.M., Starzl and Hardesty returned, carrying the precious organs in an Igloo ice chest. They scrambled onto a helicopter and were transported to the Children's Hospital operating room in which Stormie and her surgeons were waiting. The new heart was put in place by 1 A.M., February 14, the new liver an hour later. For a while afterward, Shaw, Starzl, Bahnson, Hardesty, and two dozen other surgeons and medical personnel, monitored the liver, watching carefully until they were certain that it was functioning properly and producing the golden bile required for digestion, before they began sewing the bile ducts, sealing the bleeders, and closing the chest. Stormie Jones was in critical but stable condition sixteen hours after the entire procedure started, as she was wheeled into the recovery room.

Back then, Stormie Jones's history-making surgery and her miraculous recovery—she was skipping around in the playroom at Children's two weeks later, back home in Cumby in two months—turned out to be Thomas Starzl's *pièce de résistance.* Here was a dramatic and heroic act of surgery that received unprecedented and ongoing international attention, unequaled since Barnard's "Miracle at Cape Town," and considerably more spectacular and exhilarating. This was not a middle-aged grocer hanging on for eighteen days and describing himself as a monster: here was a little girl, about to be robbed of her life, suddenly and dramatically saved by procedures heretofore thought to be impossible, appearing on TV, waving and smiling in photos on the front pages of newspapers, worldwide, in the lap of the surgeon who had orchestrated the entire procedure, a quiet and seemingly mild-mannered midwesterner who had often been criticized for his dreams.

Nearly nine months to the day later, however, on November 12, Thomas Starzl failed in his attempt to repeat his triumph, when Kellie Cochran's transplanted heart did not function and could not pump blood to her transplanted liver and to the rest of her body. She died on the operating table after four days of prayer and surgery. The biting irony of the experience overwhelmed Sandee Staschak then, and it continues to overwhelm her today, for Judy and Michael Cochran's eldest daughter, seven-year-old Elizabeth, was also suffering from the exact same incurable liver disease, entropatic biliary hyperplasia [Elizabeth did not have a heart problem, however], a situation that became so serious that Judy was forced to return to Pittsburgh only a few months after Kellie had been buried in Birmingham, to commit her remaining child to liver transplantation, once again the Cochrans' court of last resort.

"Elizabeth was transplanted," said Sandee. "Then she got pneumocystis (a severe strain of pneumonia somewhat common in patients in an immunosuppressed state; pneumocystis is actually the cause of death of many AIDS patients), and she died six weeks later." Staschak paused, looked down at the stack of papers on her desk, and nodded. "I could not imagine having a repeat performance like that; it is out of my realm of thought, how you emotionally deal with something like that. But then, when I spoke to Judy on the phone some months later—I couldn't get up the courage to call her right away—her initial inquiries were about me and my own son, Zach, and she was thrilled to hear that I was pregnant again. Do you know what kind of fortitude that takes? The courage?"

Judy Cochran maintains that she was able to remain courageous because she had no choice as an adult and as the mother of two children she brought into the world, and she credits the transplant team for its continuous and unyielding support. "Whenever I was really down and out," said Judy Cochran, "Sandee and Vicki were always the ones to cheer me up. Right before Kellie was transplanted, I was really depressed, and I went over to the office and I said, 'Sandee, what are we going to do? If we don't get a donor, Kellie's going to die.' Sandee didn't do anything special," said Judy Cochran, because there was nothing special to be done. "But she just kept assuring me, helping me over the frustration, giving me the needed support. She never made me feel like a stupid mother, as others there sometimes did. Sandee comes across to most people at first as kind of distant, 'all business,' but it does not stay that way. When you need her, she is suddenly your friend."

Judy Cochran also relied heavily on Reverend Leslie Reimer, the transplant clergyperson in residence in Pittsburgh, who as a student studying for the ministry and working at the hospital as a volunteer, first came to recognize and appreciate the special needs of the transplant community, radically different from most other patients: "People in limbo, walking a tightrope of hope and despair." Then later, after being ordained, she applied for and received a grant from the Episcopal Diocese to counsel transplant patients exclusively. Now that the grant has run out, she has remained an integral member of the transplant team, appreciative of Presby's generosity, which supplies partial funding. Mary Lou McLaughlin at Family House has arranged for subsidies through local foundations.

"At a time when you are angry and hostile and upset, you need to be able to say what you are feeling," said Judy Cochran. "Leslie made it easy. I remember this one time when Elizabeth had pneumocystis, and Mike was flying in from Birmingham, but he hadn't arrived yet. They had moved her into the ICU that previous night, and all day they were talking about putting her on a ventilator. And I said, 'You mean you can't wait just a few minutes more?' It was real frustrating, but I really knew that Mike wanted to be able to talk with her, and that would have been impossible with the endotracheal tube in her throat.

"But they said that they had to do it now, so I stopped fighting, and Leslie and I went out to the waiting room. And I guess this was the funniest experience of the whole time in Pittsburgh. There we were in the waiting room. Leslie had on her collar. And we were sitting there, and I was so upset, and she said, 'Just say it, whatever you are feeling, just say it, I know you are real frustrated, so say what you need to say.'

"And I started saying 'Shit! Shit! Shit! Shit! Shit!'—and about three people came through the waiting room during that time, and they were looking at me like I was really crazy, sitting there with a priest and carrying on something awful. But Leslie didn't mind. Every time you needed her she was there."

This is the unwritten element of the job for either the clergyperson or the coordinator—the fact that they must be available, day or night, whenever the patients or the transplant team need them. By investing so many hours a day nonstop in their work, however, and by being accessible and available, they are able to share not only the pain, but also the pleasure and exhilaration of the transplant experience. Says Fioravanti: "Sandee will sometimes call me in the middle of the night, wake me up and say, 'We're going to do [transplant] this kid; do you want to call the family?'

"Hell yes, I want to call them."

"One time she asked me, 'It doesn't bother you when I call you and wake you up?'

"You know, I told her, you know very well; that's the fun part, calling a parent and saying, 'I have a donor for your child.' You can hear them panic on the other end. They are about to go crazy. 'Now, take a deep breath and calm down. This is what I want you to do.' "

It is also wonderful to send patients home. "They're excited, and they are also scared," says Fioravanti; "they want to put as much distance between you and themselves as possible, and yet at the same time, they want to hold on to your apron strings and never let go. I feel sad when they leave, especially when they are from way far away, like Ireland or South America, but it is truly rewarding to know that you have helped them with a new start to life."

But patients are not always appreciative, especially as the wait for a donor organ goes on and on; they often become very angry and they will frequently vent their anger on the social worker or most especially the coordinator, rather than the surgeons, with whom they have cast their fate. Staschak tells of one woman, the mother of a teenage son waiting for a transplant, who "blew-up" one day at the outpatient clinic. "She just went crazy, screaming and yelling at me that we were letting her son die. She came back to my office later and apologized, but before she did that she went shopping in a supermarket, got angry at another shopper and punched him.

"Unfortunately, patients can only see their own case, they feel themselves declining on a daily basis, and they always think that they are the sickest person; they can't even imagine that there could possibly be anybody sicker than they are. I myself would probably do the same thing. If I've got ascites [swelling in the abdomen], and I was itching like crazy . . . How can you tell me there is anybody sicker? But in reality, I know we have to take the whole list into consideration.

"What makes you mad, however—it's so terribly frustrating—is when you are trying to help a patient, *trying to help them live a little longer*, and no matter how much they complain and how sick they are, they simply will not take one measure of responsibility for themselves."

Later that day, at the outpatient clinic, Sandee Staschak confronted a yellow-faced woman in her early thirties, in a lightweight denim jacket.

"Where were you on Saturday afternoon?"

"I was in my apartment."

"You were *not* in your apartment. I called you up. There was a liver for you. There was a donor that matched. You keep complaining you've been waiting so long and here, we had a liver in your blood type and size, and I called you in. But you weren't there."

"I went down for a few minutes to the grocery store."

"Why didn't you take your beeper?"

"I was only there a few minutes."

"I called you for an hour . . ."

"I was home. There must have been something wrong with the phone, because I was there."

". . . And then I got the police to dispatch a car, so someone could knock on your door. So I know that you weren't home. We can't help you here unless you cooperate with us," said

Sandee, staring at the woman, nodding vigorously, sighing deeply, tears welling up in her round blue eyes, "So how about it?"

The woman received her liver transplant soon after.

Chapter 14

THE "PATIENT-PIONEER"

Thomas Starzl, in his old wrinkled University of Colorado sweat shirt, smiled at the woman waiting for him in his Falk Clinic office. "You've got to get your son back to Chicago as soon as possible to watch some baseball. The Cubs are hard to beat."

"I plan to do just that, Dr. Starzl. Remember, you promised to release us today."

Starzl nods and smiles warmly. It isn't likely that he would soon forget the woman's fifteen-year-old son, who, before being transplanted, had suffered both from hepatitis and hemophilia "the bleeder's disease," which, because of an inexplicable absence of a substance called "Factor VIII," permitting blood to clot when it touches open air, causes its victims to bleed uncontrollably, sometimes even from small cuts and scratches. The boy had been dying from hepatitis contracted through the course of time from his frequent need for blood transfusions.

Working in his animal laboratory at the University of Colorado two decades ago, transplanting livers into dogs, Starzl had demonstrated that the liver was responsible for producing Factor VIII. Thus, he assumed, a new liver, functioning normally, would immediately eradicate the disease. Back then it was impractical for Starzl to try to prove his point clinically. The operation was hazardous enough for patients who produced an adequate amount of Factor VIII, let alone for someone who could die from blood loss caused by a simple cut. Recently, this boy's condition had provided an ideal opportunity to demonstrate that a new normally functioning liver could cure hemophilia, however.

The boy remained in ICU on the high priority list for no more than a week before the procurement people located a matching liver. The trouble projected by the transplant team in operating on a hemophiliac never materialized. The boy not only survived the procedure, but did so with less than normal blood loss, though more than 200 units had been held in reserve at the blood bank just in case. Two years later, in the winter of 1987, Hardesty and Griffith followed Starzl's lead and became the first surgical team in the world to transplant a heart into a hemophiliac. In this instance, the operation once again went smoothly, with little bleeding. The main difference between the young man who received the liver transplant and the patient who received the heart transplant, also fifteen, is that the heart patient will remain a hemophiliac, while the liver patient (because the liver is responsible for producing Factor VIII) had been cured.

Starzl and his team were not recommending liver transplants as routine treatment for hemophilia, however, because of the obvious risks entailed in the surgery, especially considering the fact that in the majority of situations, hemophilia can be controlled with drugs. "This drastic operation is justified only for end-stage liver disease because of the risks of lifelong immunosuppressive therapy [which requires costly drugs], rejection, infection, and disease recurrence," Starzl and his colleagues wrote, in reporting these findings to the *New England Journal of Medicine*. However, he pointed out that approximately 10,000 people in the United States suffer from severe life-threatening hemophilia, many of whom have livers infected by hepatitis as a result of the frequent blood transfusions they need to remain alive. Starzl estimates that there are approximately fifty patients from this group that would benefit from a liver transplant.

The lives of young people suffering from cystic fibrosis, a hereditary gland disease that causes its victims to produce a thick, sticky mucus that clogs both the lungs and the digestive system and leads, in some cases, to cirrhosis of the liver, were also for the first time in history being extended and/or preserved through liver transplantation in Pittsburgh. Over Christmas 1984, the liver team had transplanted twenty-three-year-old Daryl George who, along with his twin brother Doyle, had been slowly dying from cystic fibrosis since infancy.

Late on the evening of December 21, Daryl's mother, Connie, literally staggered into Family House after a forty-eight-hour vigil in the ICU waiting room at Presbyterian-University Hospital, praying for her son's life. She was exhausted, but glowing with excitement. She told the other residents, lining the counter in the kitchen, sipping coffee and smoking: "Before, the doctors gave him a year to live. Now, with the transplant, they say his troubles might be over. Maybe he can get on with life."

Daryl's recuperation was rapid and trouble-free and, after six months of careful observation, Doyle was also transplanted at Pittsburgh's satellite center in Dallas. Not long after, Hardesty and Griffith had also tried transplantation of the heart and lung to help a dying cystic fibrosis patient, but the recipient lived for less than two months. John Wallwork, a former chief resident at Stanford under Shumway, who today coordinates the heart-lung transplant program at Papworth in England, has had considerably more success with a cystic fibrosis sufferer, who has remained alive for two years after heart-lung transplantation.

One of the most dramatic and creative transplant procedures, dubbed the "domino donor transplant" by Shumway, took place at Johns Hopkins Hospital in Baltimore, when a twenty-eight-year-old man learned firsthand that in the unpredictable field of organ transplantation, one could both give and receive the gift of life. Clinton House, whose lungs had been destroyed by cystic fibrosis, but whose heart had remained functional, was the recipient of a heart-lung transplant in May, 1987, directly followed by a second or "domino" transplant. House's heart was sewn into John Couch, thirty-eight, who was suffering from congestive heart failure. The procedure assuaged the minds of many in the transplant community who have long believed that heart-lung transplants for patients with healthy hearts and defective lungs were wasteful, even though single lung transplants have, up to now, failed to work for extended periods in clinical trials. But with the domino donor theory, at least the good heart was utilized, they reasoned. Others, including John Wallwork, recognize ethical problems in the procedure itself, however.

Wallwork notes uncertainties relating to the long-range health of the heart after being strained by such a destructive disease. Of even more concern are the psychological implications. "The recipient will be able to speak to the donor, and if they [both] do well, that will be great. If they do badly— just supposing the heart-lung recipient lives and the person he gave his heart to dies—how is he going to feel? This is one of the reasons I haven't done it, the hidden emotion in it."

But related ethical problems become evident in the entire idea of using transplant therapy—either liver or heart-lung— for those suffering from cystic fibrosis. For in both cases, transplantation will not cure cystic fibrosis, nor curb its effects on the new lung or liver, which might also, sooner or later, be destroyed. Why waste such a valuable resource on what may well be temporary treatment?

Answers surgeons provide are obvious and sensible, considering the involved circumstances of the transplant story. At this time, it is difficult to predict when and if this—the destruction of the transplanted organ—will happen. And at least the transplant will have bought Daryl and Doyle George and Clinton House more time, during which scientists could develop a lasting cure. This idea is not in conflict with the utilization of transplant surgery for people suffering from incurable diseases such as PPH or liver cancer, or even heart disease. No one can safely predict whether the disease will return, to what extent it will damage the new organ, and how much time—"bonus miles," as Bartley Griffith has put it, the surgery will provide. An interesting and telling reminder of the literal infancy of the transplant field occurred in France a few days before the domino donor transplant, when sixty-seven-year-old Emmanuel Vitra died of heart and respiratory problems after establishing the world record for living with a transplanted extrarenal [heart] organ. Vitra had earned eighteen and a half years worth of bonus miles.

Starzl and his transplant team have also dedicated significant time and effort to the challenge of pancreas transplants with which he and other researchers in the field have been generally unsuccessful. Of the approximately 400 pancreas transplants attempted across the world, half of which have taken place at the University of Minnesota under the direction of Dr. John Najarian, one-year survival rate is only about 30 percent, considerably less than heart, heart-lung, and liver. Transplantation of the pancreas will be the primary objective of the second generation of transplant surgeons and scientists throughout the next decade.

Responding to rare incurable diseases, such as hemophilia or cystic fibrosis, and to unforeseen problems that have suddenly surfaced in real-life clinical situations, was also a primary responsibility of the residents and fellows in the animal lab—this second generation of transplant surgeons. Currently Dr. Stephen Lynch of Australia and Carlos Esquivel, who was soon to replace Bud Shaw as an attending surgeon (Shaw would go to the University of Nebraska to start a liver transplant program), were experimenting with a procedure calling for the transplantation of the entire abdominal area for diseases that infect and subsequently destroy the intestines, and lead to the gradual destruction of the liver, pancreas, spleen, and stomach.

A couple of years before, Starzl, confronted with a child who had lost his intestines in a swimming pool accident, had attempted such an emergency abdominal transplant at Children's, but the child had died soon after surgery, as had all of the dozen or so patients on whom emergency abdominal transplants had been tried since 1964. The longest survivor, a twenty-six-year-old woman at the University of Toronto Medical Center, lasted fourteen days. Recently, Starzl and David Van Thiel had decided that instead of waiting for an emergency abdominal transplant to suddenly surface, they would ask Lynch and Esquivel to prepare themselves, to be ready when and if the situation presented itself again.

Some months later, Van Thiel and Starzl jointly announced that they had in hospital a patient waiting for exactly such a transplant, a thirty-seven-year-old insurance adjuster and former prison guard from Mapleton, Utah, Herbert Glen Seal, who suffered from ulcerative colitis, an erosive inflammation of the colon. In 1981, all but six inches of his intestines had been removed (most people have about twenty-three feet of intestine), and after the operation, he was fed intravenously through most of the night and day thereafter. Van Thiel theorized that the continuous IV feeding over a prolonged period had caused Seal's liver to fail, and that, along with his overall condition, made him a candidate for a multiple-organ transplant—virtually all of the major abdominal organs, except for the kidneys.

There were also a few children being treated at Children's Hospital who might qualify for such a transplant, those suffering from what is known as "short bowel syndrome," an ailment limiting the length of the intestine, thereby prohibiting the absorption of enough nutrients to maintain an adequate nutritional level. As with Seal, children with "short bowel syndrome" must be fed intravenously a highly concentrated mixture of sugar and vitamins that frequently leads to sudden liver failure so extreme that, when diagnosed, the child is left with only a few months to live.

Even if the surgery was more successful than Starzl's and Van Thiel's wildest dreams, however, Seal pretty much knew in advance that he probably would not live for very long. He compared himself to Barney Clark, the Seattle dentist, whose life was sustained for nearly two months with the first permanent Jarvik-7 artificial heart ever implanted into a human. Seal's mother, who continued to operate the seventy-acre fruit farm in Utah, on which Seal had been born and raised, had counseled her son before he had agreed to the surgery.

"He knows his time is limited," she said. "He has a lot of faith that it is going to work. He has lived a good, clean life. He never went out and got drunk or smoked or anything like that. And he wants to be fixed up so that he can go back and live with his family and have a normal life. If he don't make it," she added, "maybe they'll find a new technique that will help someone else."

Seal's comparison between himself and Barney Clark along with his mother's statement seemed to indicate a "do or die" conception of the upcoming experience which, as Clark and his family had quickly discovered, was a simplistic and romanticized vision of the role and the prognosis of the patient in a highly experimental situation.

Fifty-four-year-old Clark lived a little less than four months on the Jarvik-7, and according to his son, although the procedure might have been justified as a contribution to research, the operation was "clearly not worth it," in terms of improving his father's health or quality of life. Clark, and William Schroeder of Jasper, Indiana, who lived 620 days—the longest ever on an artificial heart—were essentially bed-bound and handicapped for as long as they remained alive. Schroeder's experience was especially disconcerting because for the first two weeks after transplant he felt "super" enough to joke and to sip from a can of beer on national TV. He literally delighted the world when, during a congratulatory telephone call from President Reagan, he complained about delays in receiving his social security disability check.

But a few hours after the check was personally delivered by a high-ranking federal official, Schroeder suffered the first of a series of strokes that were to permanently impair his memory and his speech. For the next 600 days in which he remained alive, Schroeder required constant nursing and rehabilitative care. In both Clark's and Schroeder's cases, the results were not what the families and the patients had expected.

What they should have expected is difficult to determine, for these men were pioneers who, as their surgeon William C. DeVries so eloquently expressed at Schroeder's funeral on August 9, 1986, "pushed the seeds of a tree into the ground, knowing he may never live in its shade." What Clark, Schroeder, and the three other recipients of a permanent artificial heart did know was that Jarvik-7 implants had been often successful in laboratory animals over the years. Common belief that animals are easier to keep alive with experimental therapy than humans is untrue, according to Henry T. Bahnson, who has observed that people are not only more intelligent but more durable than animals. If, in the early 1950s, developers of cardiopulmonary bypass (the heart-lung machine) had waited until all of the animals used in experimentation lived for long periods, said Bahnson, they would undoubtedly still be waiting.

Clark and Schroeder also knew that their conditions were so critical that they did not have time to wait for a donor organ to become available for a traditional heart transplant. Without immediate action they would die. Of course, as DeVries had undoubtedly told them, they might die anyway, but at least they would have their chance at life and at enhancing science.

Although at this point Dr. DeVries contends that he plans to continue implanting the Jarvik-7, he is finding it considerably more difficult to interest participants, not only because of the many uncertainties confronted by Clark and Schroeder, but also because people, no matter how ill, are reluctant to consent to a procedure that could make them permanently dependent on a monstrous machine to provide pumping power. "An outing in the country for a patient with a permanent artificial heart," wrote Philip M. Boffey in the *New York Times*, on the first anniversary of Schroeder's implant, "could require a van large enough to transport the machine and a technician to keep running it." DeVries also has a smaller pool of patients to choose from today because of the overall success of heart transplantation. At the time of Clark's and Schroeder's transplant, most centers, with the exception of Pittsburgh, would not accept patients of more than fifty years. By 1987, patients in their sixties were accepted as candidates as a matter of course.

Many heart transplant surgeons are viewing the artificial heart, at least the current primitive versions, as a bridge to extend the life of dying patients until a human heart can be found to be transplanted. But even this compromise application raises a number of perplexing issues, beginning with the fact that the use of the Jarvik-7 as a bridge, will not save additional lives—only different lives, and conceivably not even the lives that should most appropriately be saved. A patient with an artificial heart is in such precarious condition that he will automatically get priority ahead of a waiting candidate, who might otherwise be more appropriate. In other words, a candidate waiting for a heart, who is very ill, but still strong enough to endure the procedure could theoretically get "bumped" by another candidate who had otherwise been too sick to transplant prior to the use of the artificial heart as a bridge. Now the "bridged" candidate is next in line, perhaps at the expense of the patient who had had the priority and who now might not be saved.

The situation is further complicated, according to Dr. De-Vries, by the fact that a patient who has already received an artificial heart "is not as good a candidate for a human donor heart" simply because of the trauma of the repetition of surgery. "The extra surgical procedure involved with bridging increases the risk of post-transplantation infection and other complications, thus making bridge patients less likely to have optimum long-term survival."

Not all surgeons are in agreement. Many, including Bartley Griffith, insist that the implantation of an artificial heart improves the condition of patients waiting for transplant, thus enhancing opportunities for survival. Ethical conflicts related to "bumping" one patient for another, are also nonexistent because the bridge is actually part of the overall transplant procedure. With the exception of DeVries and Jarvik himself, Griffith has become the foremost proponent of the artificial heart in the United States, responsible for more bridge-to-transplant procedures (fourteen as of May 1987) than any other surgeon in the nation. Similarly to DeVries, Griffith dreams of someday implanting permanent artificial hearts in dying patients, thus eliminating the need to bridge and the long wait for a human donor organ.

At a reception sponsored by Presbyterian-University Hospital for the artificial heart transplant team, and the patients, friends, and family members of bridge to transplant recipients, he stated: "As I stand here, I promise you that within ten years we will have a quality [permanent] artificial heart available to help others like you. There are perhaps 35,000 people in the United States alone who could benefit from such a lifesaving device."

Griffith was followed at the podium by George H. Taber, Presby's Chairman of the Board, who quoted Winston Churchill, who, during World War II, while addressing a group of sailors about to confront the enemy, declared: "Never give up. Never, never, ever give up."

This was an undefined but constant credo of patients like Schroeder and Clark, whose sacrifices advanced artificial heart technology, and for Herbert Glen Seal, who was unfortunately unable to help unravel the puzzle and challenge of the abdominal transplant. Seal waited in Pittsburgh for a viable donor for two months while his lungs, kidneys, and liver slowly ceased to function—and he died. But 3-year-old Tabatha Foster today walks in Herbert Glen Seal's footsteps, having received an abdominal transplant in December of 1987, and remaining alive and ever more healthy as the months pass by.

Chapter   15

THAT MAGIC MOMENT

For Kay Smith, the long-awaited call finally came late in February, six months after arriving in Pittsburgh, and although she had hoped and prayed for this, the blessed moment of the transplant ordeal, she experienced confusion and disbelief when it finally happened.

She was shopping at a local "five and dime" with friends from Family House "when a beeper went off. I thought it was theirs, and they thought it was mine."

"It's not mine," said Joanne Cheatham, whose daughter, Mary, would soon be Starzl's third attempt at a rare heart-liver procedure, "it's yours."

"It's yours," said Miriam, whose husband was also a transplant candidate. Miriam and Joanne carried the beepers on behalf of their husband and daughter, respectively. "You have to call."

"But I can't call," said Kay.

Kay wished that her husband Frank had been with her, for he had been guiding her since she had taken ill, and now, even at this significant instant, she felt uncomfortable acting on her own. Inadvertently, she reached for his hand, and when it wasn't there, she suddenly panicked. "But I can't," she repeated.

Miriam grasped the problem almost immediately. "We have to make a call," she said to the clerk at the front desk. She pointed at Kay. "Her beeper went off."

"Beeper? Who's got a beeper?" the clerk said.

"It's hers—she's a transplant patient," Joanne said.

"Oh, really!" said the clerk. "I hear they have a very long waiting list."

Kay dialed the transplant office. Her hands were shaking. "We think we have an organ for you," Vicki Fioravanti told her. Sandee Staschak was on maternity leave at the time.

Kay could hear Starzl in the background. "No, not 'think.' Tell her we've got one. This time it's sure."

"I had wanted so badly to get that phone call," said Kay. "But then, when it finally happened, I was scared, frozen. I just could not move. The phone stuck to my hand."

With help from her friends, Kay returned to Family House to break the news to Frank. Within fifteen minutes, Kay and Frank were heading up Cardiac Hill toward Presbyterian-University Hospital, beaming at one another in the back seat of the taxi.

Later that evening, Joanne Cheatham went to visit Kay Smith on Unit 10–3, a few hours before the surgery was scheduled, accompanied by her daughter, Mary. Because Mary was older, it was thought that she had a considerably better chance to survive the double transplant ordeal than Kellie Cochran, the two-year-old from Birmingham, who had died during the same procedure less than three months before.

Mary, however, was not particularly strong for her age, primarily because she had been sick for as long as she had been alive. She was born with strange fatty yellow deposits on her heels, which doctors initially had labeled as birthmarks. The same deposits soon appeared on her elbows, and subsequently on her hands and feet. Also, she frequently and suddenly lost consciousness, sometimes four or five times a day. Doctors speculated that she was afflicted with epilepsy, but that theory was squashed when, at nine years of age, she suffered a serious heart attack. Joanne saved her daughter's life that day when she administered cardiopulmonary resuscitation (CPR).

The heart attack had actually solved the mystery of Mary's affliction—homozygous familial hypercholesterolemia (identical to Stormie Jones)—because it was at that point that

Joanne began putting together the pieces of the puzzle. She observed that her father, grandfather, and her father-in-law had all died from heart disease, while her husband suffered from serious heart problems. Tests revealed that both Joanne and her husband carried the gene that produced the disorder. While one of the Cheathams four children is completely free of familial hypercholesterolemia, two are inflicted with a mild concentration. As a younger child, Mary had enjoyed swimming and baton twirling, but as her heart grew weaker, she was forced to curtail all strenuous exercise.

Mary was not a stranger to the operating room, however, having undergone three open-heart operations, along with one liver procedure at the University of Denver: Thomas Starzl re-routed the intestinal blood flow around her liver by building a *portacaval shunt*—essentially connecting the portal vein, which conveys blood into the liver, and the inferior vena cava, through which the blood that would normally flow through the liver drains. Although the shunt had significantly reduced her cholesterol level, it still remained about three times above normal. The shunt did not solve the problem; it had bought Mary Cheatham more time. When she arrived in Pittsburgh, however, doctors determined that she had only a few more months to live.

But that evening, all attention was directed toward Kay. "We were so excited for you at Family House," Joanne said to Kay, as soon as she and Mary walked into the room. "Nobody wanted to cook and nobody wanted to eat. We just stood around and watched the food burn."

"I still didn't believe it until the doctors came in," Kay said. On evening rounds, Starzl had told Goran Klintmalm, who was later appointed director of Pittsburgh's satellite unit at Dallas, and who was going to perform the surgery: "Mary Kay Smith is one of the easiest cases you'll ever encounter. She's thin, doesn't have a mark on her [no prior surgery]. It should go well."

Then the nurses introduced Kay to the medication that would keep her alive after transplant, and hopefully, for many years thereafter, cyclosporine. "They put it in an ounce of orange juice, shook it up, and said, 'Here, drink this.' " Later, she observed: "It makes you feel hot inside."

"Nobody at Family House is going to sleep tonight," said Joanne. "People were dancing and holding one another this evening down in the kitchen." She paused, then added: "You had confidence and faith in what they promised you, and now you've gotten what you wanted—a B liver."

"Now my hope is for Mary," said Kay.

"Not now," said Joanne. "First it is time for you."

Mary, a tall, quiet, slender girl, with skin as pale and translucent as tissue, began to cry.

"She's crying for you," said Joanne.

Kay pulled herself up out of bed and walked over to where Mary was sitting to hug her. "Remember what I told you? Just think of all the good times we are all going to have on our boat this coming summer," said Kay, holding the girl in her arms. Kay's voice was soft and soothing. "We'll both be transplanted, we'll be healthy and together, relaxing in the sun."

Sarah, another friend from Family House, whose twenty-seven-year-old daughter, Renee, had received a kidney transplant from Starzl ten years before and now needed a liver transplant, poked her head into the room. "Don't cry. This is the only operation in the world that, when it finally comes, makes everybody happy."

At the outpatient clinic the previous day, Starzl had told Sarah privately that for a while they thought they had found an organ for Renee, but at the last minute the parents of the donor had changed their minds and refused to sign the consent form. Against Starzl's advice, Sarah had decided to tell Renee about how close they had come to a donor, in order to prove to her daughter that Starzl was committed to saving her life. The plan had backfired. Upon learning of the missed opportunity, Renee had begun to kick in her bed and scream, "I'm going to die, I'm going to die!" Renee did die a couple of days later of a heart attack, brought on by liver and kidney failure.

"The one thing that this whole experience has done for

me is to make me appreciate life," said Kay. "Nothing really means anything in the long run, except for good health."

Visiting hours were just about over now. "Kay," said Joanne, "you know what you did for me when we got to Family House? You were my friend. You helped me get settled."

"That wasn't nothing," said Kay.

"Oh, you know it was, and I know it was. We were all alone when we came here, and you helped us."

"We've got to go," Sarah called from the corridor, "to catch the shuttle [bus to Family House]. We'll see you later."

Joanne put her arm around Mary and led her, crying, from the room.

"Goodbye," Kay waved.

"Give 'em Hell." Joanne said.

Chapter 16

TRAGEDY

During the two months that Mary Cheatham had been waiting in Pittsburgh for an appropriate set of organs, surgeons of both the heart and the liver teams had wavered in their determination to attempt the multiple transplant. The other option being considered was to do the transplants separately, beginning with the heart, which was the weakest of the two organs. Stabilized by a healthy heart, a liver transplant could then take place somewhere down the road. The advantages to this approach were numerous.

For one thing, a heart from a separate donor and a liver of compatible size and blood type from a second donor could much more easily be found over a period of weeks or months than simultaneously finding a matching set of organs. Equally important is the fact that although single organ transplantation is a devastating shock to the body, causing gaping wounds and multiple possibilities for infection, the potential problems and dangers inherent in a double-organ transplant in both the thoracic [chest] and abdominal areas are literally countless.

But proponents of the simultaneous heart-liver procedure countered this reasoning by pointing out that Mary, although young, was not particularly strong and/or healthy after suffering the negative effects of her disease for a lifetime—and four major surgeries as well. Under the circumstances, one difficult surgical procedure, although more dangerous initially, might be a better course to follow than subjecting her to two potentially harmful surgical onslaughts.

But in reality, since a heart-liver transplant had only been attempted twice before and only one person had lived, who could actually know the answers to these questions? It was a toss of a coin, one informed speculation versus another. And what about the unpredictable problems caused by rejection? Chances were that with a simultaneous transplant, rejection could be treated similarly. But what would happen if the heart began to reject during those crucial weeks directly following liver transplant surgery, when the body and its immune system are forced to deal with the surgical wound and the dangers of infection? In either scenario, the possibilities of unforeseen complications were too numerous to predict.

But sometimes the most difficult decisions are made even more wrenching and immediate by circumstance, such as in the case of Mary Cheatham, whose heart was increasingly vulnerable to massive cardiac arrest, which could instantly kill her. So, when a pair of organs became available in the matching blood type, but from a twenty-two-year-old male donor approximately three inches and thirty pounds larger than Mary, Starzl pondered the possibility of making an exception and extending regular guidelines in size. (As Sandee Staschak has pointed out, there is a standard ten- to fifteen-pound leeway in adults between donor and recipient.) In the back of his mind was the fact that since the day of Mary's arrival in Pittsburgh, no organs had become available that were any closer to a match than these. Also, no other matching candidates were available at that moment in as critical condition as Mary. This was her long-awaited chance—or was it?

Perhaps no other surgeon alive today has been faced with more life and death on-the-spot decisions than Thomas Starzl. Confronted with the critical nature of transplant surgery and the touch-and-go condition of the patient, there is no time to convene a committee to weigh the issues or punch the positives and negatives into a computer. The well-known sign on President Harry Truman's desk would have been equally appropriate anywhere in Starzl's cluttered office: "The buck stops here."

Starzl chose to use the available organs, and Joanne Cheatham, Mary's mother, who had lived with and cared for her daughter through the agony of a decade of waiting and hoping, watched, as a few hours later, the teenager was rolled into the operating room, giggling with relief because at least the waiting was over. Either way—perhaps she would live and perhaps she would die—but finally, something was being done.

The news that Starzl was going to attempt another heart-liver transplant literally exploded through the medical center. When Mary Cheatham was rolled into the OR at about 9 P.M., in late February, the glass-enclosed observation dome ten feet above the operating table was jammed with surgical fellows, residents, and nurses, equipped with high-powered binoculars and sophisticated 35mm cameras with telephoto lenses.

"This is medical history in the making," said Bjorn "Bo" Erickson of Sweden, "something to never forget."

Since the removal of the recipient's liver is a much longer and more tedious procedure, the liver team, led by Bud Shaw, began approximately five hours prior to the cardiac group, headed by Bahnson. The actual implant would be done nearly simultaneously. Meanwhile, Starzl and Hardesty had gone to retrieve the organs.

The atmosphere up in the dome and down in the OR was "charged" not only because of the historical circumstances of the event, but also because a four-person television crew from the Westinghouse Broadcasting Company, two in the OR and two in the dome, were videotaping the entire procedure for an upcoming documentary—"Second Chance"—focusing on transplantation. This was one of the few times that Presby's PR staff had permitted taping or filming of transplant surgery in the OR, and the first time that members of the crew had ever witnessed surgery, a situation that initially enhanced the circus-like atmosphere.

As the procedure on Mary Cheatham continued throughout the night, however, through the following morning and late into the afternoon, the devastating reality of transplant surgery, stretched to the outer limits of its potential, began to strike home.

As the hours went by, blood spilled, splashed, and squirted everywhere, until red became a dominant color in the room below, and some of the uninitiated observers began to lose both their enthusiasm and perspective. "I knew it would be long," said one member of the TV crew, "and I realized it could get pretty bloody, but I never expected it to be so endlessly gory. I thought they—the surgeons—would never stop cutting and sewing, and Mary would never stop bleeding."

"At times," said a nurse who had observed most of the procedure, "it was hard to decide whether those guys were saving her or sacrificing her."

At the end of the surgical ordeal, eighteen hours later, the prognosis for Mary Cheatham was quite positive. The heart was beating regularly and evenly, while the new liver was "pinking up," a sign that it was receiving an adequate blood supply.

But there was one serious problem developing that stemmed from the original decision to use larger organs. Generally, there is some space in the thoracic cavity to accommodate oversized organs, and it was based upon this space that Starzl and Bahnson had decided to proceed with the surgery. But soon after Mary's wound was sewn up and she was rolled into the recovery room, it became apparent that there wasn't space enough. The combination of normal tissue swelling from surgery and the larger than normal organs caused the heart and liver to press against one another, thus hampering the heart's ability to pump at full capacity. This, in turn, was creating a constant fluctuation of Mary's blood pressure.

Over the next twelve hours, the cardiac team was forced to perform two emergency bedside chest operations to provide more space for the heart to function. Neither attempt worked. Hardesty noted at the time, and Starzl later agreed, that these difficulties probably would have been avoided, if only one of the two organs were oversized, but with both the heart and liver too large, a "vicious" and inescapable "cycle" was triggered. Because the large heart was confined inside the smaller chest, it could not pump enough blood. Blood thus began to back up and engorge the liver, causing the liver to swell and to then press even harder against the heart, further limiting the ability of the heart to beat.

Starzl then directed his team to "resect" or cut off, literally, a portion of the transplanted liver. This was a surgical maneuver that had only been attempted once before in Pittsburgh at that point—ironically on Mary's best friend, Kay Smith, when the B liver that was initially transplanted into her by Goran Klintmalm did not function. After waiting a day, Kay's name had been returned to the transplant list. Under careful treatment and with adequate supplies of blood and medication, a patient without a functioning liver can theoretically be kept alive for a few weeks, but because of the buildup of poisonous ammonia and other toxins, significant and irreparable brain damage can occur in the process. To ease the danger, immediate action was required.

The irony of the situation was double-edged because, after waiting for so many months for an appropriately sized B liver, the liver that Kay next ended up with—the only liver in the entire United States available at that particular moment— came from a 200-pound male donor, and was thus not only "resected" to fit Kay Smith, but turned out to be an A blood type, as well. "After all this time waiting and praying for the B," Frank Smith said. "We could of had an A from the beginning."

(Actually, with the absence of a B, an O liver would have been a more acceptable second choice. O is a universal blood type. Because it does not contain anti-A or anti-B antigens, it can theoretically function in any patient. But transplant surgeons are reluctant to take advantage of the universality of O organs, simply because it is blatantly unfair to O blood type candidates, who could not so easily accept A or B organs. Starzl would have utilized an O at this point though, had it been available.)

Surprisingly, however, Kay made remarkable strides toward recovery with her resected A liver—at least for the first couple of weeks, during which time Starzl was quite optimistic, not only because he had extended and perhaps saved a life that might have slipped through his fingers, but also because, if the resected liver continued to work, then he would have taken one more step toward opening another door, shedding just a little more light into the riddle of liver transplantation. Potentially, it could save the lives of infants suffering and dying because of the dearth of tiny donors. (An adult liver, for example, might be cut down and used for a child in emergency situations.) In fact, the initial success of this procedure on Kay Smith led him toward the decision to provide more space for Mary Cheatham's heart by resecting a portion of her transplanted liver.

Since liver transplantation itself is a speciality in infancy, very little is known about the adaptability of resected livers used for implants, even though the procedure has been attempted in the animal lab for many years. How much of the liver can safely be cut away, and to what extent livers will regenerate in the body, are subjects of open speculation. The heart, which is a hollow muscle composed of four integral chambers, and the lungs, cone-shaped and balloon-like, probably cannot be resected, but kidneys can be trimmed down to a certain extent. Periodically, Starzl would sew two smaller kidneys together so that they functioned as one larger organ, and he would transplant them into an adult.

Kay continued to do well, but at that point for Mary, serious trouble was brewing. Laboratory analysis of the resected piece indicated that the liver had undergone too much damage. A new liver would be required if Mary could be expected to have even a bare chance to survive. And then, compounding the problem, was the discovery that the heart muscle itself was suddenly not working as well as it had upon implantation.

So here was another decision that had to be made—and quickly. Initially, there was the possibility of transplanting a new and smaller liver only, which would have been easier to find, an option toward which Starzl was leaning, but then the failing heart constituted a second serious setback. Thus, the surgeons once again needed a heart-liver set, and the Pittsburgh Transplant Foundation listed Mary Cheatham on its computer.

Meanwhile, at the Druid City Hospital in Tuscaloosa, Alabama, a thirteen-year-old boy died in the Intensive Care Unit after suffering with injuries for nearly a week when a four-wheel drive all-terrain vehicle had turned over on him. This time, the organs were a perfect fit size-wise for Mary Cheatham, but another problem then surfaced during the procurement surgery: the boy's heart had stopped beating nearly a half hour before it was removed and preserved in ice. The heart was subsequently reactivated, but there was no telling how much (if any) damage it had sustained during those thirty minutes.

The organs were rushed back to Pittsburgh where the transplant proceeded, but it was soon unfortunately apparent that the complications were too numerous for a successful result to be achieved. Mary Cheatham, who had received her initial transplant on February 26, a second implant on February 28—the first person in history to undergo a second heart-liver transplant operation—died at 3:36 A.M. on March 1, on the operating table.

Robert Hardesty pointed out that when the heart was first transplanted, it had beat strongly. This was prior to the implantation of the liver. Difficulties surfaced about two and a half hours later, when the liver was sewn in and the mechanical heart-lung machine was disconnected, thus permitting blood to circulate freely through the body. He speculated that the traumatic surgery of the past week may have upset the girl's metabolism, a symptom that would not have shown up until complete blood flow had been restored. Also, potassium levels are often considerably increased by crushing injuries, such as those the donor had sustained. Abnormal quantities of potassium in the blood might interfere with regular heartbeat.

"As I looked down at the heart then [as soon as the liver was put in], I could tell it just wasn't beating properly, and it never was able to support the body's circulation," Hardesty said.

Ross Taylor of the Royal Victoria Infirmary in Newcastle (England) was also in the OR at that time, assisting Shaw and Starzl, Bahnson and Hardesty, when the young girl died. "No one said a word to one another," he said. "We were filled with regret and gloom when we disconnected her. Even after changing clothes in the dressing room, and we all left to go to bed, no one said goodbye or goodnight."

The gloom within the transplant team and at Family House during that period of time deepened even more, when Kay Smith died a few weeks later, after her resected A liver failed and a third liver [another B] was transplanted into her, which would have functioned properly, according to Starzl, had she not, similar in circumstance to the plight of Mary Cheatham, been weakened by three major surgeries within weeks of one another.

"Last time I saw her," said Frank Smith, who had remained by her bedside in the ICU as her system slowly failed, "she had two big old tears in her eyes, and then her heart just stopped beating. I had been watching the monitor and the numbers were down in the twenties then." Kay continued to falter. "But she was conscious right to the end."

The death of both Kay Smith and Mary Cheatham cast a shadow over the liver transplant team and its leader, Thomas Starzl, as hardly any situation had in prior years. Throughout the six-day ordeal, Starzl had functioned at the hospital at his rapidly efficient no-nonsense pace without showing the least bit of wear and tear, but now, with Mary Cheatham dead, Starzl roamed the hospital, grim and unshaven, admittedly and openly depressed, uncharacteristically agreeing to a spontaneous telephone interview with the *Dallas Morning News* in which he said that he would not perform another heart and liver operation "until the collective depression wears off, and maybe not even then. It may be too much at one time," he told the reporter. "We may have just gotten away with a lot with Stormie." But on the other hand, "she [Mary] was getting sicker all the time," Starzl stressed.

But there is little time at a transplant center like Pittsburgh for surgeons to retreat into a corner and lick their wounds, for there are too many people waiting in acute discomfort or in isolation at Family House or at home, balanced on the tightrope between life and death. Not too long afterward, Starzl was able to review the events of the past two months with more perspective.

"It is actually a little harder these days to accept a defeat than it was in the days when defeats were common," he said.

"We are so close to perfection now that if you fail, it is always because of some kind of a screw-up, something that the human capacity should have been able to adjust for on a professional level. So today you are really almost looking for what you did wrong if you fail, whereas in the early days what was going wrong was that the limits of the biologic systems were being reached. That is to say, techniques for controlling rejection were not good enough to save more than 40 percent of the people, but that's no longer the case.

"It would be nice to be young again," he says, "because the fact is, I was able to do better operations fifteen to twenty years ago than I am able today. I was a better surgeon then; I had better eyesight, more strength, undoubtedly better coordination."

Starzl is generally reluctant to discuss the pain he suffers over the loss of his patients. Reverend Leslie Reimer had been in the operating room at Children's Hospital not long after the Mary Cheatham heart-liver attempt, "when they [the liver transplant team] lost a child, and I was able to kind of get Starzl to talk, actually. He actually said a few sentences at one time, at one sitting, about how hard it was to go through what they were going through in the OR. But it was hard for him to speak. It was really sad," she said, "how he squeezed those words out."

Bart Griffith will not bury his feelings about his patients as Thomas Starzl will, but he stresses the necessity of having a strong and sensitive defense system in place. "Surgeons have been described as having selective memories. I don't think that's true. I think we have *repressive* memories. There aren't many patients that you don't remember. We just repress them a little bit.

"To tell you the truth, I remember the bad times much more than the good times, the patients who almost but did not quite make it. Did you meet . . . ?" He names a fourteen-year-old girl, at that time his youngest attempt at heart-lung transplantation, who recovered quickly, was released from the hospital to Family House, and was almost ready to be sent home, when she suddenly became infected, and was rushed back into the unit. "The last time I saw her healthy, she was sitting on the porch at Family House swinging on a swing. She seemed so calm and peaceful." He shrugs. "Now she's gone. It happened—like that."

Facing him on the back wall of the office is a black and white photograph, showing a tall, dignified man garbed in old-fashioned surgical mask and gown, balancing a scalpel lightly in his fingertips, peering down at a patient on an operating table. This is Griffith's grandfather, who was a popular and successful young surgeon at Mercy Hospital, a large Catholic institution in Pittsburgh. An oil painting of this same man thirty years later now hangs in the portrait gallery on the main floor at Presbyterian, where he was subsequently named Chief of Surgery.

"I used to be very much involved in the patient's life and family," he continues. "And that became too difficult. You just can't keep absorbing those blows. You can only extend your personal feelings to people so far. You cannot keep taking it. You burn out. Dr. Bahnson says that if you can't take the heat get out of the kitchen. Well, you can only take so much heat. I learned that lesson as a resident over at Children's, doing cardiac surgery—a very high mortality business. I call it the 'Donald Duck slipper syndrome.' You go around and you see your patients before the operation, and every child, it seems to me, looks just like my kid, and they all have blonde hair and blue eyes, and they all have these little rubber ducks, you know, Donald Duck slippers? You only have to lose a couple of those kids to get a little bit hardened. Makes you a little strange. My family thinks I'm real . . ." He stops, glances at the photographs of his wife and children lined up along his windowsill. "But they know exactly what I'm going through," he says.

"A lot of things happen in this business, and slowly you begin to realize that you can't save everybody; the tools at your disposal are not good enough. So you begin to deal with statistics. Eighty percent, as in the case of heart transplantation. Well I can accept 80 percent. If I can help 80 percent, that's good. I am writing off 20 percent. If you happen to be one of those 20 percent, it's not my fault. I did everything I could to make this program as good as any place in the world so that I can offer you an 80 percent chance.

"I try to be humanistic when I visit the patients and let them know that I do care about them—and I really do—but it's not the same as having a friendship with your patient. I think you have to have a *professional* relationship with a transplant patient—or you are going to be in trouble."

Some people at Presby say that as much as he tries to deny it, as much as he rationalizes and protests, he *does* get involved with patients. He reaches out, comforts, and consoles them, and then, when he loses them, which sometimes happens, he also loses a part of himself.

"When I come into the office in the morning," says heart transplant coordinator Ann Lee, "I never ask if a transplant has taken place, and I never ask how any of our patients are doing. All I have to do is look to Bart. If he is not talking to anybody, and he continues not to talk to anyone as the day progresses, you know that you would rather not hear about what happened."

Heart-lung transplant candidate Frank Rowe had been in Pittsburgh more than a year waiting for an appropriate donor when, one evening, he and Joyce spotted Griffith at the Pittsburgh airport. They stopped to talk. "He [Griffith] said some nonspecific things about being frustrated and depressed," said Rowe. "Not enough things were going right. He didn't have enough organs to go around, and he wanted all of his patients fixed up and home. I think he was going through one of those blue periods that we all go through when things are not going the way we want them to go." Later that evening, when he returned home, Rowe sat down and wrote his surgeon a letter.

"I tried to encourage him to unburden himself of those horrible expectations that physicians place on themselves. That's a vicious Catch-22. Patients expect their doctors to be perfect, and because of that, their doctors expect to be perfect. The patients come to them in very, very helpless states and the doctors say, 'Oh shit, I have to do something about this. Christ, I can't let that person die.' Those two situations feed on each other in a venomous way. I tried to lift some of that burden from his shoulders. 'Just keep doing your best, which is far better than anybody else's best. Just keep at it.'

"Well," said Rowe, "he didn't respond to the letter. But Griffith didn't know me too well then. I think if I wrote him today, he'd answer back."

C h a p t e r 17

IS ENOUGH EVER
ENOUGH?

As a research project, Dr. Joel Frader, a tall, soft-spoken young pediatrician with a master's degree in sociology, has been interviewing parents of ICU patients at Children's Hospital during the time their children are in the unit. He has been extremely affected by his conversations, especially with fathers and mothers of recently transplanted children.

"The families are desperate, at least the ones that get themselves here and park in front of Dr. Starzl's door, and they are not the most informed and don't want to be the most informed folks in the world. They want their kid's life saved, and they don't necessarily want to know how hard that is going to be on them, or on the child. Even if there were someone who had it in his or her mind to try to convince them of how hard it is going to be, it wouldn't be someone they would want to listen to, they are so invested in the lifesaving procedure. And not just the lifesaving part of it," Frader adds.

"Many of them have seen their kids with horrible pruritis who spend all of their days scratching and suffering, and they want to see that end. Liver transplantation—either with life or death—is going to be better than that continuing suffering. Many parents have seen their children waste away.

"So it is not just that they want their kids to live, they want their kids' lives to be better," says Frader. "They know that Pittsburgh is the place where more successful transplantation has been done than anywhere else in the world, and if anybody is going to save them it is going to be 'Saint Starzl.' "

Frader is not the official Bioethicist-in-Residence at Children's, although as an active member of the University Center for Medical Ethics, Frader is considered to be the resident expert on the subject. In fact, it was Frader who was responsible for the packed audience in the auditorium at Children's Hospital one particular winter morning, for a "Grand Rounds" case presentation, subtitled "Limits of Transplantation?"

Frader began the program by reading aloud from the text he had prepared, which sketched in cold, objective medical terminology the tragic story of DK, a two-and-a-half-year-old boy from South America with end-stage liver disease, who had undergone surgery and other procedures in his home country before being brought to Pittsburgh for liver transplantation. At the time of this first transplant," said Frader, "he weighed ten kilograms," about twenty-two pounds.

"On the fourth post-op day, he developed shock from bile peritonitis with gram-negative sepsis," meaning that the membrane that covers the abdominal cavity, the peritoneum, had become seriously inflamed. "Sepsis" indicated that massive contamination and infection had set in, spreading through the bloodstream to the entire body. "He had emergency surgery to close small bowel perforations," Frader said.

"On the sixth day post-transplant, he had bronchoscopy," a tube inserted into the lung, "to remove a left upper lobe foreign body.

"On the eighth day post-transplant, he had surgery for further bowel perforations and peritoneal lavage." Once again, a tube was inserted to both wash and illuminate the abdominal cavity.

"On the thirteenth day post-transplant, the patient had bronchoscopic lavage [lung washing] to identify pneumocystis." This is the particularly destructive strain of pneumonia common to recent organ recipients whose immune system is particularly vulnerable. (Elizabeth Cochran, Kellie's sister, died from pneumocystis.)

"On the seventeenth day post-transplant, hepatic artery occlusion was documented.

"On the twenty-second day, post-transplant, a tracheotomy was performed." This is a surgically created opening into the trachea into which a tube is inserted to establish an airway to sustain breathing when blockage (due to pneumonia) occurs.

"On the fifty-fourth day, the patient was placed on the 'Status 9' list for re-transplant because of multiple abdominal abscesses," an accumulation of pus resulting from a breakdown of tissue, pneumonia, and ongoing sepsis.

"Two months after the first transplant, he developed severe bronchospasm," said Frader, meaning that the tubes that connected the airway to the lungs went into spasm, cutting off all air supply, "became apneic [without respiration] and had a seizure. Shock ensued.

"Three months after the first transplant, the patient went to the OR for a new liver, but the procedure was 'aborted' because the new organ was ischemic. Three days later, the record first notes the parents were frustrated, out of money, and having difficulty finding schooling for the patient's siblings.

"At about 100 days post-transplant, a percutaneous transhepatic cholangiogram [the patient was 're-opened' for X-ray] showed 'bilomas,' " tumors of the bile ducts, "and abscesses. Five days later, the procedure was repeated, with placement of a catheter drain externally. Four days later, this was replaced because of inadvertent removal.

"After 108 days, he had a second transplant done. In two days, the patient developed severe hypertension and bradycardia"—extremely slow heart rate—"with bilateral dilation of the pupils. Seizures ensued. A CT scan showed multiple small cortical [the cortex covers the brain] hemorrhages. Over the next week, he recovered to some response to his mother's voice.

"One week after the second transplant, a biopsy showed rejection, and experimental monoclonal antibody therapy [a very strong nausea-inducing anti-rejection drug, administered intravenously] was begun. His hypertension and neurologic status got worse. Pseudomonas and candida sepsis [very serious bacterial infection] developed. He was intermittently awake. The iliac arteries [in the abdominal area] surrounding the organs were found to be thrombosed," clotted. "A CT scan showed infarction [tissue death] in the left posterior fossa," of the brain, undoubtedly due to a stroke.

"A month after the second transplant, the patient slept through most of his third birthday party. His siblings visited for the first time in months. A social worker noted that finding translators was a problem.

"Five months after the first transplant and one month after the second, a dentist first saw the patient for the "bad teeth" noted on admission and suggested that recurrent sepsis might be related to oral infection. [The Department of] Plastic Surgery saw the patient regarding grafting for abdominal wall defects.

"Two weeks later, the patient had a 'stormy day,' as it was noted in the chart, went into shock—and died."

Frader looked up, quickly folded his papers and then retreated to a seat in the front row of the auditorium, but in the instant of silence that passed between the time Frader departed and discussion of the case began, a kind of a ripple went through the audience. It was not shock, which would be totally uncharacteristic in a medical environment, and certainly not amusement, but more of an inadvertent and instinctive chill, shared by most of the approximately 200 medical students, nurses, physicians, and social workers in attendance that morning. This was not a hostile group, not hostile to Frader at any rate, but it was common knowledge that liver transplantation, with all of the good it has done and all of the attention it has generated for the Pittsburgh medical center, was not particularly popular amongst many of the staff members at Children's Hospital, primarily because of the many situations similar to the one presented by Frader that morning.

Although medical doctors and surgeons are technically colleagues, they differ considerably—the "examiners" or the "wait-and-see-ers" versus the "cutters" or "doers." And the medical professionals involved in pediatrics—doctors, nurses, and social workers included—are one giant step further apart from physicians who deal primarily with adults. This is obviously because infants and children are so fragile, both physically and emotionally, so inexperienced with the realities of life, death, and suffering. Children are not the only patients pediatric professionals must carefully treat. With each child admitted to Children's, dying of liver, heart, or kidney disease, there are usually at least two agonizing, guilt-ridden, helpless adults.

Frader says that one of the most prevalent problems in dealing with the liver transplant team is the families' inability to "affect what is going on in the lives of their children," and most importantly, "to say 'No!' when they feel like there has been enough" treatment.

"I think those sets of concerns come out most dramatically when you see, as in the Grand Rounds, a case where for four months a child suffers in and out of the ICU and parents, estranged not only from the doctors, but from the environment generally, can't speak the language. It takes three months for the social workers to catch on that the family has run out of money, the kids aren't in school because they only speak Spanish, and there is no place for them to be in school. Plus, there is this devastated kid who is just sort of a continuous object of a technological assault.

"Or another case, where the parents, after reluctantly agreeing, because they felt they had no other choice, to a second transplant procedure in a child who had not made a neurological recovery after the first one, saying, 'Listen it has been *x* number of days or weeks since the second one. Our kid still isn't here. She has gone away. She has left us. Enough already,' and having the transplant surgeon turn around and say, 'She is not brain dead. We can't do anything about it.'

"Nobody believes that in medicine anymore," says Frader, "Very few people do. We can stop treatment in hopeless cases. There is considerable latitude in the world of philosophy and in the law to stop treatment when there is no point in treatment. And when [the transplant surgeons are] confronted with that, the response is, 'We can't do that.'

"Those are the things that grab me about the transplantation group. When people [patients] sign themselves up for it, they frequently just don't appreciate that one-third of the time, it is just not going to work. Nobody tells them that there may be kidney failure, along with liver failure, along with brain failure, along with respiratory failure . . . that all this stuff may happen, and the kid may spend three months in the ICU, get three organs, have a gaping wound in the belly with fungus growing out of every possible orifice, and that it may just be torture. I haven't quite gotten my mind around as to how to deal with that."

On the other hand, Frader admits that this one-sided story of the positive aspects of transplantation is not all that the parents are told. The dangers of the procedure and the side effects of the medications are indeed discussed, but he maintains that the possible advantages of liver transplantation are often overly emphasized. The consequences should be similarly hammered home.

"I don't want to have people coming here full of hope, and take a brick bat and hit them over the head and say, 'All of your hopes are ill-founded.' That's not true. One-third of the patients do really well. They go home and their peritonitis is cured, and they return to normal functioning, or something like normal functioning, and maybe the kids will get cancer later on [Frader is referring to the possibility that cyclosporine may be cancer-inducing], but some good times have been bought, and I don't have qualms about that. It is the other two-thirds, who either die or who have incredibly prolonged, miserable, sometimes really tortured courses, sometimes ending in good results—but not always. Those are the ones that bother me," such as in the case of the two-year-old child presented at Grand Rounds.

"Surely by the time the child was irreversibly, neurologically damaged, which was well beyond the point when the family had exhausted its emotional and financial resources, it would have been fair to say: 'We've done all we can. Even if we can save this liver or put in another liver, we are going to have a patient with a persistent vegetative state. There is no meaning in that . . .' "

On the other hand, says transplant fellow Oscar Bronsther, whose father is a pediatrician and who has had experience in pediatric transplantation, there are many counterbalancing ways to compute or measure meaning. "What I was taught in medical school, and the philosophy that is followed here, is that while you have a commitment to all of your patients on the waiting list, you have a special and unique commitment to patients you have operated on, or patients you've transplanted, which is why we will never give up on a patient, and which is why we will offer a critically ill patient a second and, if necessary, a third liver to the exclusion of another patient.

"This issue came up very dramatically and tragically three or four weeks ago. One child, Valerie, a five-month-old, about ten to eleven pounds, had received a liver a few days before, and was doing poorly. We studied her, and it became clear that her hepatic artery had thrombosed [clotted with blood]. There was another child in the ICU at the same time, of approximately the same weight, though a different age, who was critically ill and slipping into a hepatic coma and bleeding, who required a liver immediately, if he was to have any chance of surviving. A liver became available that was suitable for either Valerie or this other child, and the decision was made, without hesitation, that we had a commitment to Valerie to operate on her. She received the new liver, and the other child died the next night.

"This exemplifies the commitment you've made to your patient once you've done the transplant," Bronsther stated. "I think you have to follow that. You can't give up on your patient. You have to be concerned with everybody, but you can't save the entire world. You have to do everything you can to save the patient you've operated on; it's a commitment that you have to keep and have to make, if you are to be fair to yourself and fair to your patients. The boy's [who died] family was upset, but understood the prior commitment to the other child, although I'm sure they probably didn't agree with it on some level."

Starzl's commitment to the lives of his patients, his refusal to capitulate to the specter of death, astounded Ross Taylor of the Royal Victoria Infirmary in Newcastle Upon Tyne during his term of service in Pittsburgh. "Twice so far since I've been here, there have been patients that I thought had no chance at all, nearly no chance at all, and, I think, would have been given up at most places, but they are still alive; I never thought they would have a chance." He mentions one teenager. "When Alan kept bleeding and bleeding and bleeding, Starzl just kept taking him back to the OR time after time after time to make the bleeding stop, and then eventually when it was obvious that the bleeding didn't stop, he decided that the liver was no good, and he arranged for another liver to be put in.

"In any other transplant program I know, they wouldn't have been able to get second livers for these people, so people who've got second livers here would already be statistical failures in other centers. Here they've got a second chance because he's conjured up a second liver, and also he's established that it's not too difficult to do a second liver transplant and even a third one. In kidney transplantation, to transplant a second kidney in the same side as the first kidney is extremely difficult," Taylor said. "Alan went back to the OR seven times, and although he is not completely out of the woods yet, he is getting better."

Although he will fight to the bitter end and beyond for the lives of his patients once he has committed to them, Thomas Starzl is the first to acknowledge that his "success rate with retransplantation is not as good. I can tell you that the chances of living five years after retransplantation is only 40 percent. That's almost half of what it would be with successful primary transplants. And the cost of that 60 percent that failed is prodigious—that's where the $500,000 bills come from, and that's where the terrible suffering and the death occurs. So the cost is very high, I grant you.

"I think, however, that if you told physicians who were genuinely concerned with the humanitarian aspects of practice that they could not go forward with the next and logical step in care, then they would not practice medicine anymore, or they would not be willing to comply. There is no physician who will withdraw care from patients whose brains are alive, and if you force them to do that, they will quit their practice. The Hippocratic Oath and the bond on the individual basis between the doctor and the patient still is the fundamental credo with which medicine is practiced."

Ethicist Arthur Caplan participated in Joel Frader's Grand Rounds case study that morning: "I do feel that there is a certain obligation not to allow abandonment of patients once a commitment has been made. At the same time, in my opinion, there is totally inadequate attention to this question of 'When will we stop?' It's one thing to talk about abandonment, and I realize that that's not going to be an acceptable policy within a program of liver or cardiac transplant, but it's another thing not to raise the question of 'If this happens, and then if this happens, when are we going to be able to think about when to stop . . . ?' "

In the end, despite the heroics of Starzl and his team, the majority of the patients who are expected to die, do die, although, says veteran ICU nurse Ellen McCormick, "we have our miracles—the ones you think are just two feet in the grave and are ready to hop in—and they don't. They make it out, it's incredible."

"We had a shocking thing happen in our ICU recently," said Thomas Starzl. "It was decided by one group of physicians that a case was hopeless—the man was on a ventilator, had been there for six or eight weeks." They wanted to disconnect him. "The other group of physicians were violently opposed to this because the criteria of brain death had not been met. The first group said that they did not want the patient to feel anything, and they wanted, before taking the patient's endotracheal tube out, to obtund [deaden] the patient's consciousness with morphine. The second group said, 'we will not stand for that [the morphine].' " By deadening the patient's consciousness, you also eliminate the possibility of the patient regaining consciousness.

"So the tube was taken out," said Starzl, pausing and smiling. "And the patient woke right up, and said, 'Hi mother!'

"So there you have it," said Starzl. "One group of physicians said 'enough is enough' and the other group said 'enough is not enough.' There was a mistake made, but fortunately the ultimate solution was resistance. But how to *really* know when enough is enough, I can't answer that . . ."

Of course no one person could ever answer such a confoundingly difficult question, but Brian Broznick has pointed out that when the United Network for Organ Sharing (UNOS) was mandated by the Congress to establish a national organ-sharing network, the organization was also expected to submit recommendations in response to such questions as "How much or how many is enough?" All of the difficult dilemmas, including the use of valuable organs for liver cancer patients or for young people suffering from diseases such as cystic fibrosis, for which transplantation is only temporary therapy, are to be confronted by UNOS which, hopefully, will be considerably more successful than the God Squad.

Arthur Caplan also asked Starzl, who was present at a discussion later that same day: "Do you do as good a job getting informed consent [a patient is informed of the hazards of the surgery, and then must consent to it in writing] on retransplant as you did on the primary transplant?"

"With retransplants," Starzl replied, "it is almost never possible with informed consent involving the patient because the patient is on the ventilator and very sick. It's a transaction that takes place between the physicians and the guardians or families."

This transaction between family and physician, with the patient excluded for one reason or another, whether it is for the first transplant or the retransplant, is one of which many patients are resentful, according to social worker Lois K. Christopherson, Mary Burge's predecessor at Stanford University Medical Center. In an article in *Nursing Mirror*, a British nursing journal, she recounts the experience of a recently married man in his early thirties, the father of two children, whose end-stage cardiomyopathy was genetic. His father, grandfather, and two older brothers had all died of the condition before reaching the age of forty.

"Within forty-eight hours of the beginning of the patient's Stanford cardiology workup, however, sharp complaints surfaced from hospital staff members about the patient's general hostility and lack of cooperation. The transplant clinical social worker was asked to meet with the patient and his wife. When asked what the worker might do to help, the patient's response was pleading and direct. 'Please help me get out of here. There are things at home I have to do before I die. Everyone pushed the transplant and tried to assure me it was an easy procedure nowadays. When I told them I didn't want the transplant, I just couldn't handle being in the hospital anymore, they began to say, 'Just go to Stanford cardiology for the workup. They've developed lots of new things that might help you, and they probably won't even mention the transplant.'

" 'I wanted to believe that and I was so tired of being talked at. But it was a dumb mistake. I've known for years, I'd die young. I can't stand hospitals; I can't stand pain. A lot of times I think about killing myself so I can be in control of my own destiny. I'm a good father and husband, and I need to go home and do what's important to me and my family.'

"It was clear as the patient spoke," says Christopherson, "that his wife didn't want him to die and yet that she knew as well as he that his decision was the only one for him. The good intentions of medical personnel who wanted the patient to embrace his 'only chance' for a longer life span, and the residual feeling on the part of a few staff members that the transplant team 'should have tried harder to talk him into the transplant since he was going to die anyway,' ignored the patient's own needs and rights in the decision-making process. When he was given the psychological and medical support he needed to return home in as stable a condition as possible, a sense of calm and self-worth that had not been observed since the onset of severe cardiac failure returned to the patient."

Fortunately, this young father could speak on his own behalf, in the proper setting. But as Caplan and Starzl have both observed, sometimes these critical decisions must be made, on the spot, without patient input—and sometimes these decisions cause great heartache and suffering. Such is the case of twenty-seven-year-old Becky Little, who lay dying at Presbyterian-University Hospital months after an emergency liver transplant was performed to save her life.

Initially, Becky had been scheduled for the resection of a tumor on her liver, but when she was opened and the extent of the cancer was surveyed, a transplant was deemed as the only possibility for long-term survival.

"I knew nothing about it," said Becky, speaking in a faint voice from her hospital bed, periodically coughing and spitting blood and mucus into a stainless steel pan. She is emaciated, in great pain, and lonely. She hasn't seen her children, at home with their father in Ohio, for weeks. "My husband signed the papers and when I woke up in ICU, Dr. Starzl walked by my bed and said, 'Hello Mrs. Little. Did your husband tell you you had a liver transplant?'"

Her husband had not told her. "For a long time, I was shocked. I was angry. I cursed my husband. 'What did you do this to me for?' I kept asking." Unfortunately, Becky had been much too sick at the time of surgery to discuss the many alternatives that might become later apparent. At this time, there are no standard consent forms to cover such an eventuality, but many ethicists are pressing for such consent forms to be made available at transplant centers.

"Two months after the transplant, the cancer reappeared in my hip," Becky said. "I had to have my hip replaced twice. And now I've got it [cancer] in my ribs and I've got it in my lungs. It's hard to say now that I'm not glad I had it [the transplant] done, because otherwise I would have been dead a year ago. It did give me some extra time, and every little bit of time, I guess, helps. Yet, so often I think I would have been better off dead, and that way it would be over with. Sometimes I think that all it's done is prolong the misery. If I would have died because I didn't have a transplant, then I wouldn't have gone through all the pain I'm going through now."

A few months after Becky Little died, signs of cancer reappeared in another woman who had been rushed to Pittsburgh under similar circumstances (for a resection, only to receive an emergency liver transplant without her knowledge). For this patient, after the successful transplant, Starzl had recommended chemotherapy to eradicate remaining signs of the disease, which was effective. But because "chemo" destroys white cells of the blood, maintenance doses of cyclosporine, the anti-rejection drug that also weakens white cells, were automatically reduced. Without cyclosporine, the woman's immune system was no longer held in check, and when she rejected the transplanted liver, she was rushed back to Pittsburgh and retransplanted. (She also contracted pneumocystis.) But the transplant did not work. Not long after, a third liver was transplanted into her, but she was so devastated from the shock of two transplants nearly back-to-back—massive bleeding, infection, that she died soon after.

This was Eva King, the woman from Tampa, Florida, who, in November 1984, had been given the B liver initially promised to Kay Smith, who had similarly succumbed to the shock of surgery after three liver transplants over a period of less than one month.

Chapter 18

RETURN TO PITTSBURGH

Life continued to be difficult for Winkle and Dave Fulk, who returned to Kansas City from Pittsburgh after their November false alarm. "I had some very bad days, blue days, and I was very, very moody, and I had the terrible feeling that they had called Winifred Fulk to Pittsburgh once, so now they were going to cancel out my name. That bothered me, because after that experience, we heard nothing from Pittsburgh.

"Thanksgiving, I was sick all day long. I laid on the couch the entire Thanksgiving Day, feeling very tired, having trouble breathing, maybe feeling very sorry for myself, too, because I had hoped to, when we got the call in November, to be on the road to recovery by Thanksgiving time.

"From that point on," said Winkle, "we kinda did things with more of an urgency. It was very important that we got the tree up ahead of time, and then when Christmas was over, it was very important to get things put away. January came and I worried about getting our taxes done, and I had our taxes done by the 23rd. I really thought that over the holidays I would get called. We thought that that would be the time there would be more accidents, more people dying . . ."

Winkle fell into an involuntary pattern of using the holidays as benchmarks: "First there was going to be the Thanksgiving present (the transplant), the Christmas present (a phone call from Pittsburgh), the New Year's present, that Valentine's present—*a new heart for Valentine's Day,* and it didn't come. And then Dave had had a dream that I would go April 6." They waited. "April 6 came and went, and that was hard. Nothing happened.

"The two years that I had been given to live, according to my doctor, were up in June 1985, so I was getting a little panicky, and when I would lay at night in the bed, you know how normally you can hear your heart beat? I couldn't hear a heartbeat, I heard '*sshhhh, ssshhhhh, sshhhh; sshhh, shhhh, shhhhh.*' This is how bad my heart sounds.

"I was on home oxygen, probably about sixteen hours a day. I'd use it through the night, sometimes twenty-four hours a day. I sat in an easy chair and did handiwork, crocheting, quilting. That was about the size of what I could do. I could get up and walk to the bathroom, or get up and walk to the kitchen. We bought a Cobra phone, so I had a mobile phone, so I could always answer the phone or call for help if I felt I needed it.

"I watched the old re-runs, quiz shows, no soap operas. I never liked the soap operas. And I met with a few friends. But I did not use the time wisely, probably. I did not use it to make any final arrangements. I did not spend time teaching the kids how to carry on, in case I wasn't there. And maybe I should have, but it wasn't in my plan. I figured I would make it. But the thought of dying was always there. You can't escape that thought. Death. But you try to forget about it and to occupy your mind with other things.

"We just waited and we waited," said Winkle, "and we got two more calls on our beeper that were false alarms. The last one we got was May 1. Dave's at work and he's talking to me at home, and while we're talking, the beeper goes off. I said, 'OK, we'll hang up, you'll call Pittsburgh, and I'll wait.' And while I was waiting, I was praying, praying like crazy that it was the call.

"But, it wasn't," said Winkle. "After all that, it was a wrong number."

After her evaluation, Rebecca Treat returned to Fort Campbell, Kentucky, but, "I started to get homesick in February. My husband said, 'Well, maybe you better go and visit your parents.' And I wanted to see my parents before I died, if it was true that I only had a certain amount of time to live." Even at that point, it was very clear to her that her relationship with her husband was on the verge of shattering. "We weren't communicating too well. It just wasn't working out," she said.

Unfortunately, it is entirely possible that the shock of the diagnosis and the stress of the transplant process, which begins with evaluation and can continue indefinitely through a long waiting and recovery period, can become far too much for two people to bear.

This is exactly what seemed to be happening to a former Detroit police officer, Tom Goddard, thirty-two, and his wife—except in reverse of Rebecca Treat's situation. The spouse was not ignoring or avoiding the patient, the patient was avoiding and pushing away the spouse. Cathy Goddard remains haunted by those days and nights, when her husband drew further and further away from her. She says that Tom's isolation began immediately, with the ride home, after the initial transplant evaluation in Pittsburgh in 1983.

"We drove home. I wish we would have flown, but we drove six hours—he must have cried for four hours, and there was nothing I could do. We got home, picked up our son from my parents' house. It was like a big wall had gone up, not so much with Brian [their son], but with me. He didn't want to get close intimately, or even a hug. He was real superficial and sort of fake, 'Goodbye, love you,' and a kiss kind of thing; it had no meaning. I sat down and cried a lot, and yelled a lot, and ignored a lot. I don't know how I would feel in his position, but I think that he robbed me from some time with him. He sat back, almost like a piece of furniture, watching how I interacted with Brian, almost like he was pulling himself out of the picture and watching Brian and I function.

"I tried to talk to him about it: 'What gives you the right, you know, to tell me I am going to mourn less because I see you less?'

"He said, 'Oh, that's not what I'm doing.'

" 'Well, I don't know what you're doing.' "

Tom began to ask her to stay away from home, when he was around. "He'd call me at work, 'Do you have plans tonight?'

" 'Not really.'

" 'Well, why don't you go out?' "

She felt isolated, for she was not the person perceived as being ill or under pressure. And there were few people to whom she could talk honestly, intimately. "I tried a couple of times talking with the family, but it was not quite the same because they don't live with him. It was, 'Poor Tom, poor Tom.' And I had a lot of criticism from people, a lot of flak from my girlfriends, neighbors. One day Tom practically pushed me out of the house, 'Just get out of here, just leave.'

"I said 'Where am I going to go?' It was a weekend. I called my girlfriend up, 'Look, it's real bad here and I'm going to come over for a while.'

"And she said, 'Is Tom OK?'

" 'Yeah, he's OK. I'll be over in about a half hour, forty-five minutes.'

"I got there, you know, and the anger was just building. She had a pot of coffee on, and I said, 'You know, that son of a bitch . . .'

"And she says, 'How dare you? This man is so sick. Don't call him that. How do you know how you'd feel if you went through that?' She wouldn't let me express any of my feelings, and she never knew what happened that morning . . .''

Says Tom Goddard: "I don't know if the proper term is 'lashing out,' but I put a lot of pressure on Cathy during that waiting period, more pressure than she probably should have had to put up with. I'd get angry easier, yet I wouldn't talk about what was going on inside of me; I was kind of afraid to talk about it. I was afraid to talk about the possibility of dying, but that possibility was still eating away at me. I wasn't very communicative, didn't talk hardly at all . . . I'm not as open as I should have been; I keep things in, and that time in our lives was a bad time to keep things in. I would just clam-up and keep my feelings to myself, partially to keep from dwelling on it even more, and I just didn't want to scare her any more than she might have been scared by talking about it.

"The last couple of months were the roughest for both of us. I was becoming more and more nervous as the time went on and more and more scared. I kind of tried to prepare myself for the possibility of not making it through the surgery or the recovery period, the possibility of death. I was trying to prepare myself by doing things so my wife wouldn't be hurt so bad with the loss. I was doing more things away from the house, going out after work, staying out late, 'b.s.-ing' with the guys. I think I was probably drinking a little more, staying away from the house altogether. I think that was another way of reacting to it, saying 'The hell with it, I'm going to do what I want to do; I've put up with enough.' Plus the transplant surgery was pending and I thought, well, I've done everything I can to avoid causing problems, and that didn't seem to help [he still needed the transplant], so why ruin all my fun?"

Rebecca Treat returned to her parents' trailer in Debutante, California, near Sacramento, and for a while felt "pretty good. My mom likes to play bingo, and I can remember going to play bingo with her, but I couldn't concentrate on the numbers; it took me a long time. They would say, 'B-15', and it took me quite a while for the numbers to register in my mind."

In fact, Rebecca's recollections of most of the next few months are vague and hazy at best. "When people tell me about that time, how I looked, what I did, I'm very curious because there is very little that I can remember. Words and images come in and out, but much of it is gray. As time went on, I lost more and more of my perception.

"In April, during Easter, my mom really noticed how yellow I was getting, and she said 'Well, we better go to the VA clinic.' It was the first time I had been there. I wasn't being followed by any doctor at this time—I was waiting until November to come back to Pittsburgh. That's when they thought I might be ready, and I still had the mistaken impression that you could schedule these things. I went to the VA clinic, and we had to wait. We sat there for about three hours in

Triage, waiting for somebody to see us, and at first this doctor walked by, and he turned around and looked at me, and he looked at me like I was a *Martian* or something. I thought, 'Gee what's wrong with him?'

"But I was so tired, that I just kinda slouched there in my chair. Then this other doctor came out and looked at me, and then went back in. And more of these doctors kept poking their heads around the corners to look at me, because, I guess, I was so yellow. Finally, somebody came up to me and took me back and they started running tests on me. They sent me home, but they wanted me to come back the very next day. I came back and they sent me over to the U.C.D. [University of California—Davis] Medical Center that morning. I was put into the Medical Center, and from that time on, I really don't remember too much. I remember people came in—students—to talk to me about my illness, but not much more.

"The first week was fine, I guess, I was able to walk around, but then, I started to lose my balance. For a while, I could walk on my own and things like that, but after a while I couldn't. I'd walk and I would kinda like, tumble over. My hands would shake like crazy when they asked me, on 'rounds' to stick them out. I couldn't go and take a bath or anything; for some reason, I always wanted to take baths, and my mom would have to come and help me with that, lift me up and down, wipe me, because I was so weak.

"My brother was in the military, also; he's over in Germany. His best friend, Dutch Wood, is out of the service now, and he would come and spend all day with me; I can remember him kneeling down and praying for me. I guess I was in a coma, slipping in and out.

"Sometime around the middle of April, my mom says that the doctors came and told me that I would be leaving to go to Pittsburgh, not only because they could take care of me better there, but also because their procurement team was so much more effective, that there was a better chance for me getting a liver there. Meanwhile, I was really spacey. I called my best friend's cousin and told her that I was going to die, but that everything would be OK, just to keep in contact with my mother. My best friend had just gotten engaged;

she was going to be married in May, and she was there at this cousin's house with her fiancé, and I told her the same thing. I guess I was really upsetting people. I don't remember these things. People told me later.

"For a while there was a chance that I would be transplanted at Davis, but I developed peritonitis [an inflammation in the abdominal cavity]; they gave me everything that they knew possible to try and cure it, but they couldn't, so the surgeon didn't want to risk doing the surgery on his own. My husband was still at Fort Campbell at the time," Rebecca adds. "We didn't talk too much; if we did, I don't recall it.

"I do remember something else, though. The day. It was such a beautiful day when they wheeled me out of the hospital to take me to the airport. I remember seeing these beautiful yellow flowers, and I hadn't been out for such a long time, so I asked them, 'Can I sit here for a while before we go?' I wanted to enjoy the weather. They said there was no time.

"I can remember being in the ambulance and getting into the plane; the hospital had hired a Lear jet. We landed for refueling in Lincoln, Nebraska, and it was sunset, and again I wanted to go outside, but they wouldn't let me, but the nurse boosted me up so that I could see the snow, and they left the doors open so I could see it and feel it more clearly. And then we landed in Pittsburgh. I remember there was a lady driving the ambulance, and she and my mother were screaming and laughing at all the potholes, but I don't remember arriving at the hospital.

"My mother says that she could hear me yelling from the ER in the hospital, 'Mom! Mom!' right after we got in. I remember at the time thinking how people were talking backwards and walking backwards. But I was losing my grip. Reality was going. The world went black."

Because of the November false alarm, Bartley Griffith's office contacted Dave Fulk at work on May 2, 1985, rather than phoning Winkle at home. And then Dave called Winkle to ask: "Do you want to go to Pittsburgh?"

After all of that frightening anxiety she had endured through the previous nine months, Winkle was surprisingly calm. "Sure, I'm just waking up."

"But, this is only a 50–50 chance," Dave warned her. "They stressed that there was only a 50–50 chance that the organs would be good enough to be transplanted," Dave said.

"We'll take it."

"They called Dave at 1:35 [she is checking her journal], and at 1:40 he called me, and at 1:41 he called the airlines. And then we got a call from Griffith around 2:30, who told us that we might as well come, but we sat around a while waiting. What we were trying to do was gather all the bills and get them paid, get as many notes as we could get written."

Finally, they left the house and followed the same route to the airport that they had traveled in November. "I was much more relaxed this time because I came with the attitude that at least I knew they still had my name on the list, at least they were still looking out for me." She had vowed to herself that, "I wasn't going to let them disappoint me. I wasn't counting on the transplant. If I had it fine, and if I didn't, fine, too. At least they'd see me again and see if I had gotten any worse.

"One thought on the plane coming out was that we have a fifteen-year-old daughter, going on sixteen. Typical teenager. And when I left, I put my arms around her and kissed her. And she said, 'I love you.' And that really touched me. And on the way out, I said to Dave, 'If I don't get the transplant, it was worth it, just to get that closeness back—because we were losing it. She has been doing a lot of housework because I've been sick, and I'm sure she resents the fact that I'm sick. Typical reaction. And I was very touched just by that goodbye with her.'

"When we got to Pittsburgh, they took the blood, gave the X-ray. They put me in a room downstairs near the OR, which they had not done before. They made me wash with Betadine, scrub down. But I'm still skeptical, very skeptical. They're not going to disappoint me a second time," Winkle repeated to herself, again and again. "This time I'm ready for them.

"Then they took me to the operating room, rolled me in, put me on this little tiny narrow table. And they had a little plate on the right for this arm and a little plate on the left for this arm." They sort of strapped her down. "But they haven't shaved me yet, so I know they're not going to do this operation, at least until they shave me. And they are playing the radio and waiting. We're wasting so much time, we were just laying there waiting, and I was getting so uncomfortable.

"I was not afraid. It's amazing, but I was not afraid because I knew, 'They're not doing this. They're not going to do it.' Then one guy standing there says, 'Don't roll off the table.' "

The lights were very bright, and she was looking up into them, attempting unsuccessfully to see what this voice, this man, looked like. "And we're just making conversation. Passing the time. And I told him that I had been here before, almost. I knew of another person who had been on the operating table that they had not done. But I kept asking, 'Have you heard anything about Hardesty and the donor?'

"And then after a while, I recall the guy saying, 'Well we're going to let you breathe into this mask for a while. And that was it. I went under. But I still didn't believe that it was going to happen because they still hadn't shaved me. [She was shaved just prior to the first incision, after she had been anesthetized.] And then I vaguely recall somebody saying at about midnight—at least I thought it was midnight—that they would start."

PART V

THE PROCEDURE

Chapter 19

THE CULT

Oscar Bronsther, a tall, heavyset, balding young surgeon of thirty-one, was one of the few surgical fellows able to maintain some humorous perspective on the drama and tension constantly unfolding within Pittsburgh's liver transplant program and the members of the transplant team, driven to exhaustion by its leader, Thomas Starzl.

Bronsther, who majored in philosophy as an undergraduate and learned kidney transplantation at Downstate University Medical Center in New York, first studied in Pittsburgh under Starzl in 1984 and 1985, in preparation for establishing his own liver transplant program at the University of San Diego Medical Center. But before actually attempting a liver transplant on his own in 1986, he returned to Pittsburgh and Thomas Starzl for one final refresher course.

"When I got back here, I felt as though I had never left," Bronsther said. "I walked into the surgeons' lounge, and there was one of the fellows, Wallis, lying there, in the middle of the afternoon, exhausted after coming out of all-night surgery, fast sleep on the couch. Six other people were milling around, having been in and out of the operating room and it was like, instead of being gone for six months, it was like being out of town for a weekend."

He changed from his street clothes to the traditional blue hospital scrubs, donned cap and mask, and walked into operating room #6 with the observation dome overhead, in which most of the liver transplants are done. "Starzl was doing the case, and he welcomed me 'warmly,' by immediately reestablishing the ground rules," said Bronsther. "In a friendly, kidding way," Starzl went through the pertinent details pertaining to all of Bronsther's former Pittsburgh patients ("even I hadn't remembered all of them"), and then reminded Bronsther of "everything I had done wrong the year I was here, just to let me know he hadn't forgotten." Bronsther shrugged and laughed at this greeting, so typical of Thomas Starzl. At least, "he still knew who I was." Bronsther said that Pittsburgh was "still a crazy place, even more hectic than it was when I left. The pace seems to be overburdening the system. There are patients spread out everywhere."

There were also more surgical fellows (approximately a dozen) than ever before, not to mention a constant stream of visiting surgeons. Starzl has trained more than 250 surgeons from the United States and from approximately three dozen countries over the past six years (including Hungary, Rumania, the People's Republic of China, Germany, India, Thailand, Taiwan, Japan, Israel, Egypt, Brazil). Selection of surgical fellows, who commit themselves to one to three years in Pittsburgh, is based upon traditional standards, such as academic accomplishment, previous grants and awards, as well as personal recommendations. A key requirement is surgical experience. A candidate for fellowship should have served from three to six years in one or more surgical residencies before being seriously considered for training in liver transplantation.

While surgical fellowships in Pittsburgh's transplant program are quite competitive, Starzl, anxious to see his transplant techniques spread worldwide, will welcome an unlimited cadre of experienced visitors for various time periods. A significant distinction between fellows and visitors is that fellows are paid by Pittsburgh (they receive approximately $2,500 per month), while visitors are supported either by their home institutions or have generated some other form of outside support.

Both visitors and fellows alike seem to be as compulsive as Starzl when it comes to liver transplantation. "When you get involved in 250 liver transplants a year, it becomes almost a cult," said Bronsther. "You live and breathe and eat liver transplants. It's what you discuss, what you dream about, what you think about; it's what you are doing. It totally dictates every aspect of your life, particularly during your training."

But for many surgeons, even after their formal training, the pressurized lifestyle of the transplant surgeon and the psychological rewards that their work and sacrifice provide, are often difficult to abandon, according to Dr. Douglas Martin, an anesthesiologist who has worked regularly with both of Pittsburgh's transplant teams since the inception of the programs. "I call this 'post fellowship syndrome.' Once you have finished your fellowship and are finally done with your medical training, you are so used to spending every other night in the hospital, so used to being so deprived and having such a minimal amount of nonmedical gratification, that you really find yourself at a fork in the road. Now you are rested. You have time. You have money, usually. And you have other alternatives—such as reacquainting yourself with your wife, kids, raising your children, establishing friendships in the neighborhood or whatever other nonmedical environments you choose to avail yourself of."

But transplantation, especially liver transplantation, is not only satisfying and all-consuming, it is "the cutting edge, the 'formula one' of surgery," according to Oscar Bronsther. "It's very demanding. There's hardly any other surgery, with the possible exception of heart transplants, that is really analogous in terms of it being life and death. Other operations have to be done in a lifesaving situation, but they aren't as complex and involved as liver transplantation. It's also rare to be operating on somebody with so many pre-existing problems . . . the healthiest patient who requires liver transplant is in a total one-system failure—their liver doesn't work, which means as a baseline, they are *very* ill. Liver transplantation is the most difficult of other difficult kinds of surgery because, if for no other reason, it is such a long and tedious procedure. The average case demands somewhere between eight and sixteen to eighteen hours, non-stop."

Although the cardiac team led by Hardesty and Griffith is

a much smaller and less visible operation, it too has its devoted disciples, beginning with chief resident Dale Payne, who describes a "feeling of adrenalin in your body in an operating room and in a life or death situation, which is somewhat addicting. You enjoy that sensation after a while," says Payne, "and you look forward to the excitement associated with operating."

Payne, a very mild-mannered, soft-spoken native of Ohio, shares with Pittsburgh's liver transplant fellows their enthusiasm and motivation, while at the same time managing to be candid and realistic about his personal goals and his chosen profession. "I have often thought about why people go into medicine. A lot of people say that they want to help people get over disease, and I think that that is a noble idea and that most of us have ideas like that, giving people the best opportunity to have a good productive life.

"But there are other things involved that have to do with your life and what you want to accomplish and how important you want to feel and the type of lifestyle you want to lead. Even though transplantation surgery is time consuming, it gives you a necessary excitement, where you enjoy coming into the hospital for long hours, everyday. It *becomes* your lifestyle. It makes you feel personally important, in the forefront of medicine. To be there makes all the time and all the effort and all the years worthwhile.

"It's like walking on the moon," says Payne. "DeVries [William] will always be known as the first person to put in an artificial heart, and that's just as important as being the first man to walk on the moon. All of us are latent astronauts. All of us would have liked to walk in outer space, but if you can't do that then you do the next best thing on earth, and to me that's a transplant surgeon."

Payne and his superior, Bartley Griffith, are the same age—thirty-six—and have devoted a good part of their professional lives to medical training and practice in Pittsburgh. Bronsther is only a few years younger, and was in Pittsburgh for a comparatively short time, but "the imprint from the months here feels a lot stronger than the other years [seven years of training] I've had." When he returned to San Diego, he experienced considerable difficulty adjusting to a less-pressured, less trans-plant-oriented way of life. "I had to realize that the rest of the world is not Pittsburgh, and the rest of the world isn't committed to transplantation, and the rest of the world doesn't understand the pressures you really or artificially put yourself under."

Most of the fellows are more than capable of assisting in liver transplant surgery, but in a place as frantic and frenzied as Pittsburgh, with transplant surgery liable to begin at any time, day or night, and to extend anywhere from ten to twenty-four hours, having the honor and opportunity of being part of the team is often based upon the fellow's ability to make himself visible and available at the exact point at which the surgical team is selected.

A visiting surgeon from Germany, in Pittsburgh for a limited period of time, his efforts to scrub with the esteemed Thomas Starzl constantly thwarted, once asked Oscar Bronsther how it was that the transplant surgical teams were formed so quickly. Bronsther paused and shook his head in an exaggerated manner, cracking a bare hint of a smile. "It's a mystical experience."

Months later, Bronsther laughed when reminded of his comment to the confused and frustrated German surgeon, but he also maintained that there was a certain truth in his observation. "People just appear and things just sort of happen. The word just somehow or other gets out [that a transplant is being done], so that all of a sudden thirty people will converge in the OR to watch the case or to pitch in and help."

The surgical fellows attribute the ultimate in "mystical" powers to their mentor, Thomas Starzl, who, says Bronsther, has an uncanny ability to sense trouble anywhere in the hospital and follow his nose to it. "Invariably at three in the morning, when everything is turning to shit, and you don't know which end is up, Starzl appears. Just when you don't want to see him, in the middle of the night, and there he is, 'Hi Oscar, what's happening?' "

Starzl also seems to magically emerge from nowhere whenever one of the surgical fellows attempts to take some needed time off, no matter how many hours or how hard they might have worked previously. "It was amazing," says Tom Lennard of the Royal Victoria Infirmary in Newcastle Upon Tyne, England. "I was going to attempt to take two afternoons off when I was in Pittsburgh. For the whole time, just two afternoons off," he laughed. "The first Saturday, around lunchtime, I thought, 'Well, I've been up all night, so I will go down to the town and buy myself a local newspaper, and I will post a letter to my wife.'

"So I set off walking down towards Oakland," the area in which Pitt, Presby, and Children's are located. "I hadn't been out of the hospital or the theatre [the British term for the OR] since I had arrived just about, and who should I meet walking up the street?—I had not gone ten yards—but Starzl. And he says to me," in his maddeningly soft voice and typically polite manner, " 'What are you doing out here, Tom?' "

"And I said, 'Oh, Dr. Starzl, I am going down to buy myself a newspaper.'

"He says, 'There's a case [a transplant] on in two hours.' You know that, don't you?'

"I said, 'No, I didn't know that, Dr. Starzl.'

"He said, 'There's a case on this afternoon. You be sure to be there.' That was my Saturday afternoon—gone.

"The second occasion was equally amazing. I went to Boston for a day to look at some machinery in relation to liver transplant. I had to get up real early—5 A.M.—to get the limousine out to the airport to get the flight to Boston, and I had been up most of the night before. And I got back at 9:00 P.M. from Boston, and I was exhausted. I had to give a talk in Boston at the same time, and I was absolutely shattered, and I said to myself, 'Tonight I am not going on a procurement or watch a liver transplant. I am going to go to my bed and go to sleep for twelve hours.' I was standing outside the elevator to go up to my room, and what happens? Dr. Starzl walks by, and he says—There were three or four girls standing there with me—and he says, 'How do you get to be with all those pretty girls waiting for that elevator, Tom?'

"And I said, 'Oh, good evening, Dr. Starzl.'

"And he said, 'What are you doing here?'

"And I said, 'Well I am going up to my room.'
"He said, 'Do you know there is a case on this evening?'
"And I said, 'No, Dr. Starzl, I didn't know.'
" 'Be sure to be there, now.' So," said Lennard, "I went.
"In all the time I was there, I had only half a day off."

Unless they are nearing total collapse, which is not uncommon, the surgical fellows who participate in most of the cases go to great lengths to be included as part of the team. "The smart people who want to know what is going on hang out at Starzl's office," says Oscar Bronsther. "Ultimately, pertinent information about an upcoming transplant will work its way from one cubicle in that office, back and forth. If you hang around long enough, you usually can find out about anything. One of the things also that you can do [to keep abreast of things] before you go to bed or as soon as you get up, is to check in with the OR because they, more than anybody, will know when and what the cases are that're coming."

Jill West, thirty-two, is an RN who scrubbed for Starzl's very first case in 1981. Now, nearly a half dozen years later, she considers the fellows' constant inquiries about transplants a wearisome pain. "Every night they call the OR," she says. " 'Are you doing a liver transplant tonight?' My answer is one of two: It's either, 'Not yet' because I never tell them, 'No!' because when I tell them 'No!' fifteen minutes later somebody else will call me to say that now, suddenly, there is a transplant. So I tell them, 'As of right now, not yet' or 'Yes, we're doing one, and it's starting at such and such a time.' "

In the case of confusion or mystery about an upcoming transplant, says West, "The admitting clerk will call the OR and say that they have two [potential] recipients on the way in for organs, do we know anything about it? Well, often we haven't received the call yet. We can't help them. Then, finally, maybe one of the liver doctors will call us to tell us to get ready for a liver transplant. Or Sandee will call us. At the same time, the cardiac boys are walking around the corner, and they are standing in front of you at the front desk, and they are telling you that they are going to use the heart from the donor, too. Half the time, that's how we find out. You are sitting around doing nothing, and then suddenly the place gets crazy."

There may be one foolproof method of discerning when and if there's going to be a liver transplant. "It's kind of interesting," says West "because the running joke in the OR is 'Ask Housekeeping.' When the recipient is coming from out of the hospital, Housekeeping personnel are notified of the need for a room, so the room has to be turned over and cleaned and the bed has to be cleaned, so the recipients have a room to stay in before they go to the operating room." So, West says, when information about a transplant is scarce and rumors are running wild, OR nurses turn to their best source, other than the doctors, for information about an upcoming transplant. "We call Housekeeping."

Although the conditions and atmosphere in the operating theater will differ from hospital to hospital and country to country, the humor and irony medical personnel share is often international in scope. Derrick Wheeldon, a transplant coordinator and researcher, explains how information about an upcoming transplant will often travel through Papworth Hospital in England, where he has worked for thirteen years. "We have a set protocol [for informing people], and everybody knows what the protocol is. But odd things happen, like, for instance, the manager of Domestic Cleaning, may be having tea with the switchboard operator, and the switchboard operator might say, 'Ah, by the way, there's a donor call coming through.'

"And she, the manager of Domestic Cleaning, says, 'Well right. My staff are going off at 5:00. I better think about cleaning a cubicle (because the cubicles have to be washed; the walls have to be washed down twice). And she may appear up in the ITU [ICU] and say, 'I believe there's a donor coming through, and we're going to wash the cubicle since it's empty now.'

"And the ICU sister [nurse], and the residents, and everyone else will say, 'How come the cleaners know before us?' And then all hell breaks loose."

It would be misleading to believe that any transplant surgeon or fellow who wanted to participate in the surgical procedure at Pittsburgh could be included, simply by positioning himself in the right place at the right time. "One of the concepts that's taught here is teamwork," says Bronsther, who assisted both Carlos Esquivel and Shun Iwatsuki on Rebecca Treat's transplant, "and it really is a team endeavor. Usually two or three surgeons who have worked together before are selected by Starzl or one of the other 'attendings' to go out on the donor [procurement], which is a complicated operation, which takes at least two to three hours in the best of hands, which is a critical aspect of the transplant, because you have to retrieve an appropriate and well-preserved organ, if the liver transplant is going to be successful. And then back here, simultaneously, there's a team of four to seven surgeons involved in the recipient operation, four of them being scrubbed and at the operating table at all times, all of whom have worked together at some point in time. Anyone who participates at the table has been involved in or watched at least fifteen transplants.

"The fact that everyone in the operating room understands the nuances of the operation and understands the technical aspects of the operation, allows the surgeon actually doing the procedure to concentrate on what he's doing and not have to worry about what the other surgeons in the room are doing, and to know he's going to get excellent assistants."

Many of the surgical fellows will work in Pittsburgh for free, or supported by their home institutions, just for the opportunity to learn from Starzl. But learning is not a question of standing in line and waiting your turn. In order to participate, and to gain knowledge, you have to be aggressive. "You can't be afraid to act," says Bronsther. "One of the points Starzl likes to make—and sometimes it's hard to understand—is that you can't overintellectualize what you are doing or else you are immobilized with fear. If you believe in what you are doing and can justify it to yourself and your colleagues, then you have to have the gumption to go ahead and do it. And there isn't on this service a lot of formal conferencing.

You are supposed to learn by observation. You're supposed to be a keen observer . . ."

Which seems to be Thomas Starzl's philosophy of surgical training—to start with an excellent and somewhat experienced surgeon, to provide that surgeon with continued opportunities for observation and evaluation, to slowly ease that surgeon into the system, allowing him to gain wisdom, skill, and experience, until finally, one day, without warning, Starzl will turn the scalpel over to a favored assistant.

"When the transition from watching and assisting to being the primary force in an operation should actually take place, is a very hard question to answer," says Starzl. "We look at that question everyday now, and we try to get the cases and fit them with the appropriate surgeon. If we have a very difficult or complex case, I will either do it or else have Bud [Shaw] do it, or have Carlos [Esquivel] do it. We try to pick nice and easy cases for people coming up because we don't want their confidence destroyed by failing."

Observing and assisting is just as important at Stanford in Shumway's training program—with one major role reversal, according to Bruce Reitz. "In 90 percent of the cases, the resident is the one actually doing the surgery, while the 'attending' is standing right beside him telling him what to do.

"Shumway's quote is, 'It doesn't matter who does the surgery, it matters how it is done—the method, the technique, the sequence of 1,000 steps down the line, that's what matters about the operation, not who is actually, with their hands, doing that step or the one after. In most hospitals in the 1960s and 1970s, the vast bulk of the actual cutting, sewing, and tying was done by the attending surgeon or the professor or whatever, and the resident who was learning would be watching and assisting. But it was different at Stanford. People frequently say out there that Shumway could take the janitor out of the corridor in the hospital and have him come in and direct him successfully through that operation.

"You don't have to have any particular fantastic skill to do a heart transplant," says Reitz. "It may look that way, but that is baloney. You just have to have had the opportunity to do it. You just have to have someone with patience and with understanding, showing you how to do it, hanging in with you through all of the steps. That's how I train my residents here at Hopkins, and that is something that Shumway passed on to so many."

Contrary to Shumway's philosophy, Starzl says that he will "only hang around a little bit, and then go home" when his surgical fellows are attempting their first few cases. "When somebody starts, we like to have them to be able to do the case with their peers—not with one of us hanging over them, but with their peers. Otherwise, we are merely teaching them to be dependent. I try to put them in with an experienced crew, but emancipate them from the tyranny of faculty seniority. They're on their own." (An authorized attending must be available at all times, in case of emergency.)

Starzl is much more cavalier in theory than in practice, however, and his compulsion to be in the operating room during a liver transplant, cutting, tying, directing the procedure, working at an accelerated pace, bellowing at his assistants, is all-consuming. "I can't stand having him watch me," says Robert Gordon. "I just don't like having him peer over my shoulder. I would rather he left the room, let me do my thing, and come in later. If he wants to be in the room, I'd rather he just did it. But if he's standing there watching me, it drives me nuts. He knows that. I told him point blank. 'You want to do it, just come in and do it, but don't stand there looking over my shoulder, because that drives me crazy.' It's like having a bear around me."

Says Bronsther: "We personally get on very well and I am able to talk pretty freely. But in the OR, he beats the shit out of me. I was kidding the other night that I have two options. I either have to ignore him totally or kill him because if I took it seriously, I'd have to shoot him." His haranguing is continual. "It's unbelievable. It's relentless, totally relentless." And yet, Bronsther speculates that "it is from this harangue that he [Starzl] derives the energy to work the way he works."

RN Jill West, who has worked and battled with Thomas Starzl longer than almost anyone in Pittsburgh, observes that a man "as intense as he is, needs to blow off that steam. He cannot contain all of that and still operate the way he operates, do the operations he does. Bob and Bart are the same way. There are incredible high tension moments in all of these operations and procedures, and you cannot afford to stay tense. Sometimes, to relieve tension, they need to blow off that steam, and if it is directed toward me, what I do is, I pause and try to figure out why they are angry and what I can do to change it. The relationship that I have with them is a very special relationship. I consider them as my friends, but there are times in the operation when Bart Griffith and I will just be at each other's throats. But we always settle our differences after the operation is over.

"Starzl and I fought about a week or so ago—from 8:00 Saturday morning until 1:30 Saturday afternoon, we fought tooth and nail—and then finally at 1:30, I went into the room where he was working, and there was some visitor there, and he began telling the visitor what a wonderful nurse I was and how important I was to Pittsburgh, and I just had to shake my head and laugh out loud."

Chapter 20

FIRST CUT

"Bovie, please."

Dr. Carlos Esquivel, gowned, masked, and gloved in Presbyterian's OR #6, made "first cut" into Rebecca Treat—a long, flanged, graceful incision the shape of a Mercedes Benz insignia—at approximately 7:30 P.M.

The Bovie, an electric knife, is also known to surgeons as the "firestick" because it simultaneously cuts and cauterizes, burns right through: first a crack of skin, then a layer of yellow fat, then a thick blanket of muscle is rolled back; it all happens quickly, dramatically, gracefully, like the sudden parting of the Red Sea. There is a slight wisp of smoke, the sweet aroma of singed flesh, but at this point, very little blood.

The surgery taking place at Charlotte Memorial Hospital 500 miles away, at which Robert Hardesty and Thomas Starzl, assisted by cardiac surgeon Alfredo Trento and procurement coordinator Matt Armany, were at that very moment engaged, was extremely similar to the process Esquivel was initiating, except that the procurement team was not only about to remove the liver, but also the heart, lungs, and kidneys. Thus, not only was the incision larger—from the neck down to the lower abdomen—but the surgeons were faced with a myriad of potential difficulties in virtually any area of the body and at any given moment. The procurement surgery is made even more difficult because of the artificial nature of the situation. The brain-dead donor is usually more unstable than is the prospective recipient, who, no matter how sick or how deeply sedated, has some semblance of normal body function and instinctive resistance to danger as protection.

The stability of both the potential recipient and the donor are maintained in a relatively similar manner, however. They are ventilated, meaning that the air that they normally would breathe has been mechanically pushed at a rate of twelve times per minute into their lungs, where their blood is instantly oxygenated. Oxygen is the source of the body's energy. Each organ, vessel, and tissue must be regularly enriched or "perfused" with oxygenated blood in order for Rebecca to remain alive in Pittsburgh and Richie Becker to maintain viability as a donor. The vital pumping mechanism, providing the propulsive force necessary for circulating this precious energy is a hollow, muscular, contractile organ known as the heart.

The basic circulatory pathway is relatively simple. The blood oxygenated by the lungs travels through the heart, from which it is pumped into the body's largest artery—the *aorta*—the main branch of a twisting maze of vessels leading to every conceivable corner and crevice of the body. A number of other great arteries branch from the aorta (it is called the *thoracic* aorta above the diaphragm and the *abdominal* aorta below the diaphragm), including the *hepatic artery*, which delivers blood to the liver, and the *renal arteries*, which bring blood to both kidneys, located behind and slightly below the liver.

Blood perfuses the organs and then flows into the *vena cava*, the largest vein in the body, and the main trunk of an extremely complicated series of return vessels. The vena cava (the *superior* is above the heart, while the *inferior* is below) also collects the blood from the liver, and for a very short part of its course, it actually runs through the liver. Eventually, it delivers all deoxygenated blood back to the heart, which pumps it through the pulmonary artery to the lungs, where the process of oxygenation and subsequent perfusion begins anew.

The objective for Esquivel during this phase of liver surgery, known as the *hepatectomy*, is to slowly and carefully separate Rebecca's liver from her body without damaging or dividing any of the major connections, so that she can continue to function as long as possible on her own resources, despite their obvious limitations. Major connections in addition to the inferior vena cava, and the hepatic artery, will include *the portal vein*, which carries the absorbed products of digestion to the liver for processing. It runs into the liver, divides into branches to supply or distribute blood, which will drain subsequently into the inferior vena cava. The final connection is the *bile duct*, which serves as a passageway for bile, which helps in the absorption of fat. The bile is collected in a number of small channels, joined together like tributaries of a river, eventually forming a single channel that flows into the *duodenum*, which is the beginning of the small bowel.

In addition to the main hepatic connections, surgeons in Charlotte will also separate the heart-lung bloc from the donor's body. Connections here include the *trachea* (which conveys air to the lungs), followed by the *right atrium* of the heart (which receives deoxygenated blood from the body and passes it to the lungs), and the aorta. Because the lungs are attached to the heart, the pulmonary artery, which connects the heart to the lungs, remains connected. If this donor were to be used for a heart transplant only, then the surgeons would separate the pulmonary artery as well. Although this process occurs early in the removal of the donor's organs, the *cardiectomy* is delayed for as long as possible in the recipient so that surgeons can be certain that the donor organs are viable. It would be impossible to locate another heart-lung for Winkle Fulk right away, if the donor in Charlotte, for one reason or another, didn't pan out. However, the time needed to do a hepatectomy—a minimum of five to six hours long—necessitates that Esquivel make first cut early on Rebecca Treat.

The recipient hepatectomy is by far the most harrowing step in the transplant process. The disease has not only destroyed the liver, but it has wreaked havoc on the body's major connections to the liver. Those connections must first be preserved, then severed and subsequently bonded to the matching connections from the donor liver. For the most skillful and experienced surgeon, the liver transplant is a monumental task, for there are unexpected disruptions and complications from the first moment to the very last, each of which is life-threatening.

The portal vein, for example, which carries the absorbed products of digestion from the body to the liver for processing, is often blockaded by scar tissue caused by damage of disease, thrombosis (a blood clot), or a combination of both. This elicits a number of possible consequences, including a backup of blood, which exerts increased pressure (portal hypertension) on the walls of the connecting veins, which can become twisted or ruptured, like varicose veins, invariably resulting in serious bleeding. The congestion in the portal vein is sometimes so critical that the blood is literally flowing through the liver, and in the vessels around the liver—backwards.

The actual extent of the portal hypertension, says Oscar Bronsther, who, along with Shun Iwatsuki, assisted Esquivel that night, depends upon the specific damage and disease to the liver, "whether there has been previous surgery or not, or whether the liver is swollen, shrunken, or normal size. It is more difficult, for example, when the liver is small [as in Rebecca Treat's case]. It's harder to expose [to open up], and all the connections from the liver and body are shortened. There isn't much room to work, there isn't much room to get ties in. It is packed in, crammed in; very difficult."

Collaterals, vessels of various lengths and sizes that emerge primarily from tiny preexisting inconsequential vessels and envelop the liver in an attempt to bypass it, are a serious and ever-threatening by-product of portal hypertension. "When you go in there to do a liver transplant," says anesthesiologist Doug Martin, "it is just a mass of angleworms. All of these little venous collateral channels that provide alternate pathways for the blood to flow around the liver, represent, each and every one of them, a potential exsanguinating [bleeding to death] hemorrhage. So there is this incredible tedium of addressing each and every little possible source of hemorrhage, which makes that operation real difficult."

The surgeons maintain that they are not frightened by the prospect of delicate and life-threatening difficulties. "I don't get nervous," says Esquivel. "I just feel like I am going to do the best I can—and that's it. I'm going to go and try to help somebody, but I am not thinking about running into trouble. I can't explain it, but I have gotten into trouble in the OR before, and so far I have been able to get out of trouble. But if I begin *thinking* I am going to get into trouble, then I shouldn't go into the OR at all."

Both Esquivel and Bronsther had treated Rebecca in the ICU since she had arrived in Pittsburgh. "It was so funny," said Bronsther, "because we kept hearing about what a wonderful, warm, vibrant young woman this was, how her doctor from the military was so interested in her because he found her to be such a lovely kid. But she was just uncooperative, almost combative prior to the operation, very encephalopathic [abnormal behavior caused by brain dysfunction]." Esquivel had only one thought in his mind at first cut: "I realized that if she didn't get that liver, she was going to die."

Esquivel, a soft-spoken, dark-complected Costa Rican, now permanently relocated in the United States, is shy, warm, and friendly in social situations, but somewhat stiff in the OR, very quiet, intense, and nearly emotionless. His movements are quick and extraordinarily efficient as he manipulates the Bovie, cauterizing smaller bleeders, clamping and tying off larger ones. With each bleed successfully sealed, literally hundreds more emerge, tiny pinpoint streams of blood, simultaneously challenging Esquivel from a dozen different directions.

The liver, tucked beneath the body's rib cage, is much more difficult to reach and maneuver than are the other internal organs. "In fact, most of the bleeding from the liver is coming from the posterior [the rear]," says Doug Martin, "which makes life considerably more difficult because the surgeon cannot always see where the bleeding is coming from."

Martin and his colleagues in the Department of Anesthesia are the silent partners of the surgical team, for they alone are responsible for the "hemostasis" of the patient, the regulating of blood through the patient's circulatory system, satisfying the body's relentless requirements for oxygenation and perfusion, which are radically altered and constantly fluctuating under the onslaught of major surgery.

"Does the patient have adequate blood flow to his brain

so that he doesn't become brain dead, adequate blood flow to kidneys so that he doesn't wake up with renal failure, adequate blood flow to his heart so that he doesn't have a cardiac arrest before the new heart or liver arrives?" asks Martin. An anesthesiologist will use a multitude of drugs to enhance and balance cardiac performance, so that the heart, the body's pumping mechanism, will continue to perfuse and oxygenate tissue at all times during the surgery. "This is what we do throughout the entire procedure to achieve our first and most important goal, which is to keep the patient alive," says Martin.

Prior to surgery, Martin or one of his colleagues had prepared Rebecca Treat and Winkle Fulk for the ordeal that was to follow. "We bring them into the operating room, get them on the table. For some reason, it is always freezing cold in there, which is something that I think is ubiquitous in almost every operating room in the country. We begin by examining them, listening to their heart, lungs, evaluating their airways. We look for the superficial concerns—contact lenses, false teeth." A denture wearer, Winkle Fulk had previously given her teeth to Dave for safekeeping; neither Winkle nor Rebecca wore contact lenses, however. "We give medications, such as atropine, which will dry out the airways, so that when we are 'passing tubes' [inserting the oxygen supply through the endotracheal tube, connected to the ventilator] there are no big puddles of secretions [saliva] that might go down into the lungs." When the patient goes to sleep, Martin explains, their eyes dry out a good deal, "so much so that we often use a moisturizer. But if you have a foreign body in your eye, such as a contact lens, you could scratch a cornea."

The patients are not yet asleep, however, when Martin places two catheters (tubes) into his patients' arm veins. Because of blood loss during surgery, all transplant recipients require blood transfusions intra- and postoperatively, so intravenous access is established in advance when vessels are easily accessible. "We also place an arterial catheter—it's just like the intravenous catheter, but it goes into an artery, usually the radial artery [in the wrist]. The catheter is hooked up to a transducer that converts blood pressure into an electrical signal that is displayed on a oscilloscope [monitor] as a wave form."

To explain how and why the pulmonary artery or "Swan-Ganz" (named for its inventors) catheter is used for both the liver and cardiac transplant patients, Martin first offers a quick sketch of how the heart (or "hearts," from his unique perspective) work. "Think about the body as having two hearts and one lung rather than the other way around because, physiologically, that is the way the body behaves," says Martin. The right side of the heart only has enough muscle to pump blood into the lungs [for oxygenation], while the left side of the heart, "the left heart" pumps blood to the entire body and then back into the right heart where the cycle is repeated.

"Now let's think about the heart," Martin continues. "The heart is like a rubber band. If you stretch it a little bit, it pops back a little bit. If you stretch the heart a lot, which is usually not possible in most of the patients we see for transplant, it pops back a lot. We refer to the amount of stretch in the myocardial fibers as 'preload.' It would be nice if you could say that the right heart stretch would be exactly the same as the left heart stretch, but in these terribly sick people in whom the right heart doesn't always behave the way the left heart behaves, it isn't often true—which is why the pulmonary artery catheter is so vital."

It is a soft and flexible tube with a tiny balloon at its tip, which is inserted into the body through a large vein in the neck, and carried by blood flow to the right heart. The balloon then helps to guide the catheter to the pulmonary artery, which leads from the right heart to the lungs. The catheter is hooked up to a microprocessor," says Martin, "which, in the space of about five seconds, can measure cardiac output— the blood flow through the heart. We will take this measurement maybe fifty times throughout the operation." Once the catheter is in position, Martin will inflate the balloon sufficiently to block the flow of blood from the right heart to the lung, thus allowing the back pressure in the pulmonary area distal (furthest from the center) to the balloon to be recorded. This pressure reflects the pressure transmitted back from the left heart. "Now we have some information about the left heart, independent from the right heart."

For Martin and the other members of the surgical team, the arduous and delicate work is instantly all-consuming. "From the absolute start," says Oscar Bronsther, "you are totally fixated on the operation, absolutely oblivious to everything else that is going on. It requires intense, intense concentration, no matter what stage of the operation you are in," whether you are assisting in or directing the procedure.

During the hepatectomy and through most of the procedure, the lead or "primary surgeon," who stands on the patient's right, will do the cutting, and later, the anastomosis, or sewing—putting the stitch in and pulling it through. Opposite the surgeon, on the patient's left, the first assistant will tie knots (to cut off bleeders) and follow suture lines, holding the long tail of the suture out of the way so that it doesn't flop down and obscure the area of the next stitch.

Using hands and instruments, the second assistant, on the surgeon's right side, is "exposing" for the cutter, or expanding the surgical field as wide as possible. The large area of the first cut in both liver and cardiac transplantation is not indicative of the surgeon's actual work space, in which there is often only a couple of inches to maneuver. Thus, in concert with the first assistant's attentiveness to following sutures, the second assistant will continually enhance the surgical field by adjusting the position of whatever may get in the way, such as bowel or another vessel, etc.

Complicating the situation in liver transplantation is the fact that a significant portion of the surgeon's work takes place under the liver, where many of the arteries and veins are located, forcing the surgical team, from time to time, to work from a very difficult position. An important distinction is that the second assistant works ahead of the surgeon while the first assistant works behind. The third assistant is often responsible for retracting the liver itself so that the lead surgeon can work on the structures underneath the liver.

The scrub nurse, whose primary responsibility is to organize and hand instruments to the surgeon, and who is scrubbed, masked, gloved, and gowned just like the surgeon, is at the foot of the table, at the left, usually balanced on a standing stool. In order for a scrub nurse to see around the team, she needs to stand higher—how high depends upon the focal point of the surgeon. Most surgeons operate with the table at elbow height, but, for example, because of his short "focal point" (the distance between the surgeon's eyes and the operating field at which he or she sees most clearly), Starzl always operates higher. Also on duty in the operating room is a "circulating" nurse, who supplies materials and additionally needed instruments to the scrub nurse, replenishes supplies, helps the surgeons gown, and acts as an all-around assistant.

A good transplant surgeon, whether he is performing a liver or cardiac transplant, will platoon his assistants in a manner similar to a baseball manager, always attempting to field the best team under a variety of different circumstances. Oscar Bronsther gave as an example a situation that had occurred during a transplant led by a Japanese surgeon, Dr. Todo, who "got into trouble" during the hepatectomy—he was unable to stop a dangerous bleed—and Starzl, who had been observing, stepped in, sized up the situation, and rotated his assistants.

"He asked the third assistant to step out, while the first assistant, he made him the third assistant. He took me, originally at the second assistant's position, and made me the first assistant. He took Todo, who was really his best man in the OR, and made him second assistant, which sounds funny. But what the second assistant does is exposes—the second assistant exposes everything for the surgeon, particularly at the most difficult times. You need people who know what is going on, who aren't going to get in your way, and most importantly, who are going to expose things ahead of you quickly and properly. Which is why he put me at first assistant, so that I could *follow* what he was doing. He took Todo and made him second assistant because Todo perfectly understood the operation and would expose everything for him, immediately, without him having to direct him and waste time and break his concentration." With the team properly platooned, Starzl was then able to locate the bleeder and concentrate on tying it off in a matter of minutes.

Other factors often enter into how surgical transplant teams are positioned—or selected. "Whoever is strong that day,

whoever has gotten sleep that night and is awake and alert,"
says Esquivel. "You also always try to find a team that you
get along well with." The countries in which the surgeons
have trained are irrelevant. "Surgeons share sort of a common
language."

Usually the shape of a surgeon's hands will make very little
difference, says Bronsther, but in rare instances size could
matter a great deal. "It happened to me once with Starzl,
while we were doing a kid. I was exposing things perfectly
for him, but my hand was so big, he couldn't do what he
had to do, so in fact we switched. He exposed for me while
I did the sewing."

Surgical resident Mary Mancini says that a woman's small
hands are advantageous. "I can get into places they obviously
can't. I don't need as much room. I don't have to worry about
exposure as much as they do, or being able to see so much.
I don't have to have that chest cranked wide open all the
time." Mancini, who has been studying surgery in Pittsburgh
for eight years, would soon become one of the most experienced women cardiac transplant surgeons in the world. Over
the next year, she would be given the opportunity to perform
a half dozen heart transplants, as well as a heart-lung. There
is only one well-recognized woman surgeon in the entire transplant field at this point: Dr. Nancy Asher, who has just recently
initiated a liver transplant program at San Francisco State
University.

Although he literally created liver transplantation as it is
clinically practiced today, and he standardized surgical techniques, no one is more flexible and more experimental in the
operating room than Starzl doing a liver transplant. Ira Fox,
currently in the process of starting a liver transplant program
at the University of Pennsylvania School of Medicine, trained
under Starzl in Pittsburgh for two years.

"Starzl can take a liver out backwards; he can take it out
forwards; he can sew it in backwards and forwards. Tom Starzl
is always trying something new—always. He's never satisfied.
And as much as it drives the 'general surgeon' in us crazy,
it's an incredible thing for someone who is sixty years old
to constantly be doing something different in a field where

in surgery, you learn how to do something right once, and this is the way you do it, and you never change. Surgeons are very slow to change any technique that ever works; if it works, that's what's important. You want to get your patient home."

But Thomas Starzl realizes perhaps more than anyone else that the surgical techniques of the liver transplant have not yet evolved to a point deserving of complete standardization. There is much more to be learned, as Bartley Griffith had demonstrated to Thomas Starzl himself some four years ago. In Denver, and continuing when Starzl had arrived in Pittsburgh in 1981, liver transplant patients were too often dying on the table because of severe and uncontrollable loss of blood.

"We were just breaking the blood bank," recalled RN Frank McSteen, who manages the animal research lab. "It was a tremendous burden . . . something had to be done. You could go through from 50 to 100 units (pints) of blood, five to ten times what the body holds at any given time—and still lose the patient."

The reason for the tremendous blood loss stemmed from one of the primary challenges of liver transplant surgery: As explained previously, the major vessels or connections must be divided and temporarily clamped (closed) when the liver is removed, including the portal vein, which carries blood from the digestive tract to the liver and the vena cava, which subsequently carries the blood to the heart. When these veins were clamped, however, large quantities of blood would pool in the veins and in the abdominal cavity causing swelling, congestion, more bleeding, and injury to the tissue behind the intestines. The digestive tract was often damaged, and the kidneys sometimes failed as well. The patient could remain alive for a long time under these conditions, for the blood from other parts of the body would freely circulate through the heart, but the congestion in the abdominal area was often fatal.

After a series of experimental surgeries using dogs, Griffith, who was then a research fellow in the lab, devised an apparatus that bypassed the clamped-off abdominal area while preserving the circulatory pathway, thus eliminating the backup and pooling. A relatively simple device, the "veno-venous" (vein to vein) bypass employs a tube to detour the deoxygenated blood carried by the iliac or leg vein and a second tube for the blue blood carried by the portal vein. Ordinarily, these veins would have merged at the inferior vena cava, which would have carried the blood back to the heart for re-oxygenation. But because of the removal of the diseased liver in preparation for transplant, the inferior vena cava will have been severed and clamped. Both tubes are connected to a third tube that in a roundabout fashion carries blood up the body to the axillary, or arm vein, leading to the superior vena cava and back to the heart. The rest of the circulatory system remains untouched.

From the absolute beginning, the bypass was extremely effective, so much so that Starzl instantly adopted it as standard procedure, as did most other liver transplant surgeons in the world. A surgical equipment company now pre-packages the "veno-venous bypass" and markets it internationally.

Another surgical advance, developed by anesthesiologists at Pitt and Presbyterian to counter massive blood loss in liver transplants, is called RIS—the Rapid Infusion System—which, through a roller pump and a heat exchanger that quickly warms blood to body temperatures, can produce replacement blood flow rates of up to 2,000 milliliters per minute—more than fifteen times the flow rate of conventional blood replacement techniques. Anesthesiologists have yet to develop a fool-proof system of measuring how much blood is actually lost at any given time, however, says Doug Martin.

"If hemorrhage is slow, we can measure how much blood is in our suction bottles, how much blood is on the drapes and in the sponges [weighed by a nurse before and after they have been soaked with blood], but in liver transplantation, the hemorrhaging sometimes comes in buckets. You can't measure how much blood is soaking Bud Shaw's socks. You can't measure how much blood is sitting in the pericolic gutters [an area immediately adjacent to the intestine]. You cannot measure how much is on the drapes [on the sides of the table]. How much is soaking the bath blanket on the floor?

There may be one entire patient's blood volume sitting in these various spots that I have mentioned. To regulate inflow by how much is lost is scientifically reasonable, but practically and technically impossible. Therefore you have to measure transfusion requirements strictly in terms of intravascular pressures, which we hope reflects intravascular volume. It's a difficult proposition, however."

Beginning the procedure on Rebecca Treat at 7:30, at approximately the same time Thomas Starzl and Robert Hardesty had made first cut on Richie Becker at Charlotte Memorial, Esquivel calculated that the donor liver would arrive in Pittsburgh anywhere from 2 A.M. to 3 A.M. So far, the operating team was experiencing few serious bleeding problems, and so he was not particularly concerned about the possibility of a late-arriving liver, especially with Starzl in Charlotte at the scalpel.

Esquivel worked steadily, periodically guiding or encouraging Bronsther or other surgical assistants when they were not following or exposing effectively. At times, he would start to say something, then pause in the middle of a sentence, to concentrate while cauterizing a bleeder or asking a scrub nurse for a needed instrument. Five or ten minutes might pass before he would complete his thought. In the background, a radio played popular music, to which the surgeons paid little attention, although at times of no activity, the circulating nurse, who stood in the background, capped and masked as everyone else in the OR, would suddenly begin to shimmy and shake to a favorite tune. Now and then, a nurse would deliver units of blood or plasma, in thick plastic bags, from the blood bank. The phone, located near the head of the operating table and within reach of the anesthesiologist or anesthetist (an assistant to the anesthesiologist) rings periodically. Standing near the phone from that position, one could see Rebecca Treat's face, hidden from the surgical team by a blue drape.

Shun Iwatsuki, the senior surgeon, on duty more as supervisor than active assistant, would go in and out of the operating room quite frequently, checking on Esquivel's progress, making sure the operation was moving smoothly, then retreating to the nurse's station outside the OR door for a cigarette and some quiet conversation, or around the corner in the surgeon's lounge for a quick nap.

As the hours passed in the OR, the atmosphere became increasingly close. Even the minimal conversation existing at the beginning of the procedure gradually ebbed and died, while the sounds of surgery were exaggerated—the hollow thumping of the ventilator, the beeping of the "boob tube," its bouncing red, blue, and yellow arrows, and lines registering arterial pressure and EKG. The sound of suction, blood drawn out of the abdominal cavity through a hose and into a five-unit canister of clear plastic on the floor, periodically cut through the room like the warning of a rattlesnake. And because of the buzzing "firestick," the sweet and unsettling aroma of singed flesh continuously pervaded the air.

Sooner or later, says scrub nurse Jill West, "you lose your conscious awareness of the outside, because you are so closed in. We had windows once here—little skinny windows which made you feel sorta like you were in prison—but you could also go by those windows and catch a little ray of sunshine. Now with the windows gone, you have to try to do that on your lunch time—go to the cafeteria, and if it isn't the pitch-black middle of the night, just peek outside and see what the weather is like."

Chapter   21

THE PROCUREMENT

Charlotte Memorial Hospital is a much smaller facility than Presbyterian-University Hospital in Pittsburgh. The cafeteria closes early (Presby's cafeteria remains open twenty-two hours a day), while fewer nurses and aides and only an occasional resident or fellow walk the corridors, scribbling sleepily in charts, watching over the scattered units—trauma, orthopedics, urology, cardiology, the ER—where just twenty-four hours ago, Dick and Sharon Becker had pondered their son's fate with Sandy Bromberg.

Mike Callahan, Charlotte Memorial procurement coordinator, had an ambulance at the airport awaiting the Pittsburgh surgical team when it arrived. Thomas Starzl, who had wrapped himself in his orange sleeping bag in the tail section of the Lear Jet and dropped off to sleep the moment they had departed Pittsburgh, had also slept on the stretcher in the ambulance as they redballed the ten miles to downtown Charlotte, where the hospital was located. During the time in which cardiac surgeons Trento and Hardesty focused their attention on the separation of the heart-lung bloc, Starzl, his thick black-framed reading glasses balanced low on the bridge of his nose, kept himself busy by dictating letters into a minirecorder.

It is sometimes difficult to understand the pressure that the procurement team constantly confronts. After all, they are dealing with a brain-dead donor and not a living, breathing human being as are Esquivel, Bronsther, and the rest of the surgeons who have scrubbed in Pittsburgh for the hepatectomy and cardiectomy. If the surgery in Charlotte fails, then what could be so terrible? Richie Becker is dead anyway. But so too would Winkle Fulk and Rebecca Treat suddenly be dead, for once their organs are removed, it would be nearly impossible to find a second set of matching organs over the twenty-four to thirty-six-hour period during which it might be possible to sustain their lives, most especially in Winkle's case. That all-pervading threat, combined with the disadvantage of having to work in an unfamiliar atmosphere side-by-side with an OR staff with whom they have had little or no previous experience, enhances the tension and the extraordinarily difficult surgical challenge from the first to final cut.

But the challenge continues—in fact, it escalates—long after the procurement surgery is complete. The instant the organs are removed, their cells begin to deteriorate. In a couple of hours, the kidney will be spoiled, and within a half hour, the liver will be ruined; the heart is gone in ten to twenty minutes at the maximum.

To extend life outside of the body, organs are immediately and gently cooled (either in water or a solution of Ringer's lactate, which simulates body fluids) at a temperature of 4 degrees centigrade, just above freezing. Even then, the "ischemic" time—how long organs can be denied their precious blood supply—is limited. Kidneys, kept cold, will remain viable out of body forty hours, perhaps more, while livers can be preserved for approximately twelve hours. The six-hour ischemic period for hearts is considerably more limiting, but the ischemia of the fragile cushion of tissue that comprises the lung was thought to be little more than an hour. After this initial cooling-down period with Ringer's lactate, temperatures are maintained on a bed of shaved ice, usually in a compact and portable picnic cooler, perfect for travel.

In the early days of kidney transplantation, according to Brian Broznick, there was little long-range concern about maintaining the circulatory system. Little attention was paid to donor blood loss, blood pressure, or temperature regulation, which are of paramount importance in procurement of hearts and livers. Surgeons would quickly remove the kidneys from the body, carry them to a back table and plunge them into a cold solution. "Even then, you were getting cellular death, but it wasn't so awfully bad," said Broznick. The kidneys, after all, were preserved.

The process became more complicated when cyclosporine was introduced in the early 1980s, thus triggering unprecedented transplant activity. Of course, kidney surgeons were pleased with the success of the new miracle immunosuppressant, but now, they often had to share donors with surgeons who wanted hearts and livers. Since there is at least one kidney transplant unit in most major metropolitan areas, the kidney surgeons frequently had to wait hours, sometimes as long as a day, until a procurement team could travel from another hospital, in another part of the country. Hours more were consumed in the actual procurement surgery, before these surgeons could excise the kidneys. And at any time during this long wait, the donor's condition, unstable at best, could deteriorate. The heart could stop within seconds, thus suddenly denying the body its precious blood supply. The kidneys—all of the organs in the entire donor—could be lost.

The kidney surgeons had reason to be disgruntled for, up until the early 1980s, when medical centers throughout the country were launching heart and liver transplant programs, they had been able to do whatever they wanted with donors. Now, heart transplant surgeons suddenly had the priority. To safeguard the organ, they needed to excise the heart first. But how to do that without endangering the kidneys by cutting them off from a circulatory system whose nucleus was the heart? The answer to this problem came from Thomas Starzl.

Starzl's multiple (kidneys plus one or more extrarenal organs) procurement plan, developed in Pittsburgh with Robert Hardesty, stemmed from his early experience in kidney transplantation, long before laws determining brain death had been passed. Back then, surgeons would often use "DOAs" (dead on arrival), and they would rush into the emergency room and rapidly infuse the cold preservation solution into the area surrounding the kidneys, and subsequently remove the kidneys. The heart had already stopped, but the kidneys remained viable for transplantation. The challenge was in arriving in the ER and infusing the coolant fast enough, within fifteen or twenty minutes at most.

Ten years later in Denver in the late 1960s, Thomas Starzl developed a technique known as "core cooling," which today remains the standard way in which organs are preserved. Comparing "surface cooling" with "core cooling," Brian Broznick uses a hard-boiled egg as an example. "If you took that egg, put it in a pan of water for five minutes to cool it down, and then cracked it open, probably the yoke would still be warm, which means that all that time, that yoke, or the center of that organ, has not been protected. But if you put a needle into the middle of that egg, and started to infuse something cold, and you do it very rapidly, you would cool the whole egg almost immediately. In core cooling, through use of a cannula [a long thin tube] you are cooling the organ through its own internal vascular bed, through the capillaries, through the arteries, through the veins." Core cooling was the standard preservation method for Starzl's new procurement system.

The cardinal principle of this multiple organ procurement system is *in situ* (Latin for "in place") cooling, meaning that, contrary to current practice, Starzl was recommending that all of the organs being procured should be core cooled or preserved *in* the donor, as in his DOA experience. Thus, after the initial donor incision from the top of the chest to the abdominal cavity, the surgeons will expose both the heart and the kidneys, along with the connecting arteries and veins. They will then immediately core cool the kidneys, although the circulatory system still remains essentially intact. "Whatever complications would arise for the heart at that point, at least the kidneys are guaranteed to be preserved." Hardesty would then core cool the heart, take the heart out, and race back to Pittsburgh for the recipient stage of the operation. The kidneys could then be leisurely removed by the local surgeons. Starzl developed a similar approach for a combined procurement, in which the liver was cooled and preserved *in situ* along with the kidneys. The heart was excised first.

Immediately, *in situ* cooling in multiple procurement worked very well, and within a short time after the system was introduced by Hardesty and Starzl in 1983, almost every transplant surgical procurement team had adopted it. The challenges and difficulties were not solved, however—especially in the area of heart-lung procurement.

The ischemic time of the lung was known to be only one hour at the longest, and under those circumstances, there were only two scenarios under which a heart-lung transplant would be possible: (1) When the donor was declared brain dead at the hospital in which the transplant surgery was to occur, which eliminates travel time; (2) or when the donor, once declared brain dead, could be maintained on life support systems while being transported to the site of the surgery. In both scenarios, the donor and the recipient were then lined up, side by side, on adjacent operating tables, one surgeon harvesting the donor's healthy heart-lung bloc, while a second surgeon removed the recipient's diseased organs. The transplant could thus be completed within the ischemic limits.

Brian Broznick estimates that only one of every twenty-five heart donors will have lungs healthy enough to qualify for transplant. Further limiting hope for candidates like Winkle Fulk and Frank Rowe is the fact that most families, stunned by their loss, are unlikely to agree to extending the agony before burial while their loved one is transported to a distant hospital for surgery. In fact, Sandy Bromberg had broached the subject of flying Richie to Pittsburgh, but Sharon Becker had immediately refused. "We just couldn't. I did not want Richie to go anywhere that he physically did not know."

It was this dearth of heart-lung donors and the tragedy of so many young and vital people dying from incurable lung disease that in 1982 had initially motivated Robert Hardesty and Bartley Griffith to undertake a search for an answer—a way of extending the ischemic time of the lung so that distant procurements might be possible. At the outset of the experimentation and research, it is safe to say that neither Hardesty, Griffith, nor any of the residents, fellows, nurses, or technicians who dedicated their time and talent, ever conceived of the possibility that they would discover such a remarkable solution.

Hardesty and Griffith first tested the boundaries of ischemia in the same arena in which Norman Shumway and Thomas Starzl had conducted their early transplant experiments—the animal laboratory. Located on the ninth floor of Scaife Hall, at the end of a long dank corridor, Pitt's lab is comprised of a half-dozen connecting rooms with cement floors and bare blue-painted concrete block walls.

At the outset of the project, said Frank McSteen, an RN who, in 1965, became the first male to graduate from the nursing school he attended, they searched for the more obvious and traditional ways of extending ischemia of the lungs. They would remove lungs from laboratory dogs, store the lungs in ice, or in many different cold solutions at varied temperatures and time periods, and then transplant the lung back into the dog to see what would happen. Would the heart fulfill its vital role by feeding or "perfusing" the lung with blood? Would the lung, if perfused, "breathe" normally?

They tried, off and on, for more than a year, but "nothing worked," said McSteen. "We went on to other things, switched to monkeys, kept changing the preservation techniques, kept changing the solutions . . . it just wasn't working out; it was a bad idea."

And it was a bad time in the lab for McSteen and the residents and fellows working under him. "You would labor from 7:00 in the morning until 11:00 at night and then watch your work go down the drain, and soon you started to wonder, 'Do we really need to do this?' You would get angry about it, you would get damned angry because you just wasted what I considered a part of my life, along with the rest of the folks. After so long," said McSteen, "it started to get to me, to all of us."

But Bart Griffith refused to give up. "People on our list were dying in great numbers, waiting for transplantation. And as time went on, it became obvious that a quick fix was not possible; there was not an apparent way to store the lungs as we did the heart. We needed a totally different concept." What Griffith and his research team subsequently developed was not at all a totally different concept, but a new application of a concept developed decades before.

"About that time," said Hardesty, "we had a meeting here, focusing on heart transplants, and people came from all over the country, including a guy named Francis Robicsek, a cardiac surgeon [coincidentally, from Charlotte Memorial], known for his crazy but very often effective ideas. He's an older guy, of Bahnson's vintage, but still working, and he was here because they were thinking about doing heart transplants at Charlotte. I don't even know how the discussion started, but we mentioned that we were trying to preserve the lungs so that we could go on distant procurements, and he said, 'Well, why don't you try this technique?' " Robicsek explained that as far back as the early 1950s he had found a way of preserving animal hearts out the body and indefinitely by manually perfusing them with oxygenated blood.

"Well," said Griffith, "we figured if you could keep the heart alive, circulating blood in it, it stands to reason you'll keep the lungs alive, too, right?" Griffith explained that the transplant of the entire heart-lung bloc was widely believed to be preferable to the transplant of a single lung because the brochials, which connect the "trachea" or windpipe to each lung, do not heal very well after surgery, and also have a tendency to scar—a serious problem if ever additional surgery in that area is mandated. Also, as in the case of both Winkle Fulk and Frank Rowe: "It's difficult to find a patient who has end-stage lung disease that doesn't have significant cardiac disease caused by the initial lung problem." Griffith's view reflected the feelings of the overwhelming majority of transplant surgeons, including Bruce Reitz and Norman Shumway, although some experimentation in single lung transplantation has occurred at the University of Toronto, where as of mid-1987, nearly a dozen of these cases have lived a year, post-transplant. The University of Mississippi has also delved into the lung transplant area.

Bob Hardesty was interested in Griffith's and Robicsek's concepts, but his characteristically conservative nature prevailed. "I thought it sounded too complex, and I was not really too enthusiastic about it, and I did not see how we could carry it off. But Bart was excited, he was so excited that he started pushing . . ."

"I went to the animal laboratory," said Griffith, "and turned the project over to guys who were in my exact same position a half dozen years ago, as research fellows. They are in the laboratory to experiment and explore. 'Hey,' I said, 'let's try it.' "

Over the next few months, researchers at the lab fashioned a device that would have impressed Rube Goldberg with the creativity and ingenuity of its design. While it resembles a tropical fish tank with six translucent plexiglass sides—it is, in fact, heated with two aquarium heaters—it was officially referred to as "a perfusion device," but everyone in Pittsburgh immediately and forever thereafter called it, simply and descriptively, "the box."

In Charlotte on that day, May 2, 1985, and over the following two years in nearly four dozen procurements, it worked in essentially the same manner: During the procurement surgery, a plastic bag, outfitted with two plastic tubes, was filled with three pints of the donor's blood, and passed over to the coordinator, Matt Armany. The bag was suspended by Armany on an IV pole approximately three feet above the box, providing the pressure required for normal circulation through the heart and lungs. One of the tubes from the bag was plugged into the right atrium, the first of four chambers of the heart, which, along with the lungs, en bloc, had been excised by Hardesty and Trento from the donor. The donor's blood, compelled by gravity, traveled from the plastic bag, down the plastic tube through the heart and exited into a second plastic tube connected to the aorta, from which the blood exited the heart. The heart was perfused in the process.

Next, a third plastic tube, an endotracheal tube, was attached at one end to the trachea, which led to the lungs, and at the second end to a hand-operated bag ventilator, which would provide oxygen, thereby triggering (fooling?) the heart, now perfused and oxygenated, into beating as if it were still in the donor's chest. Finally, the pumping heart circulated blood through the lungs, providing them and itself with life-sustaining nutrients. As in the body, the blood would then re-circulate back into the heart and then again into the lungs.

The surgeons, assisted by Armany, carefully placed the

heart-lung bloc into a plexiglass housing (actually, a smaller box) containing Ringer's lactate. Temperature was maintained by the aquarium heaters, anchored to the bottom of the box and connected by wires extending up into the plexiglass housing. The heaters were plugged into an ordinary wall socket.

Meanwhile, the box was filled with twelve liters (four and a half gallons) of solution that duplicated the body's normal fluids. The housing containing the heart-lung bloc was carefully lowered into the box and immersed in the fluid. The box, sealed with a screw-on plexiglass cover, was ready for transport.

"What we've tried to do with this is to keep things as close to the way they are in real life in the body as possible so the heart-lung hardly knows that it has been outside of the body when it is sewn in," said Armany. In fact, it simulated natural conditions so well that, theoretically, it could indefinitely suspend ischemic time. In other words, if the organs accepted the artificial but "normal" atmosphere of the box, all concerns about ischemia would be superfluous.

The box was tested in and out of the lab in every which way possible. "Anything you can think of," said McSteen, "we did to test it out. We transplanted the heart and lungs of a dog and put them into the box a half a dozen times. We got an ambulance, jostled it around, drove it all over 'hell's half acre,' and the thing kept beating. Then we figured we have got to take it up in the air. Took it on a helicopter flew it around the city of Pittsburgh for a couple of hours, brought it back by ambulance, shook it up a little more, brought it back to the lab—and the heart was still beating."

Their initial attempts to extend the ischemic time of lungs had been extraordinarily frustrating, but the challenge and success of the box brought laughter and excitement back into the laboratory.

"It was just something else," he said. "When you saw those lungs and that heart out of the chest, independent of the body, with only a ventilator and that tubing going to the blood bag, all suspended in that silly-looking box, I mean, that made all the work worthwhile. 'When are we going to do the next one?' I never wanted to stop."

It wasn't the next one with which Bob Hardesty and Bart Griffith were concerned, however—but the first one to attempt clinically on a donor. "The potential recipient happened to be an air force dependent," said Hardesty, and when it was discovered that no local plane available for rental at that moment was equipped to supply electricity for the box's heating elements, "the hustlers here from the procurement group contacted the air force, which diverted a plane from San Antonio to Pittsburgh. They then flew us to Atlanta to do the donor operation, where they flew in a new flight crew to fly us back to Pittsburgh.

"I remember watching this huge gray DC-9 landing in Greater Pittsburgh Airport and 'United States Air Force' in big letters on the side, and pretty soon this ramp comes down, a huge ramp the size of my office desk unfolds, and the corpsman came running down, saluting. Lights went up on the side, a spotlight came on from above, and we sort of crept up the ramp. The boss [Hank Bahnson] went along to see the action. And he and I got inside this thing—a thirty-two-bed flying intensive care unit—and we sat down, and I was feeling awfully small and insignificant because we had this whole DC-9 to ourselves. And he leans over and he says, 'Hardesty, this thing sure as hell better work.' I figured that my hind-end was on the line," says Hardesty. "But it did work."

Or at least it worked in the sense that Hardesty and Bahnson were able to remove the heart-lung bloc from the potential donor, place it into the box, and transport it back to Pittsburgh. They were able to succeed to that extent for four of the first nine attempted procurements in which the box was employed. But in that first instance and in three of the four "successful" instances thereafter, the recipients did not survive, although Hardesty stresses that the patient fatalities had nothing to do with the capabilities of the box. Two patients died of infection after surgery, and one patient bled to death in the operating room. That patient was an attempted re-transplant.

As Griffith has pointed out, if nothing else, the transplant team learned that heart-lung surgery is such a delicate and overwhelming ordeal, causing so much damage and scar tissue, that re-transplantation, quite possible in hearts, kidneys, and livers, is simply impractical in heart-lung situations. Of the few hundred heart-lungs transplanted since Bruce Reitz's historic beginning with Mary Gohlke, only one re-transplant has been successful. Oddly enough, this was Bruce Reitz's second case at Stanford—directly after Mary Gohlke—thirty-year-old Charles Walker, transplanted in May 1981, re-transplanted in April 1984. He died on April 19, 1987 in Binghamton, New York—the longest living heart-lung recipient ever.

Hardesty and Griffith were not deterred by their less than satisfactory recipient results, for they had actually demonstrated that the box, as a procurement technique, was viable—a potential lifesaver. From that point of view, it worked. It worked then, and it worked during the next series of attempts at distant procurement, even though one or more of its jerry-rigged parts frequently failed to function. Once, in a small-town hospital in Michigan at 3:00 A.M., the tiny aquarium heaters used to maintain body temperature burned out. In desperation, Brian Broznick borrowed a car and traveled sixty miles to Pontiac, rendezvousing with the state police officer, who persuaded the owner of the nearest pet store to open his shop for early morning business.

In another instance, flying back to Pittsburgh on a Lear jet, Hardesty suddenly discovered that the plastic bag containing the donor's blood supply was leaking. Since it was in the sterile atmosphere of the box, there was no way to stop the leak. "At that point, I was so emotionally involved that I asked Matt Armany, who's a nurse, to draw the blood off me—I was the only O [blood type], or at least the only one who would admit it—they took it off me, and they put it into the reservoir bag. That was enough to hold us until we got to the airport." Hardesty is undoubtedly the only transplant surgeon whose blood has circulated through both a donor and recipient on whom he operated. In both of those cases, which occurred later that year, and most especially during that vital first attempt with Hank Bahnson, "We brought the heart-lung back," said Hardesty. This was the long-sought-after goal.

"But the hardest problem in getting the heart-lungs in the

box was maintaining a proper temperature," Hardesty explained, "and the biggest problem with maintaining temperature were the kidney guys [surgeons]. And as soon as they would start doing their exposure and dissection, the temperature would drop down for one reason or another. By the time I finished my dissection and was ready to put the organs in the box, they were too cold. The heart would fibrillate [rapid, tremulous, and incomplete contractions, which can cause permanent damage] because of lower temperature, and we would come home empty-handed."

He recalled a time in Madison, Wisconsin, that had been particularly wasteful and depressing. "The problem then, as it always is, is to prevent the temperature from getting too low and causing the heart to fibrillate. I kept emphasizing to the kidney surgeon not to start the cooling solution until I asked him to, knowing that I wouldn't hurt their organs. That day they were taking both the pancreas and the kidneys. We had everything just about ready to come out, and then suddenly the heart fibrillated, and I turned around only to find out that they had thrown ice all over the pancreas [the organs had previously been core cooled], which in turn had gotten into the chest cavity, reduced the temperature, and we lost the heart. Went home empty-handed."

These and other experiences helped Hardesty and Griffith come to realize that they needed a more reliable and skilled surgeon to make the heart-lung box work. The kidney surgeons working with them in the past had been too sloppy, Hardesty concluded, and they had also been agonizingly slow. Said Griffith: "We've been in the field where it's taken kidney people four hours [to remove the kidneys], and they've lost twelve units of blood. Under those circumstances, we can't come away with a healthy heart and lungs."

As they saw it, the one and only answer to their dilemma— the key to saving countless lives with distant procurement through their heart-lung box—was Thomas Starzl. "There's nobody else in this country with his technical surgical skills. Using the *in situ* technique, said Hardesty, "he would get the liver out in ten minutes while most of the groups around the country will spend hours." Starzl was anywhere from two to three times more efficient than any other liver or kidney transplant surgeon in the world—despite his age, Hardesty said. The surgical plan that they devised was that Hardesty would deal with the heart-lung bloc, and Starzl would take the liver for Pittsburgh, while removing the kidneys for the local program.

"Starzl has an unbelievable ability to go in the right place, no wasted movement, no fiddling around," said Dr. Robert Kormos, a visiting heart-lung transplant surgeon from the University of Toronto, after observing Starzl on a donor procurement. "No blood. No tearing apart. I was amazed when I first saw him work. Another surgeon would pick away and pick away and be very cautious, always thinking that he was going to hit something. I know it would easily take the average surgeon four hours to do what Starzl can do in half the time."

This was how Thomas Starzl came to join the procurement team in Charlotte that evening. Later, Starzl was to develop special time-saving techniques for this difficult procurement, which he taught to a few of the more skilled members of his team. But the Richie Becker procurement was the first in which he had participated.

While Armany and Hardesty were carefully planting Richie Becker's heart and lungs in their ingenious box, Starzl, assisted by Trento and a scrub nurse, was working feverishly to remove the liver and kidneys by dividing the major connections, in concert with Esquivel, who had reached approximately this same stage in Pittsburgh 1,000 miles away.

As Starzl cuts, dipping his long, slender, gloved hands again and again into a well of abdominal blood, periodically suctioned by Trento, he remains quiet and concentrated, his movements quick and precise, with no gesture wasted. His dark-framed glasses have slipped to the bridge of his nose; the wrinkles on his ruddy forehead are accentuated in the bright light, and are especially deep and pronounced at this late hour. Most transplant surgeons sooner or later discover, just as marathon runners and prizefighters learn over time, that the human body when physically stressed, can not only find a "second wind" but also a "third wind" and a "fourth wind." It has often been said that a transplant coordinator or surgeon will usually work a three-day shift—with each day taking place in the same night.

Chapter   22

THE TRANSPLANT

"First cut" on Winkle Fulk was not made until approximately five hours after Esquivel had started on Rebecca Treat and not until Robert Hardesty phoned Pittsburgh to confirm that Richie Becker's organs had been successfully removed, and were now beating safely in the heart-lung box.

"They'll [the organs] be on their way back from Charlotte momentarily," Bartley Griffith announces, as he enters from the glass-enclosed scrub area between OR #5 and OR #6, masked and capped, a small, bright light strapped to his forehead, similar to a miner's headlamp. A nurse, waiting with a towel for his dripping hands, assists him with his surgical gown and skin-tight translucent latex gloves.

Before beginning, he directs one of the nurses to adjust the three bright spotlights illuminating the surgical field, then nods his satisfaction. "This is like a Stephen Spielberg production. Did you read about him in *Time* Magazine? He's just a kid, out having a little fun." Because the heart is considerably higher in the anatomy than the liver and the surgical challenges vary, his assistants have set up differently from Esquivel's team. First assistant Dale Payne, who will both follow suture lines and expose, stands on Griffith's right side, while second assistant Mary Mancini, often rotating with Bob Kormos, will position herself opposite Griffith, the primary surgeon, helping to expose and operate the suction.

Griffith calls for the Bovie, as did Esquivel, beginning his "first cut" at the notch above Winkle's sternum—the "breast-bone," to which the uppermost seven pairs of ribs are at-tached—down to the abdomen. He then hooks the teeth of the blade of the bone saw underneath the xiphoid sternum [the very end of the breastbone], and without hesitation, switches on the saw and begins cutting. Similar in appearance to an ordinary carpenter's handsaw, the tool is equipped with a specially designed blade guard, permitting the surgeon to cut very close—within a centimeter of a specified point with-out actually harming that point.

As Griffith cuts, wisps of blue smoke and wet bone dust waft into the air, while the nagging whine of the saw's electric motor, weakening as Griffith bears down on the blade, assaults the quiet, peaceful atmosphere of the OR. Of all the sensations of surgery, this violent sound and the destruction it foresha-dows is the most disturbing. At the completion of the cut, known as the "sternotomy," Payne, who has been following Griffith and suctioning the bone dust, soupy with blood, seals the bone edge by spreading a thick layer of a gelatin-like sub-stance called "bone wax," which is actually genuine bees' wax, across the raw surfaces of bone.

Winkle Fulk's sternum is now split down the center, provid-ing access to the mediastinum, the chest cavity in which the heart sits. Griffith then requests "the retractor," a surgical device composed of two curved steel blades parallel to one another, which fit on either side of the rib cage. The retractor is also outfitted with a handle-operated ratchet that, as he cranks, inch by excruciating inch, further spreads the two halves of Winkle's sternum, thus expanding the surgical field and providing an uninhibited view of the surface of the lungs, blotched and streaked in a breathtaking myriad of pink and blue-black tones, speckled with white. (Esquivel's team had used a similar, although larger and more delicate device, to spread and anchor the abdominal area.) Working intensely and without pause, Griffith moves the lungs aside with the back of his gloved hand, and gathers in the pericardium, the sac that surrounds and lubricates the heart. Simultaneously, the scrub nurse slaps a scissors into his left hand, with which he begins to sever the pink pericardial membrane.

"This has to be dealt with very carefully," said Bob Kormos, assisting Griffith off and on through the procedure. "There are two nerves that run along the sides of that sac, and those nerves carry electrical impulses to the diaphragm, telling it when to contract and expand. So if those nerves are damaged during the cutting, she won't breathe spontaneously after transplant." At this point, second assistant Mary Mancini is suctioning blood, and first assistant Dale Payne is exposing for Griffith, and helping with difficult bleeders. There are usually only two assistants in a heart or heart-lung transplant at any one time.

Griffith drops the scissors on the scrub nurse's worktable to his right and quickly folds back the corners of the pericardium, tacking them down with facile looping strokes with a needle and thread. When finished, he momentarily raises his gloved hands, and suddenly the heart is revealed, a flexing, pulsating fist of red marble.

At this particular point in the surgery, no one says a word or skips a beat in the demanding sequence of their work, and yet there is a silent and nearly imperceptible hesitation, as everyone in their own special way pays homage to this universal symbol of existence. "I've seen open heart surgery hundreds of times," a nurse comments much later at the nurse's station during a cigarette break, "but it never ceases to amaze me. I feel something special when I first view that heart; it's only a muscle, and yet there's kind of a secret and magnificent glory to it."

Similar to the quiet steadiness in Esquivel's operating theater next door, the atmosphere surrounding Griffith's surgery is muted and businesslike. There are very few conversations during the entire procedure. Mostly, the surgeon will speak, and only then when he requires aid from an assistant or instrumentation from the scrub nurse—or if, perhaps, he wants to assure himself that his team is awake and alert.

"Winifred?" Griffith suddenly asks. "So what kind of name is Winifred?"

"How about Winnie?" says one of the nurses.

"OK, how about it?"

Later, Griffith wonders aloud: "Did God create the heart for the surgeon, or the surgeon for the heart?"

And much later, after a long, intense silence. "Adam was sort of a surgeon. He did a pretty good job operating on Eve." He is about to say something else, when he interrupts himself to address the anesthesiologist. "I think she's gasping," meaning that Winkle does not have enough oxygen to comfortably breathe.

"Really?"

"This is the third time; I'm almost sure of it. How about more O-2?"

"You got it," the anesthesiologist replies. He turns the lever on a green metal tank. Griffith was evidently correct for, from that point on, Winkle does not stir.

In addition to maintaining hemodynamics, the anesthesiologist has other essential responsibilities, prior to and during the transplant. Says anesthesiologist Martin: "The most dangerous part of the case for us is to take patients from being awake, nervous, anxious, kind of all jived up, and without any pain, to take them from that starting point and to put them to sleep, to remove all of their sensations, to remove consciousness."

With the patient asleep, the next step "is to augment the anesthetic depth to alleviate the patient from the sudden pain immediately prior to the incision of skin with scalpel. The way we do that is with huge doses of narcotics, in combination with a tiny dose of a loss-of-consciousness agent, such as valium. This is not a difficult maneuver for healthy patients, but it is an extremely dangerous balancing act for patients with severe heart disease, or with liver disease, which has exerted a monumental strain on the heart." The anesthesiologist must continually increase the dosage of narcotics in concert with the increasing pain, as the surgery continues. The challenge is often made more formidable by the patients' unwitting sympathetic nervous system responses.

"If you hit your finger with a hammer, your blood pressure goes up and your heart rate goes up," says Martin. So first the heart rate and the blood pressure have plummeted with administration of the anesthetic; the patient has also lost his "sympathetic tone"—and then the pressure and heart rate have suddenly skyrocketed with the assault of surgery. "It's the fight or flight response," says Martin. "If the patient has that kind of response, we administer drugs to reduce the blood pressure or drugs to reduce the heart rate."

Now Griffith is ready for the heparin, which will thin the blood, thereby reducing the possibility of clotting or coagulation. The scrub nurse has filled a large hypodermic which she passes over to Griffith, who glances at it momentarily before injecting the amber fluid directly into the heart. Almost immediately, the heart responds, as if in protest, by pulsing and beating in a wild and uncoordinated manner. "Now stop that," says Griffith, quietly. And then he "twicks" the heart with his thumb and forefinger, as though he were "twicking" a ball of fuzz from a woolen sweater. "Calm down. Everything will be OK in a few minutes." Miraculously, the heart reverts on command back to its normal rhythm.

"What happened there," said Bob Kormos, who had stepped out of the procedure for a while, allowing Mancini and Payne to work in concert with Griffith, "is called 'atrial fibrillation.' " There are four main chambers in the heart, beginning with the two upper or *atrial* chambers. The *right atrium* receives deoxygenated blood from the vena cava and then passes it into the *right ventricle*—the ventricles are the lower chambers—which pumps it to the lungs, where it receives oxygen. The freshly oxygenated blood then circulates to the *left atrium* and from there to the *left ventricle* and then to the rest of the body.

"The atria," says Kormos, "contain the first firing mechanism, and set the pace for the whole rhythm of the heart." When interrupted or disturbed, the heart will often start to quiver uncontrollably—or fibrillate. "So, if you 'bing' it several times, it is just like giving it electric shock, and it will put it back in the right rhythm. It becomes a game sometimes, although not in this particular instance. Surgeons sometimes like to show that they can control the rhythm of the heart, and if you hit it in the right place, you can. That's kind of a little trick that often impresses medical students." Fibrillation has many causes—loss of pressure or temperature—in addition to the introduction of foreign substances, such as heparin. Whatever the cause, however, it is a critical danger.

Perhaps the most crucial and delicate maneuver of the cardiac surgical procedure follows the injection of heparin, however. This is the process of switching the patient's circulatory system from natural resources to the "heart-lung" bypass machine, which is generally regarded as the most crucial of all technological advances in the entire realm of open heart surgery, including transplantation.

Years ago, cardiac surgeons were conducting experiments on animals which illustrated that a clear dry field for surgery within the heart could be obtained by clamping the vessels that bring blood into the heart. Their time to work effectively was limited, however, for a brain cut off from oxygen and circulation becomes inalterably damaged within five to seven minutes. During World War II, surgeons discovered that reducing body temperatures by ten to fifteen degrees (F), substantially reduced the oxygen requirement of the brain and other tissues, providing a dry field with good visibility upon which a surgeon could operate without harm for as long as fifteen to twenty minutes. The technique was achieving some limited acceptance by the early 1950s, but by that time Dr. John H. Gibbon, Jr., was about to introduce a device that would revolutionize the field of cardiac surgery: the cardiopulmonary bypass, better known as the heart-lung machine, which would, essentially, cool and oxygenate the patient's blood and pump it throughout the entire body.

Gibbon initially worked on his machine for six years at the University of Pennsylvania as a research fellow before his efforts were interrupted by World War II, after which he moved across town to Jefferson Medical College, where he had gone to medical school. Fortunately, he was able to convince the IBM Corporation to provide free of charge engineering help for the design of his machine. But even with the assistance of one of the most technologically sophisticated organizations in the world, he could not find the answers he was seeking until two of his laboratory assistants accidentally discovered that oxygenation could be increased nearly tenfold by creating turbulence in the blood as it filtered through the oxygenator. This was the final solution, the key for which Gibbon had been searching. In May 1953, Gibbon saved the life of an eighteen-year-old girl by maintaining her cardiopulmonary functions on his heart-lung machine for nearly a half hour, while surgery was being performed on her defective heart. Today, Gibbon's heart-lung machine will sustain a patient's circulatory system for many hours.

Working together, Griffith and Payne quickly complete the preparatory procedure to transfer Winkle Funk's circulatory system to the heart-lung machine. In addition to its vital life-sustaining functions, the machine is equipped with a cell saver, which will preserve uncontaminated blood. During the surgery, Payne and Mancini are actually utilizing two different suction devices, one which goes into a cannister for disposal (if they feel the blood has been contaminated) and the other which goes back into the heart-lung machine for recirculation. As part of its design, the machine will cool down the blood to reduce oxygen consumption while switching to bypass in preparation for the transplant, and subsequently warm the blood back to normal body temperature when the transplant is complete.

"Now I think we're ready," Griffith says softly to Dale Payne, who nods in response. Griffith then reexamines the connections. "Yes, I think we're ready for bypass," he says even more softly, as he once again reexamines his connections. His blue eyes above his mask go up and down, scrutinizing the machine, the masked face of the perfusionist who operates it, and the tubes that must pump and circulate the blood, oxygenated by the machine, to support the life of his patient over the next five hours. "OK," he says. "Let's do it."

The perfusionist turns the machine on. Griffith delays an instant, then "unclamps," allowing Winkle's blood to rush from the body and into the pump, which at that point automatically assumes the awesome responsibilities of Winkle's heart and lungs. Almost immediately, the perfusionist nods to Griffith—the system is working.

Doug Martin has observed that there is something "mysterious and magical" about the bypass phase of the procedure, for "essentially the patients die when they are on bypass. They aren't breathing, their hearts aren't beating: the patient is in a state of suspended animation."

Connecting the bypass and all of the other steps Griffith has taken so far throughout the procedure are exactly the same in preparing for either a heart or a heart-lung transplant. The idea is to isolate what comes in and what goes out of the heart, with the understanding that the connections (to the lung) come off with the heart connections. The heart and the lung are attached. But even after the patient is on bypass and the dissection of the recipient organs are nearly complete, Griffith will never make the critical cut, the excision of Winkle Fulk's heart-lungs from the body, until he is certain that the organs have arrived in Pittsburgh safely. He will wait as long as necessary, his patient temporarily safe on bypass.

This moment finally occurs at approximately 3 A.M., when the plexiglass box with the donor's heart-lung bloc suspended in saline solution, beating and breathing in eerily perfect rhythm, rolls into OR #5 balanced in a wheelchair, guided by Alfredo Trento and pushed by Robert Hardesty, both in green *Charlotte Memorial Hospital* surgical scrubs.

After making sure that the blood is properly perfusing the heart, while procurement coordinator Matt Armany continues to manually supply the lungs with oxygen by gently squeezing the plastic ambu (ventilating) bag, Hardesty glances across the room at his partner. "Are you ready for us yet?"

"I need about twenty-five minutes," Griffith says.

Hardesty nods, retreats around the operating table and into the tiny island between OR #5 and OR #6, lined with sinks and plastic squeeze bottles of yellow soap, where he begins to scrub. Meanwhile, with the donor heart-lung safe at Presby, the patient sustained on bypass, and her diseased organs isolated, Griffith and his surgical team move into high gear.

"OK," says Griffith quietly. "Now let's go. We commit."

With a quick series of snips with his surgical scissors, Bartley Griffith cuts Winkle Fulk's heart away, lifts it up and out of the chest cavity, and drops it into a stainless steel basin with a thud. The heart, now a lonely island of mystery and imagination, continues to beat rhythmically and peacefully in a pool of blood.

Now Griffith is poised over the patient with an oddly shaped metal instrument, somewhat similar to a staple gun, which is exactly what it is—an instrument that, when Griffith pulls the trigger, silently shoots a straight line of fifteen tiny metal staples across the root of the left lung. He then wields a scalpel and removes the pink and blue fibrous tissue of lung, which has contracted and "looks sorta like mashed potatoes," Griffith has commented. He rotates to the other chest cavity, fires another line of staples, and cuts away the second lung, depositing it into the stainless steel bowl in which he had originally placed Winkle Fulk's swollen heart, which has now and forever stopped its beating.

Bruce Reitz recalls that in his experimental work for his Mary Gohlke procedure at Stanford, he removed the heart and the lungs, en bloc. "In the monkeys, because of the shape of their chest, I could go in and easily remove the heart and both lungs together. But in the human being, it is actually easier to take the heart out first, and then go to one lung and dissect it out, and then go to the other lung, and take it out sequentially."

Suddenly in OR #5, there is a faint, high-pitched sound, like a radiator ejecting steam, and then a stream of blood shoots up, splattering Griffith's chest, staining his blue surgical gown a deep thick red, splashing onto the mask that covers his face. "Collatera?" asks Dale Payne.

"It's right on top of the trachea [windpipe]," says Griffith, nodding. He looks across the table at the anesthesiologist. "Do me a favor. Push your end of the trachea down." The anesthesiologist reaches down to Winkle's neck, draped out of sight of Griffith, to comply. As Griffith had suspected, pressure on the trachea redirects the bleeding, and muffles the high-pitched sound, which he later explained: "There are a lot of blood vessels that we call 'whistlers,' and the reason we call them 'whistlers' is because they whistle when they're cut. Noisy bleeding," he added. Griffith was able to suture this artery closed, but over the next forty-five minutes, he was confronted with a series of bleeders, some of which were quite elusive. Arteries will often snap back or retract when divided, which cause a surgeon periodically to lose control of severed vessels, which are bleeding at both ends. Working blind, Griffith would then dip his gloved hand into Winkle's chest cavity, filled with blood (from the arteries he had cut), and begin searching for them.

At one particularly difficult point, with Griffith searching and frustrated, Hardesty enters the room. He is freshly gowned and scrubbed, his hands dripping. A nurse hands him a towel. "Trouble?"

"Robert, I'm sorry I let you down here," says Griffith, "but she's bleeding pretty bad."

Dale Payne, attempting to clear the surgical field by drawing the blood out with suction, can't seem to keep up. Blood is spilling over the sides of the chest cavity, onto the table and subsequently rolling down and soaking the table drapes, and then dripping on the floor. There are bloody swabs everywhere.

"Gotta work faster, Dale," says Griffith. "No time for resting. This whole case unfortunately, you'll be working your ass off. You'll be working as hard as me."

"Anything you want?" says Mary Mancini.

"I want to be home in bed," says Griffith. "This is an elusive mother. Where the hell is it?"

With the exception of the rhythmic thumping of the ventilator, along with Payne's attempts to clear the field with suction, the operating room is now completely silent—until, finally, Griffith chooses to speak. "Well OK," he says. "Got it."

He indicates the location of the bleeder to Payne and directs and guides him to clamp and hold it, but evidently Payne is still not working efficiently enough. "Dale, I am asking you to hold this. Don't hover. All of your motions have got to be quick and decisive." There is a long pause as Griffith deftly stitches the dangerous collateral closed. True to many surgical situations, this is a quiet and anticlimactic ending to a tension-packed experience.

"I had a dream one time. Got halfway through the operation and I didn't know how to finish it," says Griffith.

"Pretty bad," says the nurse.

"You mean the dream?"

"I mean the bleeder."

"I've seen worse," says Griffith. "But I don't know when."

"What next?" says the nurse.

"That's up to Dr. Hardesty. Well Bob," says Griffith. "I guess we're ready."

Back in the rear of the operating room, Hardesty and Trento now carefully lift the precious pulsating heart-lung bloc up and out of the plexiglass box and slowly lower it into a large stainless steel basin, filled with ice and slushy saline. Their objective? To "arrest" or stop the heart. Almost immediately, the beating of the heart in the basin slows. Soon, the heart is still. The lungs decompress.

As if he is a magician with a rabbit that he has just made appear out of a top hat, Hardesty lifts the heart-lung bloc up into the air, displaying his prize. If there is a truly special moment, a triumphant instant through the transplant process, this is it. Richie Becker, a fifteen-year-old boy, who is now dead, and whose funeral will take place in Charlotte within a few hours, is giving the gift of life to a dying mother of four children, Winkle Fulk.

Hardesty then walks the heart-lung bloc over to Griffith, who, with a ceremonial flourish, embraces the whole package—the red marbled heart, the two deflated lungs, and stuffs it into Winkle's chest cavity. Now Griffith looks down at his handiwork and shakes his head with amused frustration. "If anybody tells you it's easy to know how to flip these damn things," he points down at the two lungs, "tell 'em to come and show me. I just put one in backwards."

Chapter 23

JUST ANOTHER GODDAMN MIRACLE!

In writing about the joining of blood vessels, Dr. Francis Moore in his classic clinical work, *Transplant*, states:

> For many years the joining of blood vessels seemed to be an impossible surgical mystery. Then, around the turn of the century, following the leadership of Dr. Alexis Carrel, surgeons learned to do this in a very simple way, with a needle and thread. The artery is held with a special clamp to keep the blood from leaking out, and three guide sutures are put in place. Using special small needles and thread, the two vessels are then anastomosed [from the Greek *ana*, "to," and *stoma*, "mouth"; meaning the joining of two round hollow structures such as arteries or veins] by suturing them end-to-end. The essence of the procedure is minute accuracy and delicate care in the case of the instruments and the needles. It really is very simple . . .

Simple for the skilled, experienced transplant surgeon—and simple only in comparison to the steps of the surgery that have preceded the anastomosis. In a way, says Mary Mancini, "it's like sewing two pieces of cloth together. The thing you need to be careful about is that the tissue is very delicate, so that the stitches can pull through. The type of material we use to sew is a plastic-coated synthetic thread [Prolene], which will tear cloth."

For the anastomosis, the surgeon wields a long scissors-like clamp that holds a threaded, semicircular needle, the size and shape of the edge of a dime. This is the manner in which the surgeon must sew. "You've got a curved needle in a straight instrument working down in a deep hole. It takes a little practice," said Mancini.

It also takes patience, and a high tolerance for the meticulous. The hepatic artery in an adult, for example, is less than a centimeter in diameter, and in an infant it may be just three millimeters. Surgeons use a circumference stitch, meaning that they run the sutures around and around, rather than taking one bite [tying and cutting]. They will also wear special glasses for the anastomosis which magnify the surgical field two and a half times for adults and three and a half times for pediatric cases.

This stage of the heart-lung transplant differs from the same stage in a heart procedure because there are three rather than four anastomoses. In the heart-lung transplant, the *trachea* (which conveys air to the lungs) is usually sewn first, followed by the *right atrium* (which receives deoxygenated blood from the body and passes it to the lungs). And finally the *aorta* (which returns blood, now freshly oxygenated, back to the body). But because the lungs are attached to the heart, the pulmonary artery—the artery that actually carries the deoxygenated blood from the heart to the lungs for oxygenation— remains connected.

Eventually, Griffith allows blood to be gradually transferred from the bypass machine back into Winkle Fulk's circulatory system, and within a few minutes, Winkle Fulk's new heart is suddenly quivering—fibrillating. Griffith immediately calls for the "defibrillators," a set of two long-handled paddles with circular heads. "Just as a mechanical tap will sometimes set the heart in motion," says Kormos, "an electrical discharge [with the defibrillators] will reset all the cells in the heart to zero all at the same time." Then the defibrillators are discharged again. "When that happens, the first cell that fires will then reset the rhythm for the rest of the heart."

Now there is a long period of silence as Payne, Mancini, Hardesty, Griffith, and the rest of the cardiac cadre hover in the anonymity of their masks and their blue surgical garb, watching with weary satisfaction as the heart beats, the lungs breathe, at first sluggishly, but gradually with more authority, until "it almost pops," said Doug Martin. Now Winkle Fulk, whose prognosis was almost certain death, actually begins to feel once again the rich sweet juice of life. It is 4:15 A.M.

Dr. Eric Rose, a cardiac transplant surgeon at Columbia Presbyterian Hospital in New York, finds himself sometimes confused, emotionally, at this climactic point in the transplant because "after doing so many of them, the transplant is both amazing and at the same time rather routine. I always think about what Keith Reemstma [Chief of Surgery] usually says at this point in the operation."

Reemstma, a Starzl contemporary, is a tall, gaunt, gray-haired gentleman, with a gruff but gentle manner. He will clear his throat, shake his head, and announce, according to Rose: "Well, it's just another goddamn miracle!"

Next door in OR #6, the miracle for Rebecca Treat is much longer in coming. "A lot of people come here, watch the liver transplant, see the graft sewn in, the clamps released, the liver [which has turned grayish-brown in ice] pinks up—and they leave the room," says Robert Gordon. "But at that point, the case is only half over.

"That mundane part, which they didn't stay to see, which is spending several hours, even more, just stopping the bleeding, making sure the patient is what Dr. Starzl calls 'bone dry,' is every bit as important as what has gone on before. Three of the four last patients who bled postoperatively, died. You lose patients if you close them wet. So we spend a long time cleaning up the mess and just looking after details, making sure that everything is right, and that's an important part of the operation, just as important as what's gone on before. It doesn't always take that long—on the average, the entire procedure is ten to twelve hours, but it can take as long as twenty."

Postoperative bleeding is not a frequent problem for the cardiac team, says Griffith, but when it occurs it is more serious. "The liver group faces terrible odds with respect to bleeding, but because they are implanting an abdominal organ, there's no problem if they put pressure and 'pack' [with cotton or gauze] it. You can't 'pack' a chest because the heart's got to function, and you can't put pressure on either the heart or the lungs." Also, says Griffith, "Once you get the heart and lungs in, you have no access to the areas that are bleeding because where it is bleeding is generally in the posterior [the back part] chest."

Now OR #6 is relatively silent. Back in the corner, Starzl, his hands folded in front of him as if he is praying, his glasses balanced on the bridge of his nose, is hunched forward, unmoving, on a stool. His eyes are closed, but his ears monitor the activity at the table. With the exception of occasional catnaps, he has been awake at least forty-eight hours.

At 5:35 A.M., Griffith leaves OR #5, next to where Starzl is now quietly sitting and contemplating, to go on his first break since surgery began. He drops down wearily on a soft sofa in the surgeons' lounge, joining Shun Iwatsuki, who is silently smoking a cigarette. The two men greet each other with a nod, and sit staring stonily out into space, digesting the reality of their exhaustion for the first time. After a few minutes, Iwatsuki comments casually that in his next career, he is going to do brain transplants. Griffith counters by saying that he might just as well transplant the whole head, rather than just the brain.

Iwatsuki shakes his head, inhales deeply, and shoots smoke out of the side of his mouth. "I have often threatened to transplant Starzl's head to another body, but even if I did, he would still be screaming at me. That will never stop." Griffith and Iwatsuki shatter the silence by laughing out loud, then they slump back in their seats, now even more exhausted than before because of their outburst.

Back in OR #6, even with Starzl sitting in siege in the corner, Esquivel is beginning to relax. "I go through different stages of emotions and energies during the liver transplant," he says. "It's interesting that the first part of the operation, it could be just a bloody mess, and it is when your adrenalin goes sky high. And then you take the liver out, and you sew the new liver in, and that's when you have to be peaceful, calm, sew these vessels delicately. The case changes completely from something where you are forced to work fast and remove the old liver, to something where you have to have complete control. Then, after you get the new liver in, there is another stage, and that's when you have to stop the bleeding from all the raw surfaces. That's the most boring part of the operation. A little buzz [with the Bovie] here, a little buzz there, a suture here and there. That can go on for hours. The last part is when you try to hook up the bile duct to the recipient's bile duct and to test it, and again you have to be careful and try to do it right, and that's when you are exhausted and it's at the end of the operation.

"The last part is the nicest when you see the new liver working. It makes you feel good. And you know something else; you know that now you can go find a bed somewhere and sleep for a few hours."

Next door in OR #5, Bob Kormos has stepped back into the procedure, replacing Mary Mancini, who has gone for a cup of coffee. Dale Payne is doing most of the closing. With Griffith gone and with the tension of the procedure significantly eased, the two men talk quietly and comfortably about the difficulties and joys of the surgical experience. They agree that surgery is a "creative and artistic experience," a comment that Kormos later explains. "There's a certain flow and motion during an operation that is similar to choreography, and there is a certain amount of choreography that goes into an operation. How you direct your assistants, how you control your nurses; the rhythm and flow can be very different between two surgeons, and I like to think that if I do an operation, it is not only the best I can do, but it is as good as the next person's, if not better. And all of that depends upon how you set up the operation, and how you orchestrate what happens.

"And there is also something aesthetically pleasing about the operation if it is done correctly. If you create a graft that lies just the way you want it to lie, there is a certain artistic quality to it. I've worked with wood and soapstone and a lot of times you get the same kind of satisfaction at the end of the operation, as you would after working on a piece of art."

As the activities in OR #5 and OR #6 begin to gradually decrease, the suspense in the dark overheated room one floor below—the ICU waiting area—in which Rebecca Treat's family and Dave Fulk have been camped since before "first cut," also slowly ease. "After Winkle and I said goodbye at the door to the operating room, I was tired," said Dave, "extremely tired, and I felt that now the entire situation was out of my hands. I had done everything I could. Now it was up to the Good Lord and the doctors."

"Not that we weren't scared," said Ethel Thompson, Rebecca's mother, "we were all real scared down there through the night, but I realized that if the doctors didn't come to see us right away, that the transplant was going on as planned. The nurses in ICU told me that it was about eight hours to twenty-four hours before I would know anything. In the end, it was about fifteen hours before I heard."

"When they turned the lights down and everybody settled down," said Eugene Thompson, Rebecca's father, "I was awake. I couldn't go to sleep, I *wouldn't* go to sleep, but no one was talking in the waiting room itself. Some people would step out in the hall and say a few words, then come back in and sit in the dark." Rebecca's husband, Michael, had also come up with his mother and father from Fort Campbell to be close to his wife during the operation, but according to Ethel Thompson, it appeared that the brief marriage between the two unfortunate young people would probably not last much longer. They had been separated for too long by distance and by the heartless mystery of disease for the relationship to have been sustained.

"We smoked a lot of cigarettes down in that waiting room," said Ethel, "all of us there together; we drank a lot of coffee, said a lot of prayers, and just waited. After eight hours and no word came from the doctors, I figured we had it made."

Winkle Fulk was rolled into the recovery room at about 7 A.M., May 3, where she was thoroughly bathed before being transferred to a private glass-enclosed room in the Intensive Care Unit. Bartley Griffith reported the results of the surgery to Dave Fulk in the ICU waiting area at approximately the same time. He and Dave then proceeded, separately, up to the Presby cafeteria for breakfast, where they both ate eggs, sausage, toast, and coffee, also at separate tables. At 9 A.M., Dave was permitted to visit with Winkle who, barely conscious, refused to believe that she had really been transplanted, no matter what her husband told her. "I was certain that they had opened me up and then closed me up, without the transplant," said Winkle later. "I simply wouldn't believe what Dave was telling me until he got a nurse to confirm it."

It was nearly 3 P.M. before Carlos Esquivel walked into an ICU waiting area to report the results of Rebecca Treat's transplant. Mrs. Thompson says that she had been getting scared and a little "miffed" because the liver team had taken so long "to tell us anything—any message whatsoever. But as soon as we learned that Rebecca was alright, out of recovery, and safely back into ICU, all our resentment was immediately forgotten."

Less than twenty-four hours after opening her eyes in the ICU, Winkle Fulk was once again anesthetized and rolled back into OR #5. Surgeons had discovered the formation of a clot inhibiting the flow of blood and causing her temperature to markedly increase, which meant that she had to be reopened so the clot could be eliminated before serious damage could occur. Three days later, Rebecca Treat, like Winkle, was also briefly reopened because of an infection to her wound. Both procedures, representing minor problems, went smoothly.

P A R T VI

LIFE AFTER TRANSPLANTATION

Chapter   24

THE LONG ROAD HOME

Reality is elusive during the first few postoperative days in the Intensive Care Unit, more so for liver than cardiac transplant recipients. Because the liver has yet to adjust to its new body, narcotics and other mind-altering drugs administered by the anesthesiologist will usually linger in the bloodstream longer than normal—which is also the reason liver transplant patients must endure pain without medication: The new liver may not efficiently process the medication (usually morphine). Liver patients are also in danger of suffering kidney failure due to the shock of surgery and the influx of cyclosporine and other medications and anesthetics. More than a week went by before Rebecca Treat's kidneys began to make urine.

Rebecca Treat's struggle for emotional clarity was especially severe in the ICU because of her intense encephalopathic condition (her brain was dysfunctioning) prior to surgery, which had been caused by ammonia poisoning. "During those first few weeks, she would just be burning up to the touch with fever," said her mother, Ethel Thompson, "and I was taking ice and washcloths, and constantly cooling her down. She wouldn't eat, wouldn't speak for maybe five hours at a time, and then suddenly she would grab and hold on to me, screaming for dear life. Her hands would shake. Her fingers were spastic. She had to be fed, couldn't do much for herself at all."

Complicating the situation was the fact that Rebecca also experienced an unusually severe bout of rejection (a "first rejection" episode can be predicted within the first few weeks) for which she received Orthoclone OKT3, a monoclonal (a group of cells, derived from a single cell) antibody developed in the laboratory to precisely focus on the body's killer T cells. After being tested in Pittsburgh and at other transplant centers, OKT3 has become very effective in combatting rejection after transplantation. There is at this time no replacement for cyclosporine, which must continually be used for maintenance immunosuppression, but Thomas Starzl has called OKT3 his "silver bullet, a one-time treatment used in crisis situations, when it's likely that a patient is about to lose a newly transplanted organ." The Pittsburgh transplant team has also been experimenting with what some believe to be the antirejection drug of the future, a Japanese product known only as FK-506, which has proven to be much more effective than cyclosporine at preventing organ rejection in animals. The drug will not be used in humans for at least another year, however. For the immediate future, cyclosporine remains the primary maintenance immunosuppressant, with OKT3 utilized for serious situations.

During the prescribed fourteen-day treatment, Starzl's "silver bullet" successfully fought off the rejection and gradually, as Rebecca's liver began processing waste and cleansing her body, eliminating infection, her mind began to clear. Said Rebecca: "I remember that there was a calendar on the wall, and one of the doctors, a man from Greece, Andreas Tsakis, would come in and say, 'What's today?' But I could never answer. Finally, my mother would come in before rounds, and she would tell me, 'Now today is such and such. Can you remember that?" And she would say it over and over again so that when he came in and asked me, I would be able to tell him."

"Meanwhile, we kept trying to get moved up to the tenth floor, unit 10–3," said Ethel.

Rebecca laughed and pointed at her mother. "She would sit there and she would tell me, 'Well, you can get up and walk around on 10–3. You can eat whatever you want on 10–3.' "

"I wanted to get you excited and motivated," said Mrs. Thompson.

"It seemed crazy to me. I remember finally arriving on 10–3," said Rebecca. "I couldn't walk, I couldn't do anything, I couldn't even keep my hands still enough to press the button for the nurse's call station. And I thought, 'What am I doing up here?' I remember laying on my bed and looking at my roommate. She was sitting up and talking on the phone. 'Am I ever going to be able to do that?' "

Unlike Rebecca, Winkle Fulk did not experience a serious or extended hallucinatory period. But the trauma of the initial surgery, combined with the second surgery for the blood clot, considerably inhibited her progress, causing the onset of an unshakable feeling of irritation and depression. Even when the ventilator (transplant recipients remain intubated for a day or two after surgery) was finally disconnected and the tube was removed—an event she had anxiously awaited—she did not enjoy the elation she had expected. Her breathing was weak and shallow. "Panicky," was the way she described it to Dave.

As the days went by, Winkle began to fear that maybe Hardesty and Griffith had made a mistake and not provided a heart and lungs large enough to accommodate her size. She complained bitterly to Dave, who consulted with the nurses and was assured that Winkle's depression was more or less normal. It takes time to make the emotional transition from the point of inevitable death toward an elusive but considerably more optimistic outlook—especially while bedbound, surrounded by a maze of tubes, wires, machinery.

Her feelings stabilized when she was finally transferred to cardiac care, unit 7–3. Six days later, when asked to describe her physical condition, she commented: "I'm still not breathing as well as I think I should be. But I'm thrilled to death with being able to walk. The last couple of days my legs have ached—also the bottoms of my feet—and I am thrilled that they hurt. But I'm really looking forward to walking around outside. I'm just dying to get out there in the open. So far I have walked up twenty-seven steps. I'm looking forward to going home and walking down into the basement just to see what it looks like, because I haven't been down in the basement in two years. We have a pool table there, and we used to play pool every night."

She paused and sighed deeply. "God, how I am homesick. I never have been away from the children for this length of time, and I miss them. I miss my house. I miss being home. We are very much 'home people,' and this transplant business is no vacation."

With the ICU behind them, most patients will experience a honeymoon period, a feeling of being reborn, augmented by an immediate awareness of their physical improvement— despite the trauma of surgery. The steroids, which have an initial euphoric effect, will often temporarily enhance this positive outlook. But because both Rebecca and Winkle had remained in the ICU for three weeks—much longer than the average patient—neither experienced the glee of a "new lease on life" until much later. In fact, after five weeks in ICU and on the cardiac care floor combined, Winkle Fulk's depression seemed to deepen, while her mood swings grew more intense.

"They won't let me leave," she complained. "I want to go out on a pass. I want to have dinner with Dave at Family House. I want to go home to my kids. But the doctors are cautious. 'Don't do this, don't do that. Don't get a cut. Don't get a cold,' they tell me. You know, I don't want to be a fanatic about it. I don't want to become a person who stands around with a little can of Lysol and squirts everyone. I will be as careful as I can be—within reason."

Home was becoming an obsession. "I am terribly homesick," Winkle said. "I am so homesick that I really don't even want to talk to the kids when they call. It hurts too much. It has gotten to the point, I don't even want to get out of bed or walk around. I know I am hurting myself, but I want so much to get out of here."

But when she was finally released to Family House, she suddenly didn't want to leave her "great protection" on 7–3.

"What if something happens? Who is going to take care of me?" Her hesitancy vanished very quickly, "I never expected to be so physically attached to this place. That realization took me by surprise." Finally and mercifully, two weeks later, Winkle departed Pittsburgh and Family House for Kansas City—perhaps the happiest moment in her entire life.

Depression and mood swings are only two of the many emotions suffered by the transplant recipient during the recovery period. Down the corridor from where Winkle Fulk was located, John (Ted) Allen, thirty-two, a resident of Williamsport, Pennsylvania, whose cardiomyopathy (heart muscle disease) was discovered fifteen years before while in the army, was recovering from heart transplant surgery. Four weeks after his transplant, he suddenly began crying, wringing the shirttails of his powder blue pinstripe pajamas in his pale skeletal hands.

"Initial feeling when I got out of surgery is that I haven't felt this good in years. Felt great. It was worth every minute of the hell and suffering. If today is the last day, it was worth it all. But as time goes on, you get used to it," says Allen softly, referring to the good healthy feeling that the transplant brings, "and you get to like it, and the first thing that comes into your mind is, 'Is it going to last?' The next thing that comes to mind is the same thing. It's just constant. 'Is it going to last?' And every little thing that happens, you worry. But every time I ask a question, everybody says, don't worry about it. They put you down right away to make you stop thinking about it. Then they leave the room.

"Well, after everybody cruises out of here, the wife goes home [Susan Allen is staying at Family House], I'm here by myself in this room. And there's all kinds of ghosts in here with me. Over on the wall. On the floor. I took a sleeping pill at 10:30 last night, and I was tired, but I was awake at 1:00. Nobody came in to disturb me or anything. I woke up on my own. And I sat up drinking soft drinks and eating crackers until 4:30 or 5:00 before I could fall back to sleep. It's been like that almost every night. Constant. That's the way I am. I don't know if everybody's like that. If they say I can go home next week, or the week after, or the week after that, I am just going to be so happy. Just getting out of here is going to be really something."

Allen seems stunned by the fact that he has actually received a heart transplant, and somewhat traumatized by the realization that he has lived through it. "I told them in the beginning that I could do it standing on my head. But I was wrong. From the medicine, I have moments of euphoria, where I'll be laughing for no reason at all. Then, in another half hour, depression. I wonder sometimes if I can ever adjust to this. Boy, if you've ever been in battle—I never have—but I've been in the service and been around many a guy that's been in battle. If this is what it's like, I'd turn my tail and run like hell. I wouldn't stay there for one second. I wouldn't care if they shot me or not. If I didn't have to do it [have the transplant], I wouldn't have done it. And I'm not kidding there. I'm telling you the truth. If I didn't have to be here, buddy, I'd be out, I'd be home, I'd be gone. I try to be strong about it. But it is very hard."

"You *are* strong," says Susan Allen, who has come into the room, just as her husband has been speaking. Susan is very slender, freckled. At Family House, she will often appear in the kitchen after Presby's visiting hours have ended at 9:30 P.M. in a long quilted robe, where she will sit alone in a corner, smoking, sipping coffee, and writing intensely in a journal for long periods of time. She is very soft-spoken, almost to the point of sounding meek and ineffective. But she is a high school social worker in Williamsport, and knows very well how to support the frightened man she loves. "You are very strong," she repeats.

"If I can just get through this . . ." says Ted. He is still crying, off and on, as he talks. He too is slender and small in stature. In bed, frail from surgery and years of sickness, he looks much like a teenager with an old man's face.

"You are well; you are on your way." Susan tells him.

"That's what they say. But I don't know if I am or not. I don't know if they are telling me the truth."

"They said you would be the first to know if something goes wrong," says Susan.

"They don't tell me everything. One minute they say I'm a member of the team, we're all team members around here, and you're part of the team, but I'm the last man on the team that learns anything. That's why I'm so emotional. If there's something wrong with me, I want to know. Come and tell me."

At that moment, as if on cue, a nurse, her face also masked, comes in. "What do you think about that?" Ted asks.

"What? I didn't hear what you were talking about."

"One minute they tell me that I'm alright, and the next minute they're taking blood."

"But you are alright. You are doing fine."

"You see, that doesn't mean anything to me."

"You are doing very well. It's just that your 'H' and 'H' has never gotten caught up from the surgery. That's hematocrit [a measure of the volume of red cells in the blood] and hemoglobin [that part of red blood cells that transports oxygen to the whole body]."

"He doesn't know what that means," says Susan.

"See, I don't know these things," says Ted.

"Well, he lost some blood through surgery, and he was never able to build it up on his own. Now we're just replacing it, which isn't unusual."

"Yeah, I know, but it's just that nobody tells me that."

"I just did."

"I know, but . . ."

"I told you this morning, too."

"No, you didn't explain it like that."

She laughs. "Oh, c'mon."

"No, you didn't."

"When he asked me this morning . . ." she turns to Susan.

"Why didn't the doctors explain it to me?" Ted asks.

She shrugs. "Eh."

Once again, he begins to cry. "This is hard on me."

"Yes," the nurse replies, kindly.

"I want somebody to tell me the truth. I want to get better."

"You are getting better."

"It wasn't too long after the operation that all the boogie men came out at night," says Allen, "and they were right here in this room. Last night I had to sit outside with the nurses at the station for three hours like a baby because I thought I might be infected."

"You're getting yourself all upset for nothing. You are doing fine," says the nurse. "Goodness gracious, you were out galavanting in the halls the first day up from ICU."

"I know."

"Well?"

Now he smiles. "I was showing off."

"Well?"

"I felt good."

"Well? And you still feel good."

"I can't walk."

"Today you are tired." She points to the IV pole above his head. "You can always hold on to Sally for moral support. Say hello to Sally. All my IV poles are 'Sallys,'" she says.

"Sally?"

"Yeah."

"I'm not going to call this one Sally," Ted says, tapping the pole above his head. "This one I am going to name after you."

Heart and heart-lung recipients must return to Pittsburgh at regular intervals, at first approximately every six weeks for both a biopsy and a lavage (for heart-lung transplants only), a process in which a catheter is inserted into the nose and down through the throat to both wash out the lungs and monitor for infection. Later, Hardesty and Griffith want to see patients once every three months, and then, after a year, every six months.

"I have not even started to tackle housework," Winkle said when she returned for her first visit. "Nor do I have the desire yet. The cooking, the baking, and just looking around the house and yard, that's all I've wanted to do. I am savoring the fact that I have finally made it back home. Pretty soon, I'll get down on my knees and pull out some weeds in the garden. But the biggest thrill was going to the grocery store. Just walking into the store. Getting anything off the shelf I really wanted, being able to reach it. Not being in the wheel-chair. How elating!"

Her elation continued for the next visit in September. "I went to see my old doctor, and he put me in the room and every secretary and every doctor in that whole place came in. I had to show them my scar, which is nicely healing. They all asked questions. They were truly amazed." She paused, and then said: "And that is exactly how I feel about myself—almost all the time. Amazed. Truly amazed. I feel like just going outside and screaming at the top of my lungs, 'Hey, look at me, I'm a living, breathing, honest-to-goodness miracle!"

Chapter   25

SETBACKS AND
DISAPPOINTMENTS

Unfortunately, despite the rapid recent advancement in organ transplant technology, the questions surrounding postoperative patient care far outnumber the available answers. This is an evident and troublesome reality in the highly complicated and delicate process of balancing symptoms of rejection and/or infection with an array of possible treatments, an exhausting task represented on unit 10–3 in the large charts taped on the wall beside the patient's bed and the "numbers" each chart will reveal. The charts list the results of a blood analysis, repeated and updated for most patients on a daily basis.

Early each evening, the liver transplant team will "round" to analyze the charts, which tell them, among other things, the "trough" level—or the lowest possible amount of cyclosporine remaining in the body—eleven and a half hours after the medication has last been taken. Unless the patient is on IV cyclosporine, which is not the standard postoperative practice, cyclosporine is self-administered twice a day, drunk down in apple juice or milk, usually at 10 A.M. and 10 P.M. Thus, the blood samples for 10–3 are drawn at 9:30 A.M.

The patients realize how important these "cyclosporine rounds" are (for at the very baseline the surgeons are monitoring for rejection), but they are steadfast and bitter in their resentment of the dehumanizing experience it creates—a situation in which the surgeons, en masse, will enter the patient's room, nod at the patient curtly, and proceed to discuss the patient's "numbers" for five minutes or more before turning and walking out of the room, with hardly a word to the person about whom they are so intensely speaking.

Albert Lilly, a thirty-six-year-old computer specialist and liver recipient from Scranton, Pennsylvania, suffered intermittently from opposite afflictions: cyclotoxicity—too much cyclosporine—and rejection—an indication that perhaps he was taking too little of the precious medication. Lilly grew to be extremely hostile to the surgeons and coordinators, angered by their impersonal and insulting style. "I don't know why in the hell they even come into my room. What the hell do they do when they get here? Stare at the wall?"

In Lilly's admittedly depressed state of mind, the surgeons may seem to be ineffective, but in truth, the men and women who so intently study the wall chart each day, are attempting to solve a perplexing and ever-changing puzzle. How to create stability in the transplant patient, how to establish a proper and lasting balance between the medications the patient receives to stave off rejection and the harmful side effects of those medications? The complicating factor of this situation is that no patient's numbers are apt to be identical, and thus, no patient's treatment will precisely mirror the treatment of any other patient. The surgeons literally "cook up" each day a specially designed immunosuppressive recipe for each patient on the floor.

If, for example, Al Lilly's bilirubin count has suddenly increased (indicating rejection), while his cyclosporine levels are high (indicating low absorption), the surgeon can increase the cyclosporine dosage, thereby increasing absorption that might, in turn, halt the rejection, thus lowering the "bili."

Other numbers lead to other complications, however. Considering the nephrotoxicity of cyclosporine, if Lilly's BUN (blood urea nitrogen) and creatinine (a byproduct of urine and blood) levels, both of which provide rough estimates of kidney function, begin to climb, the treatment described above might be impractical, since increasing cyclosporine would in turn increase BUN and creatinine, thereby weakening and perhaps endangering the patient's kidney function. On the other hand, the surgeons will have to consider the other medications Lilly is taking that could affect BUN and creatinine. Some antibiotics are extremely nephrotoxic, for instance, and often the diuretics (drugs that increase urination) that patients receive will dry them out too much, thus elevating BUN and creatinine. Theoretically, then, if it is determined that the increase in Lilly's BUN and creatinine is caused by other factors, the surgeons will probably take a chance and increase cyclosporine dosage as a first-line defense against rejection.

At this point in his treatment, if Lilly continues to reject his organ (which is eventually what happened), a surgeon might then attempt a heavy ballast of steroids (prednisone)— a course of action in Lilly's case that resulted in a terrible case of herpes. For three weeks, Lilly, now quarantined in a room on 10–3, was riddled with large red herpes lesions, leaking a malodorous pus and itching maddeningly. Subsequently, doctors also tried the new miracle rejection medication OKT3, to which Lilly also had a very harsh reaction.

Rebecca Treat had experienced great success with OKT3, but the doctors had extreme difficulty finding her proper trough level for cyclosporine. Even after being released to Family House, her body, for some unexplained reason, could not retain enough of the precious medication to adequately control rejection. Each week, doctors continued to increase the dosage until levels of cyclosporine became so intense she began to vomit it up. She was subsequently hospitalized for three days. Soon after, a trough level was established.

As time passed and his condition worsened, Lilly's depression and bitterness grew more acute. In the hospital, he slept through most of the day or sat in the dark in his bed, thinking, sometimes talking: "I've been back and forth to Pittsburgh several times [he was transplanted five months before], and it seems that now the thinking is that the liver I got was bad. There's nothing they can do to fix it once it's inside, so now you just go and get another one. You hear terminology about, 'Well, if it doesn't work we can just slip in another one.' That kind of stuff. I just often wonder what the doctor would think if he was sitting here and I was standing there," he pointed up at the doorway, " 'cause I've been through hell."

Although Oscar Bronsther acknowledges that the constant balancing act that the surgeons must perform for each patient, daily, is often frustrating, it is also a "very exciting thing about transplantation. Nothing is written in concrete. There is no Rosetta Stone to unlock the mystery. Things are very much in flux . . . vis à vis the use of multiple drug therapy, vis à vis the use of new drugs, vis à vis the amount of immunosuppression you can give a patient and not kill him, vis à vis the complications of immunosuppression. What we do here is not exactly 'off-the-cuff'; it is based upon the background of [Starzl's] twenty-five years of clinical and research experience, but it is often formulated on the go, on the run. You have a problem, you don't have time to go back to the lab or to textbooks or to look it up in the library [as in other medical and scientific disciplines], you say here's the problem, now let's figure out a solution, and that's—whatever the solution is—what you do. That's exciting and challenging, but yeah, it's a little bit shooting from the hip."

Although Al Lilly went home and then returned to 10–3 a half dozen times (once, riddled with herpes, he was permitted to fly into Scranton for his father's funeral, and then fly back the following day) before the desired immunosuppressive balance was finally established, he was released near the late spring of 1985, and mercifully has not needed to return. But Lilly remains acutely aware of the ever-present insecurity of life as a transplant recipient, an awareness that Terry Avery, an engineer for Boeing Aircraft Corporation in Seattle, Washington, will never escape.

Released from the hospital early in 1985, Avery spent two additional weeks at Family House. He was feeling so well and his recovery was progressing so smoothly that his wife, Maureen, felt it was safe enough to leave her husband—the family was cramped into one tiny room—and to take the children and return to Seattle, readying the house for Terry's arrival.

The day that Maureen left Pittsburgh, Terry Avery wandered the streets of Oakland, looking lazily into shop windows, stopping for snacks of pizza and ice cream, listening to the loud and happy voices of the students, hanging on the corners in front of the fast food joints that ring the cluttered inner-city campus. "I was experiencing life again," he recalls.

By the time he returned to Family House, however, he was beginning to feel somewhat sluggish and depressed, and when he touched his chilled hand to his forehead, he was convinced that he had a fever. In addition to fatigue and fever, Sandee Staschak has identified other signs and symptoms of rejection: lethargy, abdominal tenderness, light-colored stools, dark-colored urine, and yellow eyes and skin. Fever and fatigue are also signs of infection, such as flu, the common cold, or childhood diseases such as measles, mumps, or chicken pox, which are extremely dangerous to patients who are immuno-suppressed. Staschak insists that recipients, no matter where they are located, contact their local physician or (preferably) phone the transplant center if any of these symptoms persist. But because rejection and infection represent such a monumental threat to their future well-being, many patients will deny the existence of the symptoms, or delay the inevitable contact with the transplant team, hoping that the problems, with time, will pass. Luckily, however, Avery complied immediately—and not a moment too soon.

On the phone, Sandee Staschak told him not to worry, just "hustle up to the ER." When she hung up, her face was grim, however. "Emergency admission, Terry Avery," she called to a secretary in the outer office. Then she said, almost to herself, and shaking her head in disgust: "He's got pneumocystis. Damn." Immediately, Terry was transferred into ICU.

"If you would have asked us what Terry's prognosis was the day he came back," said RN Mollie Curran, a three-year ICU veteran, "we wouldn't have been too positive. He looked real bad." In retrospect, he was even worse than he looked.

Caring for Avery and the other immunosuppressed patients suffering from "opportunistic infections"—infections that take advantage of the immunosuppressed status of transplant recipients—is always a difficult and sometimes a fruitless juggling act. In order to treat the pneumocystis, the maintenance doses of cyclosporine, which had been holding the killer T cells at bay, had to be decreased, for the T cells would protect the patient from the pneumonia. But without an adequate amount of cyclosporine, the patient is no longer protected from the danger of rejection, and soon, predictably, as the virus began to clear up, Avery lapsed into rejection.

Meanwhile, Maureen returned to Pittsburgh from Seattle—she was home for about twelve hours in total—and began waiting in siege at her husband's bedside. Each day, she came to the hospital and sat beside him, clutching his hand, listening to his delirious, mumbling ramblings, nodding intently and making comforting and responsive sounds, as if he were actually speaking real words and expressing real ideas to her.

At the time, Maureen got to know another woman living in Family House, whose husband was also in the ICU unit. Darlene and Bill Huff had come to Pittsburgh from Reno, Nevada, in early September to wait for a liver transplant, but as the months passed and no liver had been made available, Bill became dejected and angry. Their children were also experiencing trouble adjusting to a new school they had to attend in a suburb of Pittsburgh—enough trouble, when combined with the empty frustration of waiting, to justify a return to Reno.

"I was just too healthy to get a transplant," Bill Huff had concluded angrily. "You have to be near dead to get transplanted here." Huff returned to Pittsburgh some four months later, weakened and submissive, apologetic to Sandee Staschak for leaving so suddenly. He was transplanted within a month, but his liver rejected, and so he was transplanted a second time. The surgery went smoothly, and his initial recovery went beautifully, so much so that the nurses decided to allow him to sit up just a few days after surgery.

Darlene walked out of the ICU as the nurses were moving her husband to the chair beside his bed. She promised she would return in a few minutes. It was the last time she would see her husband alive.

"Bill took my hand last night before I went back to Family House, and he squeezed it real tight," she told Maureen, whom she met in the corridor. "He said that he felt real good about the surgery. 'This time we got it made.'"

It was at that moment that Maureen Avery and Darlene Huff heard the code alert coming from the loudspeakers, witnessed the doctor on call and the support staff go into action in the ICU. But despite a considerable effort, it was too late. Bill Huff had arrested (had a heart attack) as the nurses had eased him into the chair by the bed. The strain of the back-to-back surgery over a period of just a few weeks had simply been too much for him.

Even before her husband's death had been confirmed—just minutes after the code had been sounded—Darlene Huff, strong and calm throughout the transplant ordeal, had turned to her friend, Maureen Avery, whose face had turned white. Darlene saw the fear telegraphed in Maureen's dark brown eyes. She raised a finger and pointed: "Don't you even think it," she stated. "This won't happen to Terry. Terry is going to make it."

Darlene's valiant assurance was warranted. Slowly and steadily, Terry Avery began to improve. In a few weeks, the doctors had been able to treat and eliminate his pneumonia, which then made it easier for them to administer the proper medication to overpower his rejection. After almost six weeks in a coma that many nurses thought would lead to almost certain death, Bud Shaw told Maureen Avery for the first time and with a great deal of conviction, "We think your husband is going to be alright." Three months later, Terry and Maureen returned to Seattle together.

Chapter 26

SYNDROME OR DISEASE?

Rebecca Treat continued to ride the transplant roller coaster after returning home to Debutante, California, for she immediately caught a mild case of pneumocystis that kept her in bed for a couple of weeks. But Rebecca, even as she lay in bed, recovering in her parents' trailer, realized that now she had to worry not only about her physical health, but also her emotional well-being. Although her husband had come to Pittsburgh the night of May 2 to wait out her transplant surgery, he had not visited her since she began her recuperative period. She had not actually seen him since February.

"After the transplant I didn't know what type of life I would be able to live," she said, "so I came back to stay with my parents for a while." Some months later, the two agreed to divorce. "The separation from my husband," said Rebecca Treat, "is really more hurtful than the transplant itself."

According to Jack Copeland, a cardiac transplant surgeon from the University of Arizona who recently completed a major psychological study of forty heart transplant recipients, two thirds of the married patients had marital problems, and more than half of the men over thirty years of age experienced phases of sexual impotency. Women recipients also reported a loss of their sex drive.

Similar results have been computed by Dr. Norman Levy, a psychiatrist at New York Medical College, who launched a systematic study of the sexual problems of kidney recipients.

Levy attributes some of the difficulty to hormonal changes associated with kidney disease. He says also that the steroids patients must take also contribute to the problem. Mostly, however, he blames the "precariousness they experience about the possibility of [organ] rejection. Sexual functioning is often an outlet in which difficulties in other areas of life are expressed."

Although his liver transplant ordeal (two transplants in fourteen months) was the most directly attributable cause of the breakup of his seven-year marriage, Tom Goddard, the Detroit police officer introduced in Chapter Eighteen, maintains that the economic and social pressures exerted by government and society, actually established the gruesome atmosphere that led to his divorce.

The pressures for the Goddards began with the police department, which he had served loyally for nearly a dozen years. Although his insurance covered inpatient and outpatient hospital care, once he returned to Detroit to recover at home, Goddard was informed that he was on his own, financially. With his wages cut off and their savings eradicated, Tom and his wife, Cathy, were forced to rely upon the generosity of other people for some of their living expenses. Friends sponsored benefit programs and fund-raising campaigns netting approximately $6,000, and co-workers took up collections about "a half dozen times." Cathy's employer paid her salary for a number of weeks as she waited with Tom in Pittsburgh. But, all together, this was simply not enough to cover their financial commitments (mortgage, car payments, etc.), which had been based upon two salaries.

To make matters more difficult, however, the Goddards soon learned that Cathy's salary, ironically, was too high to qualify the family for food stamps (welfare). Thus, although their income was reduced suddenly by 60 percent, they received no government assistance.

As a rule, the Detroit Police Department did not pay into the Social Security system, so Tom was ineligible—even though he had contributed through other employers before joining the force. In desperation, the Goddards sold one of their few remaining possessions—a wooded lot in northern

Michigan where they had once dreamed of putting up a trailer and having a summer home. Their only asset now was the tiny house in which they lived. They also approached Detroit's United Fund, but were ineligible, as individuals, to collect. Since Tom was recovering from his first transplant and then subsequently being treated for Hodgkin's Disease, responsibility for battling with the Police Department administration (which led to the Mayor's office), the union, which had failed to protect Tom, fell squarely on Cathy's shoulders. The pressure from all of these different directions became very difficult to endure. The state of near poverty into which Cathy and Tom had sunk, two working-class people who had earned a regular wage for all of their adult lives, was a great shock to both of the Goddards.

The Goddards' situation was not unique, but in their minds and in the minds of the hundreds of other families trapped by similar circumstances, the inane illogic of the situation was unfathomable. It is the ultimate of depressing and destructive ironies that federal and state assistance programs, private insurance companies, and Blue Cross and Blue Shield organizations will, often without question, invest as much as a half million dollars to save the life of a dying man or woman, but provide absolutely no assistance to help the people whose lives they have preserved return to the mainstream of productive life.

After all options were exhausted, the Goddards finally concluded that one way yet remained that would enable them to survive financially, to save their house and care for their adopted child. They separated, which meant that Tom would then be eligible for welfare payments. As long as he was with Cathy and she was working, Tom did not qualify for assistance. Their separation, compounded by all of the other problems they had experienced over the past two years, eventually led to divorce. "I think that if it would have just been the health problems," said Tom Goddard, in retrospect, "we could have coped with them together, and made it through. But all the other, outside things—the money, the fights with the department and the union, the rules and regulations, the red tape in every conceivable direction—were too much."

Not that Goddard or many of the other transplant recipients who find themselves in similar situations do not want to work. After all, they have not suffered through the debilitating gauntlet of transplantation just to remain alive—they clearly want to be productive contributors, and have an improved post-transplant quality of life. According to Roger Evans, project director of the National Heart Transplant study, conducted by the Batelle Human Affairs Research Centers in 1983, only 34 percent of 152 living heart transplant recipients had returned to the work force, either on a part-time or full-time basis one year after surgery. By the fifth year, only 20 percent were employed, while before the transplant, 80 percent had been in the labor force.

"Most transplanters are reluctant to acknowledge these figures," according to Evans. "But the fact is that most patients continue to have the same problems as any individual with a chronic disease." Evans estimated that 60 percent or more of the people on kidney dialysis are dependent on disability benefits. "If that is what we end up with in the heart transplant program, we will have just created an increasingly dependent portion of people in our population." William Van Buuren, the world's longest living heart transplant survivor (as of autumn 1987), has not been able to work in the entire seventeen years since transplant surgery.

A subsequent study conducted by the University of Arizona, however, indicated that many more heart recipients between the ages of twenty-six to forty-three very much wanted to go back, but they have been effectively stonewalled by frightened prospective employers.

Such has been Winkle Fulk's experience since returning home to Kansas City more than two years ago. Even before departing Pittsburgh after her surgery, Winkle had written her former principal, asking for her job back. "He never even answered," said Winkle. "After all I went through, I was crushed."

At first, Winkle had been content to stay at home and put the house back in order, happy to cook and garden and get to know her children once again. But within six months, she had accepted a part-time teaching position at a local junior college, teaching mathematics. In order to qualify for a full-time position at the college, Winkle subsequently enrolled in a master's degree program at another college. "Right now," two years after transplant, "I am taking nine credits at school per term—and I am teaching six." She commutes many miles a day, three days a week, often beginning her day at 7:20 A.M. and arriving home at 8:45 P.M. And yet, she says, "There's a lot of discrimination. No one will consider me for full-time teaching, although I continue to actively apply for positions."

Winkle asks an interesting ethical question: "Do I tell prospective employers that I have had a heart-lung transplant? I think it would be wrong not to tell—and it really shouldn't make any difference. I should be hired anyway, if I qualify and if I am the best candidate. I do almost make a point of informing them of the transplant, but then, during all this time, despite my many years of teaching experience, I never get the job. I know in my heart that the transplant, more than once, has been the deciding factor."

To be fair, employers' doubts about the strength and endurance of organ transplant recipients, especially those who worked (and must continue working) a labor-intensive blue-collar job prior to their illness, are understandable. Can Tom Goddard's body, wounded by two devastating transplants, withstand the sudden spurts of action and the physical and emotional abuse inevitable in the line of duty as an officer of the law? Because Goddard is one of only 1,500 survivors of liver transplantation, worldwide, there is probably no easy answer to that question at this particular time. But history demonstrates that there have been thousands of kidney recipients and a smaller number of heart transplant patients who have been able to endure a great deal of physical stress, running marathons (a "transplant Olympics" competition has been operated for three years) returning to construction work, painting houses, etc. As a heart-lung recipient, still considered an experimental procedure, Winkle Fulk is in a much smaller minority than even Goddard, but two healthy years post-transplant clearly demonstrate that she has proven her physical abilities. Must she wait until heart-lung transplantation becomes commonplace in order to be permitted to return to her profession?

Brian Reames, only the fifth patient to be transplanted by Hardesty and Griffith (in May 1981) is today a visible and outspoken symbol of the potential of transplant surgery, as well as the disadvantages and disappointments to which transplantation might lead. Reames, a captain in the U.S. Army when inflicted with heart disease, who now lives on a disability pension, has led an extraordinarily active life since transplantation, commuting four or five times each week from his home in Greenville, Pennsylvania, sixty miles north, to the University of Pittsburgh, where he has been working toward a doctorate. He has also become a recognizable and important presence at Presby for he, along with Mary Lou Michel, executive vice president, have founded TRIO, Transplant Recipients International Organization.

As president of TRIO, Reames regularly visits candidates waiting for transplantation, to answer their questions, allay their fears—and to demonstrate the energy and vigor that can result from organ transplantation. He and other members of TRIO are especially important and effective ministering to candidates frustrated by the long wait for a donor organ. Although he tries to appear as a positive role model, Reames is always extremely forthright about the many dangers and drawbacks inherent in life after transplantation.

The complications Reames has confronted just as a result of his medications include gout, bleeding ulcers, constipation, cataracts, hearing loss, weight gain, and warts. Recently, Reames suffered a stroke while having a cardiac catheterization, a process in which a tiny plastic tube is passed into the heart through a blood vessel, from which blood samples are taken for testing. The catheter that is used for a "cardiac cath" is designed for a heart in a normal position, but "my heart apparently had twisted because it is not attached in the same manner that a normal heart is. As a result, a blood clot formed on the end of the catheter," which subsequently caused the stroke. "So I was unable to move my left hand

and my left leg for a period of about four days. It's back to normal now, luckily.

"This past February, I went into a very bad case of rejection," Reames continued, "the second serious episode of rejection since transplantation, and it was kind of unusual because it had been five years since my transplant when I had my first episode. So I have come to understand and accept the fact that no matter how much time elapses, rejection will always be plaguing me."

To protect him from future rejection, Hardesty and Griffith have put him on a higher dose of prednisone. "But now I am experiencing such things as I bruise much more easily, and it takes a long time for the bruises to heal." The extra boost of steroids have given him a great deal of nervous energy. "I can't seem to sit still. I know how a hyperactive child feels. There are times when I have to come into the house and force myself to sit down and watch TV or read. Just to stop moving." And he remains troubled by his body image. "I look in the mirror," says Reames, who is blond and six feet tall, "at the round hairy face and the big pot belly, and even after six years, it's sort of embarrassing. I can't believe that that strange person staring back through the glass is me.

"Other things that I do notice is the weakness in the muscles caused by the prednisone. I don't have the strength—the physical, brutal strength that a person probably my age would have or could develop. I don't have stamina. I know I could probably dig a ditch, but I know it would probably take me a week longer than it would take another person my age who was in good health. I have noticed a change in my eyesight. Some days, I have a lot of difficulty reading, even with my glasses. Soon, I will have to have surgery for cataracts. I've noticed a significant change in my memory. I'll meet somebody and in two seconds I can't even remember their name.

"People ask me what I do for a living," says Reames, laughing, "and I say I am in medical research. I ask them [Hardesty and Griffith], 'What are the long term effects of cyclosporine?' They look at me, and they say, 'You're it.' It's the guinea pig syndrome, and I am the guinea pig. I may be six years down the road, post-transplant, but I am still on the cutting edge."

Reames is similarly forthright about the dilemma of the transplant recipient and full-time employment. Could he and other heart transplant recipients work a regular forty-hour-a-week, fifty-weeks-of-the-year job? "I am sure that there are some transplant recipients who can do that," says Reames, "but I don't know for how long. I find that I can do pretty much what everybody else can do, but I have to be very flexible. There are times when I reach a point where I can't go any further, and I have to stop, have to rest because this body just can't take that. I guess it depends upon what kind of job you are doing. Is it high stress—mentally or physically? Is there a built-in flexibility?"

Because of this fact—what might happen to them at any given moment in time—the transplant recipient is a different sort of animal, Brian Reames stresses. "You do not lead a normal life. You have to say, sometimes, 'Gee, I can't be at work today because I have to go for these tests now. Or you get the gout, which makes it difficult for you to do something, like a lot of typing because it gets into your fingers. So I would find it very difficult to say that everyone can go back to a forty-hour-a-week job. Some can, some cannot. But almost all of us can be considerably more productive members of society, if only we were given the opportunity."

As to the transplant teams' continued assertions that transplantation is not a panacea, but a disease, which will remain with the recipient forever, Reames agrees—and disagrees. "Transplantation is a lot of things. Number one it's commitment—you are committed to do certain things, to take care of yourself. You have a commitment to take the medications on schedule. You have a commitment to keep yourself active, your body working and exercising, and your mind alive with ideas. You can't sit home and do nothing because if you do, you will die.

"I would say that transplantation is more a syndrome than a disease because it is actually *many* diseases. You are trading one disease—the one you had before transplantation—for many others. But these others are treatable. Gout is treatable.

Pneumonia is treatable. Ulcers are treatable. Sinus infections are treatable. What I had before transplantation, cardiomyopathy, wasn't treatable. But the question that it comes down to on the bottom line is, 'Is it worth it?' That's a very good question, and I am sure that if you ask different people, you are going to get different answers. It's been all worth it for me, but not everyone is going to say yes quite so readily, especially those people who have been bogged down in financial difficulties caused by the transplant experience."

For the recipients to whom Reames refers—people trapped by money problems in a manner similar to the way their initial disease had trapped them in a downward slide toward death—there is no escape. The expenses for medication after transplant (cyclosporine alone can cost more than $400 a month) will require an extra $7,000 to $10,000 per recipient. Social worker Helen Michalisko of Johns Hopkins Hospital in Baltimore explains the ever-frustrating Catch-22 situation: "Someone requiring $7,000 a year for medication, plus food and other living expenses, while earning only $20,000 a year cannot support a family. That's obvious. So what are they forced to do? Under the present welfare system, they must quit their jobs and eliminate all of their assets, property and savings included, and go on medical assistance. That's the one and only way for them to survive.

"In essence, we are forcing these people to remain on the disabled list forever—despite the fact that they have had surgery that eliminates their disability. You are putting those people in a no-win situation. They are now living on public welfare with a very, very low income. But if the government would help them a little bit by subsidizing their medications while permitting them to seek employment and be paid a reasonable wage, they would become again much more productive members of our society."

Although in 1984, a Senate subcommittee recommended that cyclosporine be included under the 1972 legislation for kidney dialysis and transplantation compensation, the Reagan administration, fearful of establishing a precedent that could lead to compensation for all extrarenal transplants, a proposition they adamantly oppose because of the potentially prohibitive cost, has been reluctant to support such a resolution. Most state legislatures, when presented with the problem, have responded similarly.

Judging from the experiences of patients in Pittsburgh, white-collar workers have a definite advantage in receiving help and cooperation from employers both before and after transplantation, however. Whereas Tom Goddard lost his salary soon after transplant, Boeing continued paying Terry Avery's substantial wages long past the point at which he legally could have been forced to accept disability, a much lower rate of pay. Avery's health insurance, provided by Boeing, also covers the costs of medication post-transplant—indefinitely. Frank Rowe's employer, Philadelphia Electric, has so far paid Rowe's salary through all of his waiting time. The company has in addition provided the Rowes with a brand new rental van, a $600 per month value, free of charge.

Also, after transplant and recovery, the white collar professional will usually have his or her job waiting for him, as did Avery, who was permitted to ease himself back into a comfortable work schedule, by beginning with half-days, and generally determining his own hours. Avery, whose position required a great deal of world traveling for Boeing prior to his illness, has been able to resume the same position without travel, and without any pressure to resume travel from superiors. After a year and a half back on the job, he felt he was ready to venture beyond Seattle, so he flew to visit with a Boeing client in Japan. His travel schedule is gradually increasing.

Avery realizes how lucky he is, considering what might have happened, as does Rebecca Treat, who at twenty-one years old, divorced, with a high school diploma, and from a family of only moderate means, might have lived out the rest of her life on welfare or assistance. However, she was retired from the military, where she undoubtedly picked up her hepatitis infection, at full disability, along with an education bonus exceeding $17,000.

"I think that this in some ways may be a good thing that has happened to me," she says, in retrospect, "because I am one of those persons that tend to fall into a rut and never get out it. If I hadn't of become sick, I probably would have never gone to college. I probably would have stayed in the service and never used my college fund. Now it's like I've just graduated from high school and started all over again."

In 1987, Rebecca married a young soldier from Oklahoma and soon became pregnant. This was not a first by any means in the world of organ transplantation—a few dozen extrarenal recipients have fathered or mothered children over the years— but it remains a very unusual and in some ways a controversial occurrence, not only because of the precariousness of a recipient's future, but also because of the danger of transferring the side effects of the drugs into the fetal circulatory system. Rebecca, however, remains confident and feels strong, in control of her destiny.

"I am often involved in a situation where another person, considering what has happened to me, might assume that I am not strong. But I can sit there and think, 'You don't know what kind of hell I have been through. I have survived, and I am a lot stronger than you think I am.'"

For Tom Goddard, after a long and difficult series of setbacks, the future looks brighter. At some point, his union's president had suggested that Tom look back into the history of his disease to determine, possibly (as in Rebecca Treat's case) if it was a work-related problem. Goddard subsequently reexamined his medical file and discovered an incident that shed light on his past, and brightened his future prospects. "About six months before I started having liver problems, I had been stuck with a dirty hypodermic needle while searching a drug addict that we had arrested. I had forgotten all about it, but I had made an injury report on it, and when I went through my medical file, I found it. We contacted the doctors in Pittsburgh, and Starzl in a letter to the pension board, confirmed that my original liver contained evidence of hepatitis. With this information, documented by Starzl, Goddard was soon awarded a pension equal to one that a police officer might receive after serving twenty-five years on the force.

What will he do next? "Go back to school, and pick up another trade. I was a cop for twelve years and that's all I know. I still miss it, but I have been thinking about looking for a counseling type position with people who are going through what we have already been through. But I'm still a little leery of something, infection, rejection—whatever—anything could happen," says Goddard. "But I am feeling safer lately. It's been almost a year since I've been in the hospital, and I haven't had a bit of problems since I've been home."

That one-year mark is an ideal guidepost. Episodes of infection and rejection decrease by 75 percent after the first twelve months. From a mental-emotional standpoint, according to psychologist Ralph Tartar of the University of Pittsburgh who, along with gastroenterologist David Van Thiel, is in the process of studying the long-range recovery periods of 100 liver transplant recipients, a year is also a landmark of achievement. "We're finding that the mental capacities seem to be returning to normal within one or two years after transplantation. There are some persistent emotional issues, but not all people have them. These people have had chronic liver disease for years, and to expect them to reverse quickly is totally unrealistic. We are finding progression of improvement, but it is not perfect after one-year post-op."

According to Van Thiel, "This is a good news/bad news finding. The good news is that they were better than they were. The bad news is that they're not perfectly normal. But they are getting steadily better."

Terry Avery can feel the steady improvement in his health, as time slowly passes. He says that he has been playing a lot of golf since returning to Seattle, and exerting himself around the yard, "moving railroad ties, doing heavy work. The funny thing is, that before the transplant, I was to the point where I was having a terrible time with back problems, muscular aches, joint problems, knee problems, shoulder problems. And all of a sudden now, my golf game has improved by about five strokes. I am experiencing no back pain, and I have developed a tremendous backswing! To me, it's fantastic, the difference. I had four nine-hole rounds of forty over the past few weeks, and I haven't had a round in the forties before, since I was eighteen years old.

"The other startling fact is that, in the same league I play in, there's a guy, about sixty years old, who had a bypass operation about three years ago. A very nice guy. But unluckily, he had a bad blood transfusion and he got hepatitis from it. Last spring, they gave him five years to live. So he's retired now, and maybe too old and at this moment too healthy for a liver transplant, and I have watched his golf game deteriorate like mine did. It's been ironic because I never really noticed it when it happened to me. I really wasn't realizing what was going on, but progressively I could not hit a ball as far. I was taking more iron shots, and my eyesight was getting bad. The same thing is happening to this guy. His skin is getting yellow, an increasing amount of discoloration. It's just ironic and uncomfortable to watch it happen."

Memories of those terrifying days of fear and uncertainty seem to haunt Maureen Avery much more so than they do Terry, however, because she is the one who endured the reality of the experience, while he languished in a deep and dangerous coma. "I still think about the whole thing a lot," she says, "not the liver part, but the six months with pneumocystis, that relentless siege in ICU, probably because I know it can happen again, and real fast, like it did before. When the kids sneeze or anything, or if somebody has the flu, or when flu season is starting, I get upset and scared that Terry might catch the infection. I still spend a lot of nights waking up and thinking about going through the ordeal in ICU. The years will go by, but I can tell you one thing: I'll never forget it."

Indeed, organ transplantation is an ordeal that cannot be forgotten, not only because of the long road of pain and suffering through which the patient and family must travel prior to the transplant experience, but also because of the gauntlet of danger that is awaiting them forever thereafter. No better example of this situation exists than Brian Reames, who suffered a sudden heart attack in September 1987. Today, he remains at home, bedbound, Status 1 on the Hardesty-Griffith transplant list, waiting, just as he had waited seven years ago, for the magic phone call that will summon him to Pittsburgh for retransplant—a further extension to what has become for Reames and for many others, the unavoidable reality of the transplant experience: a beautiful, but often-flawed, second chance.

Epilogue

THE MIRACLE

In discussing his approach to his work, the journalist Gay Talese has said that it has always been his ambition to remain with the characters about whom he was writing long enough to see their lives change. When I began this book four and a half years ago, it was my ambition to remain with my characters—candidates for organ transplants—long enough to see their lives saved. In the process of my work, I was able to see how their lives changed because they were saved, and I saw, perhaps even more clearly because of my long-term period of observation, the lives of the people who saved them change as well.

In Pittsburgh, the most visible, although not necessarily the most dramatic change, has occurred in the area of organ procurement, where the Pittsburgh Transplant Foundation, with Brian Broznick replacing Donald Denny, has disconnected itself from its original home base, the University of Pittsburgh, purchased its own building, and moved two miles down the road. Meanwhile, a rival cross-town hospital, Allegheny General Hospital (AGH), was granted permission to launch its own kidney transplant program and that institution and Pitt, Children's, and Presby are the constituencies that the Pittsburgh Transplant Foundation will serve from its new headquarters. (Some months later, AGH was granted permission to do heart and pancreas transplants as well.)

The fact that Broznick has actually moved the Pittsburgh

Transplant Foundation to neutral territory is also indicative of great change. Even though physicians still dominate the expanded nineteen-member Board of Directors, the expansion and relocation symbolize rather dramatically a gradual separation of church and state (procurement and the hospitals in which the transplants are performed) in the world of organ transplantation. That bold step, combined with the recent governmental funding and subsequent formation by UNOS (United Network of Organ Sharing) of the national organ distribution network, will eliminate any potential conflicts of interest.

I am not at all certain that the procurement coordinators are completely enjoying their newfound freedom from the health center, however. The building the Foundation now owns is spacious and well-equipped, as are the coordinators' individual offices—much more comfortable and prestigious than the tiny closets in which Hardesty, Griffith, and Starzl must sit. Broznick has also hired a fifth coordinator—their first woman—and a number of technicians (RNs) to accompany the surgical teams on long-distance procurements. Now coordinators handle all local donor referrals and coordinate in the usual manner out-of-town procurements, but with the "techs" now available, their presence is no longer required to surgically assist. This new system has permitted a substantial improvement in their private lives, but it has also led to a partial loss of that "adrenalin high" to which many coordinators had become addicted. The physical tension and emotional excitement on which Bob Duckworth, Matt Armany, Broznick, and Denny once fed are not completely missing, but are certainly less intense and thereby less rewarding.

It is important to point out, however, that I am describing the look of the future in organ procurement—in fact, in the entire world of organ transplantation—and not the reality of the present. As you travel to and from transplant centers in the United States and England as I have done, you begin to realize how far advanced Pittsburgh really is—not just technologically, but administratively, as far as the size and capability of its personnel. The gap in experience is tremendous. Throughout most of the country, organ transplantation is revolutionary—high-tech medicine at its purest and newest form. In Pittsburgh, organ transplantation is not only high-tech and constantly changing, but it is also business—the biggest business the university and the health center have ever experienced.

AGH's attempt to launch its own transplant operation in the literal lap of the largest and most prestigious organ transplant program in the world is evidence not only of change but also of the potential future of organ transplantation. In 1983 and 1984, when Mary Katherine Smith, Terry Avery, Kellie Cochran, and the other patients whose stories were told in this book learned that they needed a liver transplant, they could choose from only two medical centers (Pittsburgh and Minnesota) across the United States, and Cambridge in England. Today, there are thirty-five such centers. A similar evolution has occurred for hearts and heart-lungs. First there was Stanford, and then Stanford and Pittsburgh, and now Winkle Fulk could go to any one of a dozen medical centers for evaluation for heart-lung transplantation, while Brian Reames would have more than 100 options across the United States for the less dangerous, less challenging heart transplant procedure. These days, it is not unusual for candidates for extrarenal organ transplantation to have been evaluated and wait-listed by two or even three transplant centers.

Although it is very costly in terms of facilities and support staff to launch an organ transplant program, the most formidable challenge for AGH and other institutions expanding into transplantation is in locating and attracting competent surgeons with enough training and experience to perform the highly technical and continuously demanding surgery, followed by the even more delicate and difficult task of managing the constantly tenuous immunosuppressive regimen. To find an experienced surgeon for their new transplant program, AGH reached 1,000 miles into the Midwest to the University of Iowa Medical Center for Dai D. Nghiem, a Vietnamese refugee who had immigrated to this country nearly twenty years ago. Indeed, had Nghiem not been willing or available, AGH could have and would have extended its search 3,000 or even 10,000 miles if so required. But the fact of the matter is that wherever

AGH would have searched and whomever they might have selected, the surgeon they recruited would probably not only be coming to Pittsburgh to start an organ transplant program, but also he or she would be *returning* to Pittsburgh and/or to the womb of his or her mentor—the person who made a career in transplantation possible: Thomas Starzl.

It would not be incorrect or overly dramatic to state that Thomas Starzl towers like a tree in the transplant world. There are other trees, such as Shumway, Cooley, Barnard, but no tree stands taller than Starzl, no tree's roots reach out and embrace so many patients and enrich so many disciples, such as Nghiem at AGH, who trained under Starzl, and many of the other surgeons discussed extensively in the book. In the field of liver and (in a modified form) renal transplantation, Thomas Starzl has fathered a second generation of transplant surgeons to follow in his footsteps, to turn the trail he has blazed into a modern medical highway of lifesaving.

It would be fair to say that Hardesty and Griffith are in the forefront of that second generation of transplant surgeons. Over the past year, they have pioneered the use of the artificial heart as a bridge for transplant patients waiting for an organ, and in so doing have preserved many lives that would have been otherwise lost. Their miraculous heart-lung box was recently put to rest, incidentally, eighteen months after Winkle Fulk's procurement, with the inevitable emergence of a new method of lung preservation developed simultaneously in England and by Stanford in the United States, which extends the ischemic time of the lung to three hours—nearly equal to the heart—through a simple adaptation of Starzl's original core-cooling technique. But the strange and jerry-rigged box to which they and their associates had dedicated so many hours and such superhuman effort, can be directly linked to the salvation of nearly two dozen lives.

At the International Organ Transplant Forum in Pittsburgh in September 1987, the largest and most prestigious gathering of transplant specialists and recipients ever organized in the United States, a ten chemical potassium-rich solution called UW-lactobionate, was unveiled by the University of Wisconsin, which potentially could preserve donor livers for twenty-four hours—or longer—thus providing surgeons with more valuable time to match and transplant donors and recipients. There were other glimpses of the future provided at the forum. Although the areas of fetal and brain transplantation seem to be attracting the attention of the national media, a more widespread scientific interest was indicated in *xenografting* and in the transplantation of body parts.

In Pittsburgh, researchers have transplanted hands from one set of baboons to another. In the Netherlands, thumbs from macaque monkeys have been traded, while in Belgium, kidneys have been transplanted from pigs to baboons—a few with moderately good, albeit temporary results. Cyclosporine has been used to combat rejection in the experimental work of Dr. David Furnas of the University of California (Irvine), who illustrated in a slide presentation how forelimbs, jaws, noses, and ears have been transplanted successfully from black Dutch rabbits to white New Zealand rabbits. Dr. Zhan Bing-Yan of Hubei Medical College in Wuhan, China, reported that he has conducted thirteen living related procedures, successfully transplanting testicles in men suffering from sexual dysfunction.

Throughout the forum, scientists stressed that the purpose of the animal-oriented studies, especially, were not to create bizarre composites, but to serve as a testing ground for future transplants of limbs and facial bones from cadavers to people severely injured in fires and traffic or industrial accidents. These studies show the real direction of transplant technology in the coming decades—a slow transition from the "lifesaving" procedures of hearts, livers, and heart-lungs to surgeries similar to those detailed above, with the potential of enhancing "life quality."

But indeed, the vast majority of discussions and papers focused upon the ever-pressing unanswered questions in the world of transplantation, which included the side effects of immunosuppressant medications, the social, economic, ethical, and cultural problems resulting from transplant technology as discussed in this book, and the most critical of all unsolved issues: the unyielding dearth of donor organs—a depressing fact of life that I personally could never quite evade because of my long and close relationship with a man who has observed the evolution of the world of organ transplantation for almost as long as I have, but with a more unique perspective: Frank Rowe of Philadelphia, now a transplant candidate for three consecutive Christmases.

As I have indicated before, during his time in Pittsburgh so far, waiting for an organ donor, and waiting to become close enough to death for Hardesty and Griffith to be willing to take the chance with his life, Rowe has lived and breathed transplantation, working tirelessly, and with all of his remaining and steadily depleting energy, for the cause of organ donation. Despite the fact that his health continues to erode, Rowe has steadfastly maintained his faith in the transplant system and held firm to his optimistic philosophy of opportunity: to live a high-quality life with his loyal and dedicated wife, Joyce, for as long as humanly possible, and to help people in circumstances similar to his by "ministering" this philosophy of opportunity to them. Part of Rowe's ministering includes talking with other people who, like him, are facing the specter of inevitable death.

At a quiet dinner at his house not long ago, I told Frank that one of my very oldest and dearest friends would soon be visiting me who, at forty years old, was recently diagnosed as having incurable lung cancer. Depending upon the effectiveness of her chemotherapy treatment, she was given only one to three years to live. It was at this point that Frank volunteered his assistance. "I would appreciate talking with her," he said. "I might be able to help her since this—dying—is something I have been, obviously, repeatedly contemplating."

I told Rowe that I thought that I could arrange a meeting, but I hastily and naively pointed out that the circumstances of their situations were considerably different, first because his transplant could potentially save or significantly extend his life, whereas there was no window whatsoever to my friend's future. I also commented that she was only recently diagnosed, and so had had only a few months to think about her fate, while he had had three years to mull it over. To him, in a manner of speaking, this was an old story.

Frank and Joyce Rowe, incidentally, were the last of a group of approximately thirty patients and families that I had be-friended in 1984 and in early 1985, while I lived at Family House, whom I chose to follow through the organ transplant ordeal. Each of those patients had had some ending come about to their transplant stories, either by being transplanted (and living or dying in the process) or dying while waiting for a donor organ. Frank Rowe was the only candidate of that initial group I had selected who was still waiting.

The Rowes had faced a difficult up and down battle to remain courageous and positive during this unrelenting ordeal, an often embarrassing and personally revealing process that had, without exception, been made open to me. I must say that most of the patients and families with whom I became close were also very forthcoming. Their need for concerned companionship, for a sympathetic yet somewhat removed and objective listener, is overwhelmingly evident. I filled that void for them sometimes, and in the process, I learned a great deal about how people, necessarily brave and obviously fright-ened, viewed life—and faced death.

Frank paused for a while after I had made my comment that evening and looked across the room at me. It was a week before Christmas, and I was dining, ironically enough, at the Rowes' new house in Pittsburgh, one that they had just pur-chased at Thanksgiving time. They had always wanted to pick out a new house together, Frank had explained (in Phila-delphia they lived in Joyce's parental home), and they had come to realize that waiting for a donor organ and subsequently enduring the process of transplantation, when and if the donor organ arrived, made little sense. "If I die," Frank had said, "at least Joyce will have a home which we selected and shared together, however fleetingly."

The lights had been dimmed in the homey dining room as we finished dinner. Christmas decorations and evergreen boughs salvaged from their church's recent Christmas party, where Frank had read from the scriptures to the entire congre-gation, were hanging from the mantels and draped around the windows and sills. Handmade quilts and the many other early-American crafts that Joyce and Frank had so carefully and diligently collected over the years, now covered the walls.

"The prospect of dying can never get old," Frank said to me quietly, in a near whisper. "You think about it all the time—it continuously pervades some part of your consciousness. After a while, I guess you come to accept the notion that tomorrow you might not wake up in the morning—you might be dead—but you never get used to it. Never once. Not ever. The knowledge and the thought constantly haunt you."

Similarly, Dick Becker, Richie's father, has never gotten used to the death of his only son, to whom he was so faithfully devoted; never once has the weight of that loss been lifted from his consciousness. This unfortunate and pervasive reality was especially apparent one Sunday in Charlotte, North Carolina, when I brought together, all in one room, Richie Becker's parents, Dick and Sharon, along with the recipient of Richie's heart and lungs, Winkle Fulk, and her husband Dave.

As it turned out Richie had been an amazingly productive donor—perhaps the most productive in the history of organ transplantation. In addition to a liver and a heart-lung, there were two kidney recipients, a young man from Saudi Arabia, who had subsequently returned to his country to further his studies, and a twelve-year-old Egyptian boy, whose family had relocated in Pittsburgh, where he attends school. One of Richie's corneas had not been successfully transplanted, but the other cornea had improved the sight of a twenty-five-year-old mother of two from Charlotte, Glenda Alexander.

The fact that Ms. Alexander is a black woman, while Richie Becker is a white male, and that two of the five recipients are foreign nationals demonstrates the universal humanitarianism of organ donation—a gesture that Rebecca Treat will extend one generation further when she gives birth to her child, who is due late in 1987.

Rebecca, and the other recipients were, unfortunately, unable to participate in the extraordinary "reunion" in Charlotte. Only Winkle was in attendance, and she continues to be recuperating very nicely. For their frequent papers and presentations demonstrating the accomplishments of the cardiac transplant program, Bartley Griffith and Robert Hardesty often utilize slides of Winkle Fulk, horseback riding, bowling, enter-

taining guests, or working in her garden. This, and other relevant facts about her past and her hopes for the future, including
her ongoing lack of success in finding full-time employment,
she nervously and hesitatingly explained to Dick Becker and
his wife Sharon, who held their one-year-old daughter, Erica,
on her lap that warm summer evening.

If anyone in that room was more nervous and more excited
than Winkle Fulk, however, it was Dick Becker, a short, conservative, and soft-spoken man, who does not seem, at first
meeting, to be a very easy-to-get-to-know individual. But after
we all got comfortable in the Beckers' new suburban lakeside
home, Dick loosened up and began speaking very directly
and honestly, and in a seemingly uncharacteristic and impas-
sioned manner.

"I'll tell you what, I'll be very truthful with you," he said,
directing most of his conversation that evening toward Winkle, exclusively. "This week has probably been one of the
longest weeks of my life. I didn't think this weekend was
ever going to get here. I kept looking at the calendar, and it
always seemed to be Wednesday. Yesterday, we went grocery
shopping, and when we got back I told Sharon I was tired—
we had stayed up late Friday night—so I sat down on the
couch, and I wanted to watch a movie on television, thinking
it was 10:00. I turned the TV on, turned the right channel
on, but the movie I wanted to see wasn't on, and for a while
I couldn't figure out why. I got the *TV Guide* out to see if I
had the right night. Then I looked at the clock. It was 8:30—
only 8:30. I tried everything to get the time around sooner
to when you would arrive," Dick Becker emphasized. "I was
very nervous about seeing you, but I was also driven by it.
So was Sharon, I think."

Across the living room, Sharon Becker sat on the floor,
comfortable in Levis and a T shirt, as she tended to Erica,
and listened intently to the conversation between her husband
and the woman who had been blessed with her stepson's heart.
Right before this particular conversation had begun, Dick had
lifted Erica up into his arms, carried her out into their spacious
backyard, and disappeared for some time behind the trees
that encircled their home.

"A lot of times," Dick Becker said, now continuing, "like I did this evening before dinner, I'll take Erica out in the backyard about at sunset. She likes to watch the sun sink down through the leaves at night, all the silhouettes and such. And if she doesn't go to sleep out there, with me sitting in the hammock or something like that, we'll come in and we'll walk around in our bedroom, listen to a little music box we have. Well, the other night, while Sharon and Erica were in the bedroom and the music box was playing, I went into the bathroom down the hallway, and I heard Sharon talking to Erica, as she was walking around trying to get her to fall asleep. This was like Tuesday or Wednesday night, and she was kind of whispering to Erica, patting her on the back and everything, and saying, 'You gotta be good Sunday because Richie is going to come and visit for a little while.' Later on, after she put Erica to sleep, I asked Sharon what she meant by that.

" 'Well, she said, 'I don't believe that Richie is actually coming back, I just think *part* of Richie is returning.'

"You know," said Dick Becker, "it sounds damn silly, but I think that, in a way, she was right. We could both feel that something special was happening this week. We really, really could. This, your visit here, was a homecoming to us," he told Winkle, as he leaned forward. He seemed to be edging closer to her, as if he wanted to reach out and touch her, as if there were hundreds of thoughts he wanted to communicate to her, if only he could find the exact words with which to say them. "I don't believe that Richie in his death could have given us anything that we could have or would have cherished more than seeing you, alive and well, being able now to take care of your family," he told Winkle. "For us, Sharon and me, it is great solace."

At the end of the evening, just as we were about to say goodbye and return to the motel—we were going back to Pittsburgh the following morning, where Winkle was scheduled for a biopsy—Dick Becker stood up in the center of the living room of his house, paused, and then walked slowly and hesitantly over toward Winkle Fulk, who had once stood alone at the precipice of death. He eased himself down on his knees, took Winkle Fulk by the shoulder and simultaneously drew her closer, as he leaned forward and placed his ear gently but firmly first between her breasts and then at her back. Everyone in that room, including Richie's godparents, who had also come to visit, was suddenly and silently breathless, watching as Dick Becker listened for the last time to the absolutely astounding miracle of organ transplantation: the heart and lungs of his dead son Richie, beating faithfully and unceasingly inside this stranger's warm and living chest.

Afterword

MANY SLEEPLESS NIGHTS, 1990

The expansive scope and persistence of Thomas Starzl's vision has led to the formation of more than seventy liver transplant centers in the United States alone. Some of the most prominent of these are the University of Nebraska at Omaha, initiated by Byers (Bud) Shaw and Patrick Wood; Baylor University in Dallas with Goran Klintmalm; and Pacific Presbyterian Hospital in San Francisco, directed by Carlos Esquivel (Rebecca Treat's surgeon), who also recruited transplant coordinator Vicki Fioravanti and anesthesiologist Douglas Martin from Pittsburgh.

In the cardiac transplant field, Robert Kormos, originally from the University of Toronto, and John Armitage, a surgical resident at Presbyterian-University Hospital during the same period, are now attending surgeons in Pittsburgh, spearheading heart and heart-lung transplantation. Robert Hardesty and Bartley Griffith are pursuing new avenues in clinical and laboratory research, most especially on an implantable left ventricular assist device (LVAD) called Novacor designed to work in tandem with the biological heart. A long-range goal is to develop a totally implantable artificial lung, perhaps by the year 2000. Pittsburgh's first woman cardiac transplant surgical fellow, Mary Mancini, who scrubbed on Winkle Fulk's procedure, is now director of cardiac transplantation at the Medical College of Ohio. The rapid proliferation of transplant centers throughout the country has been most dramatic in the cardiac area, with approximately 150 programs to choose from—nearly four times the number in existence five years ago.

With costs which can exceed one million dollars for chronic and complicated liver and heart-lung patients, it should come as no surprise that organ transplantation has evolved into big business, often breeding heated competition. This rivalry occurs not only because of economics, but also due to the aggressive and hyperactive personalities of the surgeons who have pioneered transplantation from dream to reality over thirty-five years. This competitive tradition was aptly illustrated by Henry T. Bahnson, former chief of the Department of Surgery at the University of Pittsburgh, in a presentation at Tulane University:

In Paris in 1951, Marceau Servelle had experimentally transplanted kidneys in about twenty-five dogs. He learned that a murderer was to be guillotined and obtained permission from the judge to remove for transplantation one kidney just after execution. When he arrived just before the execution, he found a resident from a competing service expecting to do the same thing. The issue was decided by the fact that the resident had neglected to bring sterile linen. For allocation for this resource in the future, we must have better criteria than who remembers to bring the linen.

Over the past few years, the major problems concerning the distribution of available donor organs—a considerably more complicated task than assuring sterility of equipment and supplies—essentially have been solved. The more serious and long-range problem, however—and perhaps the real failure in the organ transplant movement in this country—is the crisis brought about by the continued shortage of organ donors. In January 1990, according to the United Network of Organ Sharing, seventeen thousand patients were awaiting kidney transplants, with an additional three thousand requiring heart, liver, pancreas, heart-lung, and lung transplantation. During 1984 and 1985, Winkle Fulk waited a little more than a year after being accepted as a candidate; today there would be a good chance that she would die while waiting for a matching heart-lung bloc.

As of this writing, the federal government's new and well-intentioned "required request" legislation, which mandates that hospitals ask families of potential donors to consider donation—or be in jeopardy of losing federal funds—has been generally unsuccessful. No mechanism exists to enforce required request, and attorneys speculate that any attempt at coercion could be entangled indefinitely in litigation. What is so frustrating to transplant coordinators such as Brian Broznick and other members of the North American Transplant Coordinators Organizaion (NATCO), is that many more people would be willing to donate if only they were properly approached and asked. Results of a study conducted by the Pittsburgh Transplant Foundation indicate that six hundred potential organ and tissue donors were bypassed in 1987 in the state of Pennsylvania alone.

Although reimbursement for kidney (covered by Medicare since 1972), heart, and liver transplantation is not as much of a problem as it was five years ago, ethicists and legislators have recently refocused attention on the economics of transplantation, especially those lifesaving attempts which lead to three, four, and even five liver retransplants. In addition, the experimental "desperate measure" procedures, such as the multiviscerals (total abdominal), may well be, according to the esteemed historian and retired distinguished professor at Harvard University, Francis D. Moore, "the most expensive form of hospitalization known to humanity."

Who will carry that financial burden in the future, Moore wonders—a burden which, he estimates, far exceeded one million dollars alone for Tabatha Foster, who died after living for six months. How are such expenditures justified, considering the inequitable distribution of the health care dollar in this country? There has been one recent development which, hopefully, is an aberration and not a sign of the times. In April 1989, in order to decide which health care service to finance, the Oregon state senate established a commission to prioritize categories covered by Medicare. Organ transplantation was listed on the bottom rung, along with cosmetic surgery.

As I have indicated repeatedly in this book, many surgeons believe it is not their responsibility or their right to make decisions for or attempt to influence society and their patients. Just as the military is bound to leave politics to elected officials, surgeons more often than not abstain from the economic and psychosocial problems created by the excellence or the limitations of their work. Now, however, may be the time for surgeons to become more active, both within the transplant community and throughout the nation at large, not only in an effort to stimulate organ donation, but to preserve and protect the future of organ transplantation.

Who else but the transplant surgeon can lobby and testify influentially for legislation permitting the use of anencephalic babies as donors? Who else can push authoritatively for establishing acceptable incentives to donate—including tax credits or compensation for funeral or burial services, an idea supported by many surgeons? Who, other than the leading men and women in the field, can more effectively help unite the transplant community into one large and powerful organization committed to protecting the rights and interests of recipients such as Winkle Fulk and Tom Goddard, and other men, women, and children who have been bypassed for employment and government assistance simply because they had had an organ implanted in their bodies?

In an interview, surgeon Keith Reemstma, an early transplant pioneer at Columbia Presbyterian Hospital in New York, marveled at Thomas Starzl's foresight and presumption in lobbying for liver transplantation in Washington with the National Institutes of Health (NIH) in 1982–83 and testifying at congressional hearings—even going so far as to discuss the topic with Mr. and Mrs. Reagan. (One of Starzl's mentors had been Dr. Loyal Davis of the University of Utah, Nancy Reagan's father.) What was so ironic to Reemstma was that heart transplantation was a much more sophisticated and accepted procedure at the time, with a one-year survival rate significantly better than liver transplantation. Yet because of

Starzl's one-man lobbying effort, liver transplantation became an approved treatment modality by the NIH, which essentially meant that insurance carriers would pay for the procedure—months before heart transplant recipients were accorded the same benefits. "I don't know why we [cardiac transplant surgeons] weren't also out beating the bushes in Washington," Reemstma told me. "In retrospect I have to admit that we should have been more aggressive. Starzl beat us to the punch."

When I began researching this book in 1984, one of Pittsburgh's liver transplant attending surgeons, Robert Gordon, remarked that Starzl normally pushed his surgical team to perform two or three transplants a week for three or four months at a clip—and then would back off for a couple of weeks to allow for a much-needed recuperative period before starting up again, full-throttle. Less than five years later, in stark and incredible contrast, Pittsburgh's liver transplant program performed sixteen procedures—twelve liver transplants and four "organ cluster" operations—in one typical week in July 1989. Pittsburgh will perform more than six hundred liver transplants in 1989 alone.

Not yet even a gleam in Thomas Starzl's frenetic eye when I began this book, an organ cluster operation is a procedure, developed for patients suffering from pancreatic and/or hepatic cancer, in which the liver, pancreas, duodenum, stomach, spleen, and colon—all areas affected by cancer—are resected and partially replaced. Pittsburgh's transplant team has also invented a "modified cluster" (also called an upper abdominal exenteration) in which the spleen, stomach, pancreas, liver, and part of the small bowel are removed and singularly replaced by a donor liver. In the spring of 1989, Starzl told the *Journal of the American Medical Association* (JAMA) that eleven of the thirteen adults who had received an "organ cluster" transplant remained free of cancer for as long as six months. After nearly a year, most of those patients have remained cancer-free, and Starzl, true to his transplant obsession, continues to orchestrate this new procedure at an ever-increasing rate, although he admits that even a year may not be sufficient time to adequately and accurately gauge conclusive results.

Anyone who has ever had the privilege of observing or interacting with Thomas Starzl to any significant degree will admit without hesitation that he is the most perplexing, frustrating, driven, argumentative—and brilliant—human being they have ever encountered. His advancing years (he will be sixty-five by the time this edition is published) and his recent success have not altered his personality or his shoot-from-the-hip style to the slightest degree. If you talk to staff members at Presbyterian-University Hospital or Children's Hospital or to his fellow surgeons from around the world, they will tell stories of fiery temper tantrums which enrage and embarrass subordinates and colleagues alike; incredible kindnesses which soothe frightened and miserably sick children; and sincere humility with strangers who seek his autograph or the opportunity to shake his hand. In my interviews and discussions with nurses, doctors, and patients, Starzl has been called charming, maniacal, charismatic, egocentric, heroic, and humble, as well as "the ultimate human being," a "Clint Eastwood incarnate," "the man who talks to God," and "the slickest snake oil salesman to ever be put on this earth."

Although none of these descriptions are completely accurate or fair, there is probably a measure of truth in most everything that colleagues, detractors, and objective observers have said about him. To a great extent, Starzl seems to lack an understanding of the complexities of his personality and of how his actions and reactions—positive and negative—will significantly affect a great many other human beings.

I do not want to mislead anyone into believing that Thomas Starzl has been and continues to be oblivious to the many honors and awards that have been bestowed upon him or to the criticisms under which he has had to function, especially during the past few years. There is no question that the stories generated by the *Pittsburgh Press* concerning transplantation of foreign nationals hurt him a good deal—an injury and an insult that he will not soon forget. With time, however, Starzl has come to be more accepting of such situations, continuing to believe in himself with an unbending passion and to conduct himself with confident spontaneity. In fact, the grand jury investigation into Starzl's alleged abuses was eventually and quietly dropped, clearly signifying a victory for the pioneer surgeon.

Robert Hardesty and Bartley Griffith were not visible personalities such as Thomas Starzl was, but I always enjoyed watching the two men in the late afternoon as they rounded in the cardiac care units. They seemed so comfortable with one another, like soldiers who knew the same war stories and had fought the same battles side by side, trusting each other implicitly, yet aware of and willing to respond to each other's weaknesses.

In *Many Sleepless Nights*, I focus more attention on Bart Griffith's thoughts and personality primarily because of my own personal interest in and fascination with the heart-lung procedure, and also because of my relationships with Winkle Fulk and Frank Rowe. Clearly, Griffith was the prime mover in the heart-lung transplant area; Hardesty, as I have indicated, had his doubts about such potentially devastating and, at that time, experimental procedures. The two were in every way partners, however, sharing equally in the glory, the responsibility, and, in some instances, the depression, anger, and emptiness of defeat.

Of all the heart-lung transplants the Hardesty-Griffith team has performed since the initiation of their program in 1984, Winkle Fulk's post-transplant course has probably been the most positive. Although Winkle has experienced many complications over the past four years which necessitated hospital admissions in Pittsburgh and in Kansas City, she has managed to avoid the most serious bouts of rejection and infection which have complicated and often destroyed the lives of many heart, heart-lung, liver, and kidney transplant recipients. As already noted, Winkle was also a victim of society's ignorance of organ transplantation's potential. The principal of the junior high school where she had taught for ten years not only refused to restore her position, he did not even offer Winkle the courtesy of acknowledging her request.

Winkle plunged herself back into life's mainstream after

transplantation. Within six months after returning to Kansas City, she persuaded a local junior college to offer her a part-time position in mathematics. Subsequently, Winkle took classes at another institution—at one point taking nine credits per term and teaching six—and earned her master's degree in mathematics in 1989. For an entire year, she commuted many miles a day, three days a week, continuing to care for her family and apply for full-time high school teaching positions—with no luck and little encouragement.

Winkle also remains in contact with her donor family, Dick and Sharon Becker—who, she reports, are now busily raising their two young children—and with her "special sister," Rebecca (Treat) Adkins, who recently gave birth to her second child, a ten-pound baby boy. Winkle also counsels a number of heart-lung transplant candidates and recipients, helping them to cope with the waiting period and the challenges of life after the transplant. Winkle's hard work and continued persistence were finally rewarded when Johnson County Community College offered her a full-time position. "The mathematics department actually hired three people," said Winkle, "but they gave me the worst schedule of all because they figured I could handle it. Their confidence made me feel real proud."

I wish that all of the stories told in this book ended as happily and triumphantly as Winkle Fulk's, Rebecca (Treat) Adkins's, and even Richie Becker's, whose unfortunate death made Winkle's and Rebecca's second chance at life not only possible, but also so very positive. But Tom Goddard, the Detroit police officer, a victim of the legislative and bureaucratic system in Detroit and in the nation's capital, died of Hodgkin's disease early in 1988. Brian Reames, the founder of Transplant Recipients International Organization (TRIO), also died in early 1988 after undergoing retransplantation. Of all the transplant recipients I had ever met, Brian was the one recipient most willing to recognize and intelligently discuss both the positive and the negative aspects of organ transplantation. Brian harbored no illusions; he realized and accepted the bitter reality of organ transplantation—a life in which the prospects of staying alive for each succeeding tomorrow would always remain in doubt.

Frank Rowe did receive the phone call for which he had so longingly and faithfully waited early in December 1987. The heart-lung transplant surgery, with Bartley Griffith presiding, went smoothly, but his postoperative course was riddled with a series of unavoidable and irreversible complication. Frank fought valiantly until his heart and will gave out in February 1988. He was buried in Philadelphia, his hometown, but there were two memorial services for him in Pittsburgh where, because of his commitment to transplantation and his courageousness in the face of impending death, people perhaps knew him best.

When I first started this book, I vowed not to become involved with the people about whom I was writing—not to make friends—because I knew that some of my characters would die, and I would hurt and feel empty and alone because of their loss. Frank Rowe was incredibly persistent, however; we shared a passion for the intricacies of organ transplantation just as other men share avid interests in football, golf, or their professions. Frank would telephone me almost every day to talk transplantation and to update me on his health and personal feelings as he edged closer to "the end of life's rope." He was incredibly hungry for details about the progress of my book and made me promise that he could read the finished manuscript as soon as it was ready. He believed that if and when he died, his memory and his courageous struggle would be recorded forever within these pages. I regret that Frank did not live long enough to read *Many Sleepless Nights*, but I have tried to present both him and Brian Reames, who were quite close, as truly and honestly as I know how.

My most vivid and lasting memory of the three of us together took place, ironically, in a popular Pittsburgh restaurant called Froggy's. Frank and Brian should not have been drinking, obviously. But it was a rare and special night, and even men as sick as Frank and Brian may choose to dispense with caution once in a while and have a good time. We had a couple of drinks before dinner, then thick, juicy steaks; afterwards, we adjourned to the bar to continue our conversation.

As it turned out, I knew one of the waitresses and introduced her to Frank, and in the spontaneous way in which conversations often flourish over drinks, they became involved in a long discussion, with the waitress attempting to convince Frank that holistic medicine (her area of expertise)—not organ transplantation—would eliminate his PPH and save his life. Meanwhile, Brian had cornered two young women, budding actresses, to whom he was showing a series of recent photographs of his children, discussing their accomplishments in school.

It was nearly 2 A.M. when we finally said good-bye and left Froggy's. None of us were drunk, but we were in marvelously good spirits. Frank was driving, with Brian beside him; I was in the back seat. The city was dark and sleepy as we headed home. An "oldies" station was playing on the radio, and almost immediately Frank began to hum—and then sing. Brian soon picked up the words—I can't remember the song—and they began harmonizing, barely in tune, but softly and together.

It occurred to me then, as I watched the lights of the city whiz by and listened to the two men crooning up front, what a wonderful evening it had been—not because we had talked to women and drank a little too much, but because this experience had been so commonplace and unexceptional. For a few special hours in their very difficult, stressful, and frighteningly insecure existences, Brian Reames and Frank Rowe were suddenly not a heart transplant recipient and a heart-lung transplant candidate, respectively; they were just two ordinary, middle-aged guys, singing an old song, feeling good, and having fun as they headed for home. Whatever were to happen in the coming months, they—*we*—would always have this intimate moment of normalcy together.

Index